Pediatric Skeletal Scintigraphy
With Multimodality Imaging Correlations

Springer

New York
Berlin
Heidelberg
Barcelona
Budapest
Hong Kong
London
Milan
Paris
Santa Clara
Singapore
Tokyo

L.P. Connolly, M.D.
Staff Physician, Division of Nuclear Medicine
Children's Hospital, and
Assistant Professor of Radiology
Harvard Medical School

S.T. Treves, M.D.
Chief, Division of Nuclear Medicine
Children's Hospital, and
Professor of Radiology
Harvard Medical School

Pediatric Skeletal Scintigraphy

With Multimodality Imaging Correlations

With 195 Figures in 547 Parts

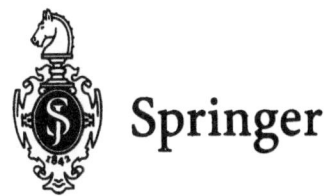

Springer

L.P. Connolly, M.D.
Staff Physician, Division of Nuclear Medicine
Children's Hospital
and
Assistant Professor of Radiology
Harvard Medical School
Boston, MA
USA

S.T. Treves, M.D.
Chief, Division of Nuclear Medicine
Children's Hospital
and
Professor of Radiology
Harvard Medical School
Boston, MA
USA

Library of Congress Cataloging in Publication Data
Connolly, Leonard P.
    Pediatric skeletal scintigraphy / Leonard P. Connolly, S. Ted
Treves.
        p.   cm.
    Includes bibliographical references and index.

    1. Bone diseases in children—Radionuclide imaging.   2. Fractures
in children—Radionuclide imaging.   I. Treves, S. T.
II. Title.
    [DNLM: 1. Bone Diseases—in infancy & childhood.   2. Bone
Diseases—radionuclide imaging.   3. Radionuclide Imaging—in infancy
& childhood.   WS 270C75p   1997]
RJ482.B65C66   1997
618.92′7107575—dc21
DNLM/DLC
for Library of Congress   96-29796

Printed on acid-free paper.

Production managed by Terry Kornak; manufacturing supervised by Jacqui Ashri.
Typeset by Best-set Typesetter Ltd., Hong Kong.

9 8 7 6 5 4 3 2 1

ISBN-13: 978-1-4612-7444-5   e-ISBN-13: 978-1-4612-2174-6
DOI: 10.1007/978-1-4612-2174-6

To my parents Madeleine and Edward

LPC

To Nancy, Erik, Alex, Blake and Olivia, and to my parents Catherine and Elias

STT

Preface

Extensive use of skeletal scintigraphy for a wide scope of clinical applications in children and young adults has resulted from its enabling early accurate diagnosis and prompt treatment for a number of disorders. This became possible with the introduction of technetium-99m (^{99m}Tc) labeled phosphates in the mid-1970's. These agents, such as ^{99m}Tc labeled methylene diphosphonate (^{99m}Tc-MDP), have permitted high quality scintigraphic imaging at reasonably low radiation exposures and short imaging times. Agents employed before (strontium-85 and strontium-87) lacked the favorable characteristic of a relatively short physical half life and emitted photons with energies less optimal than that of ^{99m}Tc for imaging with gamma cameras. Therefore, the use of skeletal scintigraphy in pediatric patients was more limited than at the present time. Dramatic improvements in nuclear medicine instrumentation have also significantly contributed to the success and acceptance of skeletal scintigraphy in children. Favorable characteristics of modern nuclear medicine instrumentation include excellent spatial resolution (in the order of 5 mm) and field uniformity. These inherent features plus pinhole magnification scintigraphy, which can achieve spatial resolution in the range of 1-2 mm, contribute to optimal scintigraphic imaging of children. Other favorable features of modern instrumentation include large area detectors that permit imaging of larger body parts in shorter time than smaller instruments. Multiple detector systems allow for more rapid imaging than single detector systems. Detector systems currently provide high quality single photon emission computed tomography (SPECT) with spatial resolutions in the order of a few millimeters (i.e.: 5 mm).

As skeletal scintigraphy has advanced over the past few decades, radiographs have remained essential tools and new methods for evaluating the skeleton have been developed. These new techniques involve radiopharmaceuticals, such as thallium-201 and metaiodobenzylguanidine (MIBG), as well as the structural modalities of computed tomography (CT), magnetic resonance imaging (MRI), and ultrasonography. In contrast with radiographs and the structural modalities, scintigraphy produces functional images. Scintigraphy can show early and subtle changes in blood flow, cell metabolism, membrane transport, cell character, and cell population that are not detectable by other imaging modalities. One of the most wonderful aspects of nuclear medicine is that by the use of different radiopharmaceuticals, scintigraphy provides images depicting several different processes that involve or affect the skeleton. Changes demonstrated scintigraphically are not dependent on gross anatomic alterations as are the changes depicted by radiographs, CT, MRI, and ultrasonography. This unique view of the skeleton in terms of perfusion and regional function makes scintigraphy so highly valuable. While the spatial anatomic resolution of scintigraphy is much lower than that of radiographs, CT, or MRI its functional resolution and sensitivity are very high.

The goal of this work is to serve as a concise reference that highlights skeletal scintigraphy while providing a direct correlation (in words, figures, or both) between what skeletal scintigraphy depicts and what other techniques demonstrate. The book is designed to illustrate valuable characteristics of skeletal scintigraphy for evaluating disorders that affect the musculoskeletal system in children as well as to convey advantages and pitfalls of skeletal scintigraphy and other modalities. It is hoped that the reader will gain an understanding of the role of scintigraphy relative to other imaging studies in answering clinical questions. The work is not meant to replace nuclear medicine textbooks regarding general principles and techniques. Those are reviewed only briefly to serve as a reminder for readers who are experienced in nuclear medicine and as a general overview for readers who are not.

The book contains a relatively short text that is supplemented with abundant illustrations of case material. It is divided into five chapters dealing with general principles as well as peculiarities and important aspects of pediatric nuclear medicine (Chapter 1), infection (Chapter 2), trauma (Chapter 3), benign lesions (Chapter 4), and malignant conditions (Chapter 5). The work is derived from over 27 years of experience at Children's Hospital in Boston—an institution that, for well over a century, has earned a world-wide reputation of excellence in patient care, research, and teaching and served as a referral center for pediatric diseases ranging from the common to the esoteric. Its facilities include state-of-the-art imaging equipment and resources.

The opinions and technical preferences throughout the book reflect the work and experience of the authors. We do not pretend that our ways and assertions are the only correct ones but do submit them for the reader's review, noting that they have proved to be valuable over the years. The authors enjoyed working on this book and hope that it becomes a useful and valuable resource for practitioners who evaluate the musculoskeletal system of children.

L.P. Connolly, M.D.
S.T. Treves, M.D.
Boston, 1997

Acknowledgments

We extend our gratitude to numerous individuals who directly or indirectly made this book possible:

Zvi Bar-Sever, formerly a fellow at our institution and now at the Rabin Medical Center in Petah-Tikva, Israel. His assistance in selecting scintigraphic images and his understanding of pediatric nuclear medicine and clinical pediatrics proved invaluable.

Diego Jaramillo and Tal Laor at our institution and Susan Connolly of Massachusetts General Hospital. By sharing their extensive knowledge of pediatric skeletal radiology, they have prevented numerous factual gaffes and enabled us to choose appropriate correlative images.

The fellows in nuclear medicine from the Harvard Joint Program in Nuclear Medicine and the fellows in pediatric radiology from Children's Hospital, who have worked in our division during the writing of this book. Their help in preparing many cases included in this book was essential and their interest in nuclear medicine provided the authors with the inspiration with which we worked. We especially thank Kimberly Applegate, Ariane Staub Neish, and Gabriel Soudry for their efforts.

Our colleagues, particularly Don Kirks, Tom Hill, and Jim Adelstein, who have provided us with support and encouragement during the writing of this book and at other times.

The many referring physicians who have relied on our services to help in their assessment of countless patients over the years.

Lucy Willoughby, who assisted with all phases of manuscript preparation, and Emily Feinstein, who has helped with the final stages. They consistently handled the challenges presented by our work habits with pleasant professionalism.

Karl Mitchell. His expertise in information systems and clinical data base research allowed us to find the cases needed to illustrate this work.

Don Sucher, whose skills in radiologic photography meet the highest standards.

Bill Day, Editorial Director at Springer-Verlag, New York, who supported this work from its inception onward, and the production staff at Springer-Verlag, particularly Terry Kornak, who worked meticulously with diligence and patience.

Our deepest thanks go to our technical team, headed by Royal T. Davis: Dianne Itrato, Nancie Keane, Maryellen Mannting, Tracy Tetrault, Jim Ulanski, Terri Wilson, and Jennifer Winfield. Their superb technical skills, dedication, compassion, care, and patience are highly appreciated.

Contents

1
Scintigraphic Evaluation of the Pediatric Skeleton

This chapter reviews the methods for studying the pediatric skeleton with radio-nuclides. Factors that make skeletal scintigraphy different in children than in adults are emphasized. These include radiopharmaceutical dose adjustment, personnel issues, choice of instrumentation, patient preparation and sedation, considerations regarding examination techniques, and the normal appearance of skeletal scintigrams related to patient age. The chapter concludes with a brief review of other scintigraphic studies that are useful for assessing suspected skeletal pathology in children.

Skeletal Scintigraphy: General Considerations

Technetium-99m Phosphate Compounds

Skeletal scintigraphy is performed with technetium-99m (^{99m}Tc)-labeled diphosphonates.

Technetium-99m, the most commonly used radionuclide in nuclear medicine, has excellent physical properties for imaging: a physical half-life ($T_{1/2}$) of 6 hours, a predominant 140-keV gamma ray, and no particulate emission. A convenient molybdenum–99(^{99m}Mo)–^{99m}Tc parent–daughter generator system allows on-site production of ^{99m}Tc at imaging centers worldwide (Fig. 1.1). This system employs an alumina column on which ^{99m}Tc is absorbed. Elution or washing of this column with physiologic saline readily removes ^{99m}Tc, in the form of ^{99m}Tc sodium pertechnetate with ^{99m}Tc in the +7 valence state.

The diphosphonates are analogues of pyrophosphate, a normal constituent of bone (Fig. 1.2). Labeling of these substances with ^{99m}Tc is accomplished by reduction of ^{99m}Tc from the +7 to the +4 valence state by stannous ions. In this form, ^{99m}Tc binds to phosphonate groups ($H_2PO_3^-$). Following intravenous injection, ^{99m}Tc-labeled diphosphonates concentrate in amorphous calcium phosphate and crystalline hydroxyapatite, localizing in lines between osteoid lining marrow cavities and the more peripheral bone. The greatest localization of these tracers occurs in areas of high blood flow, active bone growth, and reactive bone. Between 40% and 60% of administered tracer localizes in the skeleton at 2 to 4 hours following administration. The remainder is cleared by the kidneys (Fig. 1.3). The most commonly used agent is ^{99m}Tc-methylene diphosphonate (MDP).

The biodistribution of administered radiopharmaceutical may be altered by factors related to radiopharmaceutical preparation and by various medications. Although these variations are rare in practice, it is important to be aware of their existence. During radiopharmaceutical preparation, care must be taken to avoid the introduction of air into the kit vial. This, as well as the failure to use the agent within 3 hours of preparation, can result in reoxidation and release of unbound (free) ^{99m}Tc pertechnetate. The resultant images demonstrate radionuclide in the normal distribution of ^{99m}Tc-pertechnetate as well as in the skeleton. The stomach (Fig. 1.4) and, to a lesser degree, the thyroid, salivary glands, and choroid plexus

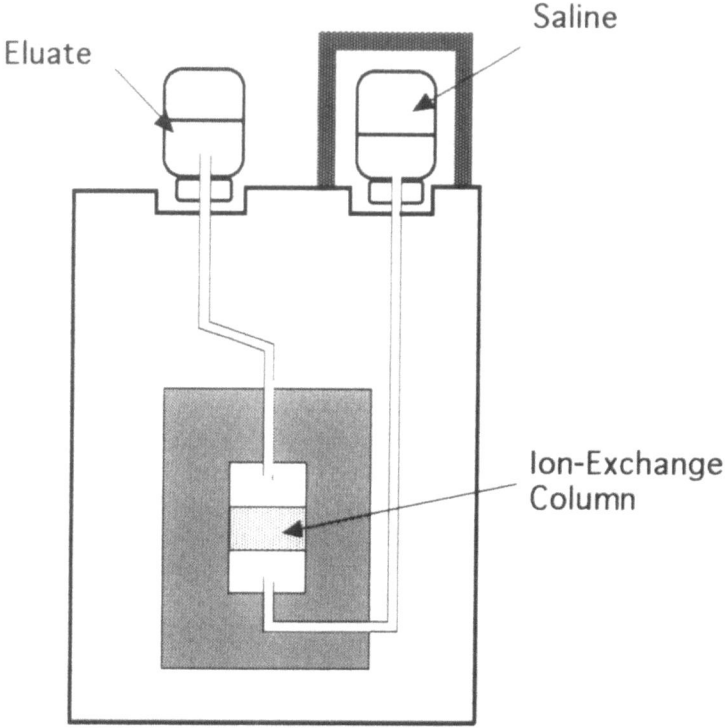

Figure 1.1. Elution of the ^{99}Mo-^{99m}Tc generator system with physiologic saline (the eluant) removes ^{99m}Tc, in the form of ^{99m}Tc sodium pertechnetate, from the alumina ion exchange column on which it is absorbed.

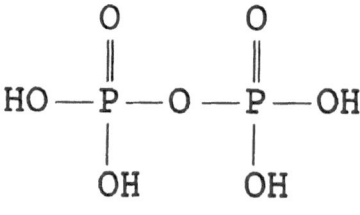

Figure 1.2. Chemical structures of pyrophosphate and methylene diphosphonate.

may be identified. The small or large bowel may be depicted due to ^{99m}Tc-pertechnetate released from the stomach. Hydrolysis during radiopharmaceutical preparation or excess aluminum in the generator eluate can result in colloid formation. Visualization of the liver and, occasionally, the spleen occurs secondary to colloidal phagocytosis in reticuloendothelial cells (Fig. 1.5). Radiographic contrast agents, gentamicin, various chemotherapeutic drugs,[22] and iron-containing compounds are agents that children may have received, which can increase renal retention of ^{99m}Tc-MDP (Fig. 1.6).

A number of physiologic states not related to the skeleton may affect the appearance of the study. Decreased cardiac output, inadequate hydration, and impaired renal function can result in slow clearance of tracer from the blood, decreased skeletal localization, and increased soft tissue localization. Bone-seeking tracers may localize in soft tissue lesions in which there is high blood flow, increased capillary permeability, high calcium metabolism, or calcification. In children, this is most frequently seen with neuroblastoma (see Chapter 5). Ischemic or infarcted tissue, such as the infarcted spleen of a sickle cell patient,[14a] may show abnormal tracer localization (Fig. 1.7). Bowel visualization may be caused by necrotizing enterocolitis, protein-losing enteropathy (Fig. 1.8), intestinal infarction, vesicoenteric fistula, or urinary diversion.[11,32] States associated with metastatic calcification may result in tracer localization in any organ. In the rare case where significant extravasation occurs at the injection site, regional lymph nodes may be visualized secondary to lymphatic absorption of the radio-pharmaceutical (Fig. 1.9). Due to normal renal excretion of diphosphonates, abnormalities of renal number or position may be demonstrated. Parenchymal retention, hydronephrosis, or bladder deviation may provide evidence of a pathologic condition (Figs. 1.10 and 1.11) that, in some instances, is unsuspected.

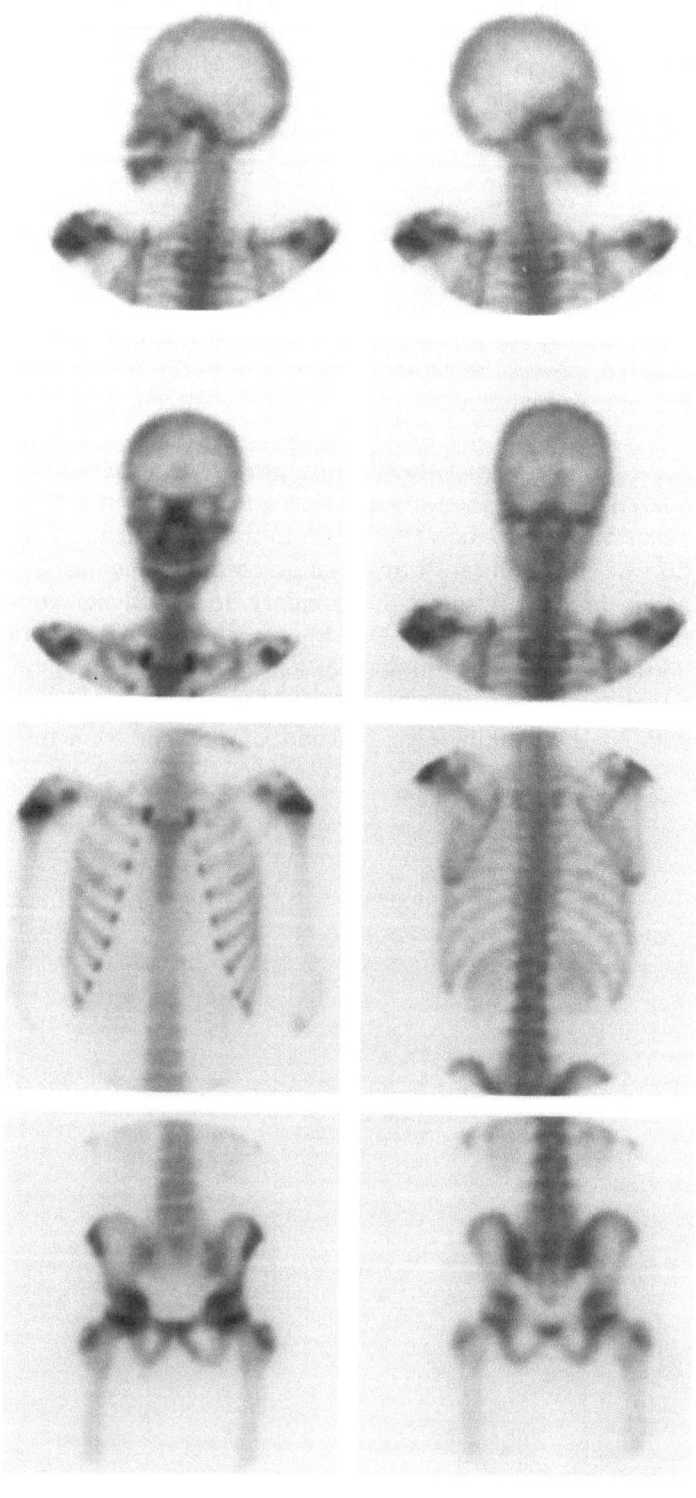

A

Figure 1.3. Skeletal scintigraphy, multiple-spot technique. Note the normal intense localization of ^{99m}Tc-MDP at growth centers. The kidneys are faintly visualized. Images of the thorax, abdomen, pelvis, and hips were obtained in anterior and posterior projections. The skull was imaged in both lateral projections as well as in the anterior and posterior projections (A).

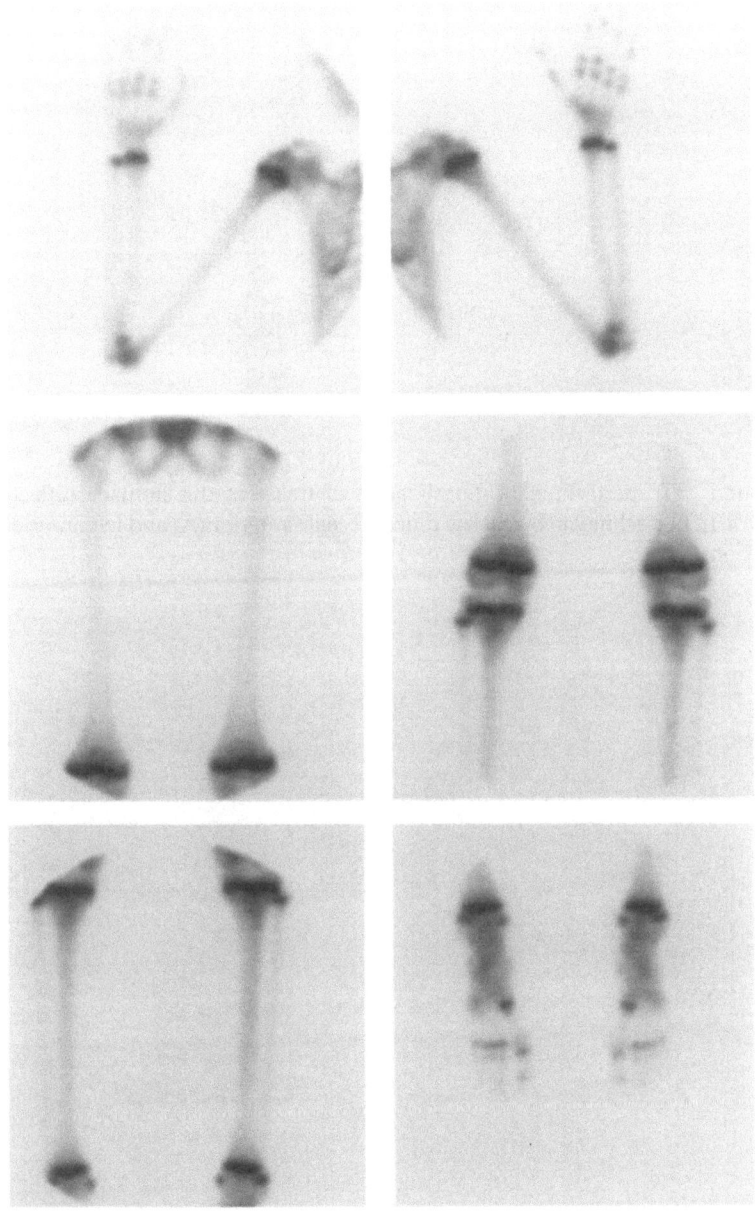

B

Figure 1.3 (*cont'd.*) The upper extremities were imaged in a posterior projection and the lower extremities in an anterior projection (B).

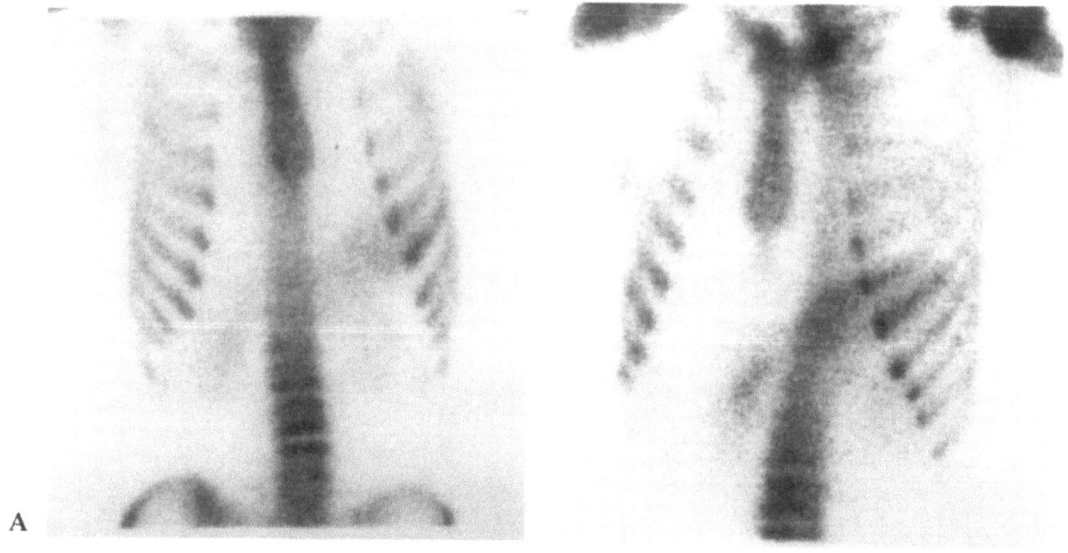

A

B

Figure 1.4. Unbound ^{99m}Tc pertechnetate. Localization of tracer in the stomach reflects uptake of ubound ^{99m}Tc pertechnetate by gastric mucosal cells: anterior (A) and left anterior oblique (B) projections.

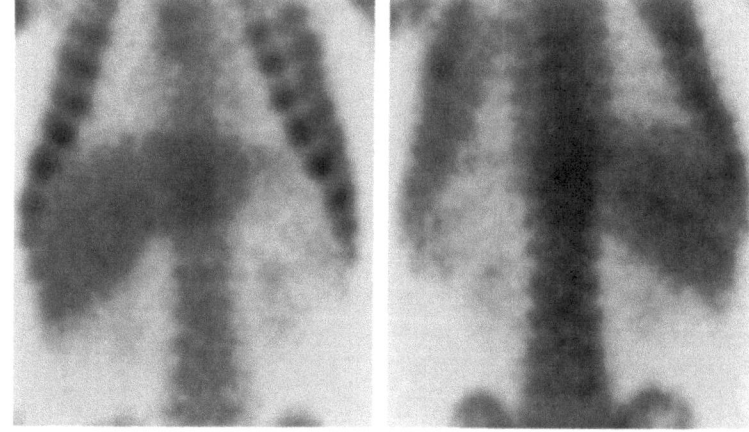

Figure 1.5. Hepatic radionuclide localization. Visualization of the liver may result from colloid formation during radiopharmaceutical preparation (anterior and posterior projections).

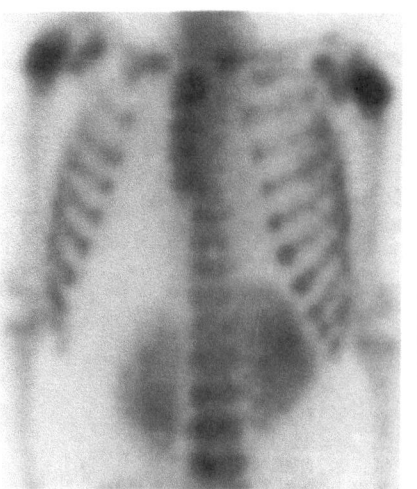
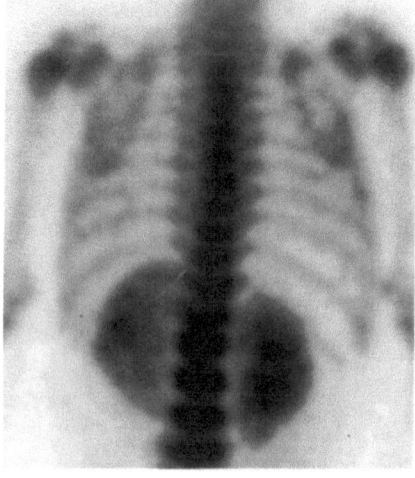

Figure 1.6. Increased renal localization of ^{99m}Tc-MDP. There is higher than normal concentration of ^{99m}Tc-MDP in the kidneys of a child following systemic chemotherapy.

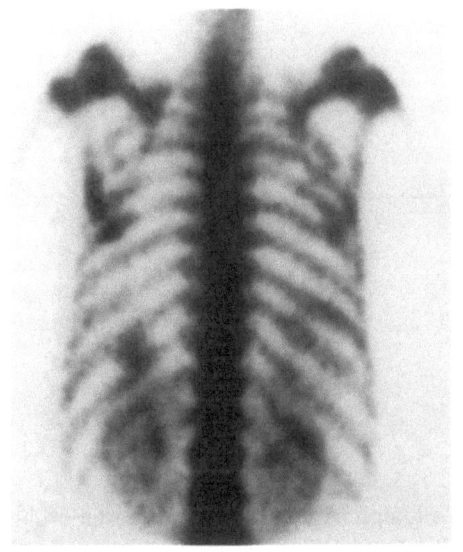
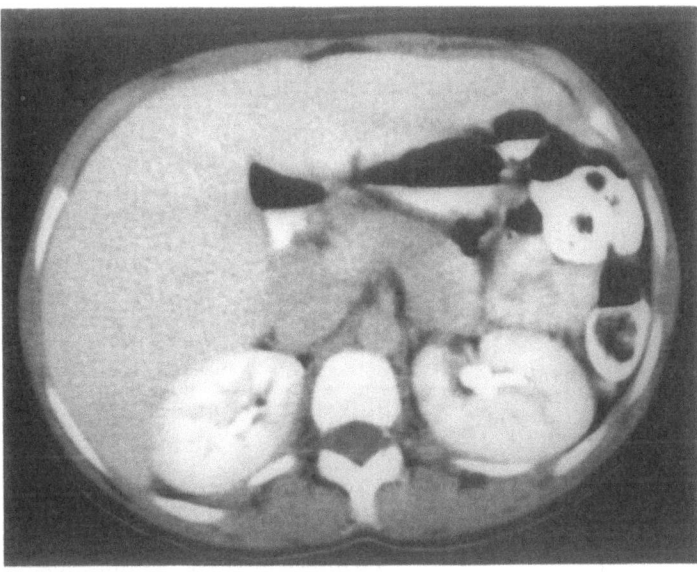

A

B

Figure 1.7. Sickle cell anemia. Concentration of ^{99m}Tc-MDP overlying the ninth left intercostal space is within an autoinfarcted spleen (A; image windowed to enhance contrast). The spleen is not identified on computed tomography (CT) and the splenic bed is occupied by the colon (B).

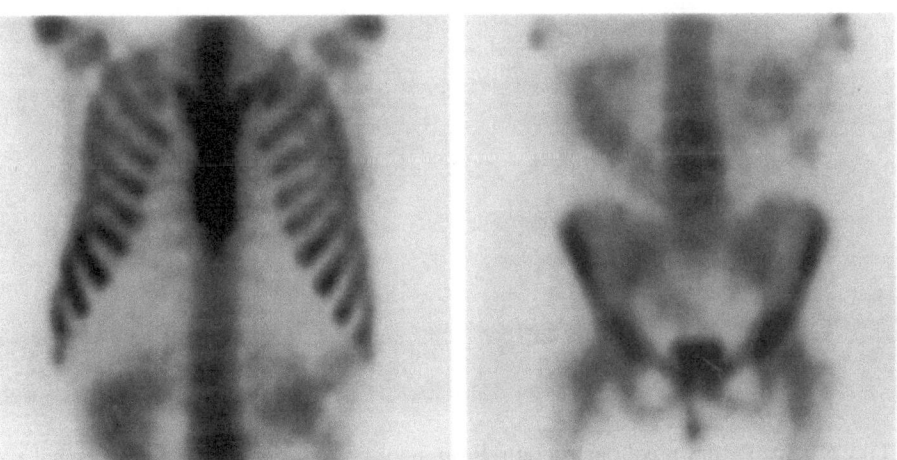

Figure 1.8. Bowel visualization on skeletal scintigraphy. Excretion of tracer into the colon has occurred in a child with protein losing enteropathy.

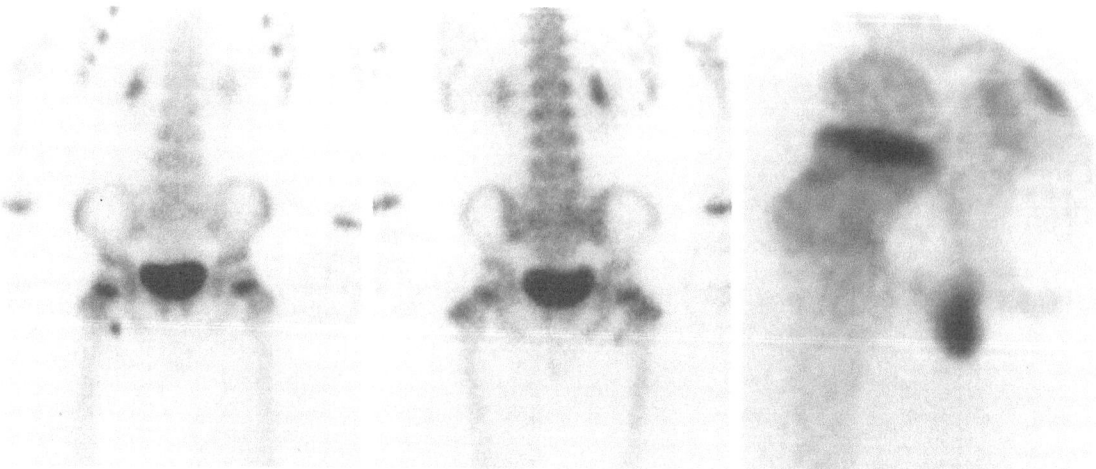

Figure 1.9. Localization of ⁹⁹ᵐTc-MDP within a lymph node. Anterior and posterior high-resolution planar images and a pinhole magnification image depict accumulation of ⁹⁹ᵐTc-MDP within a right inguinal lymph node secondary to extravasation of a portion of the administered dose at the injection site in the right foot.

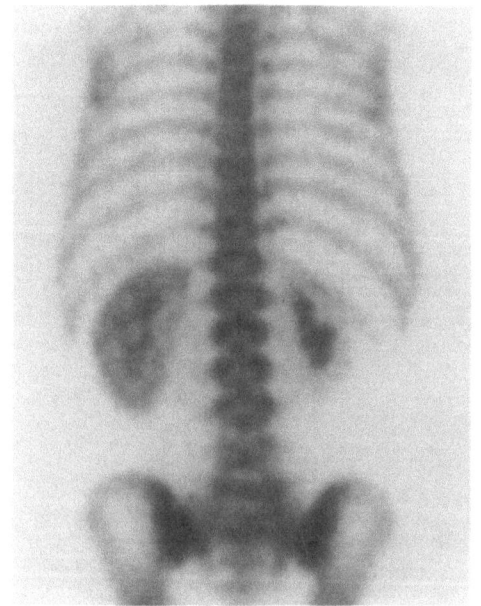

A

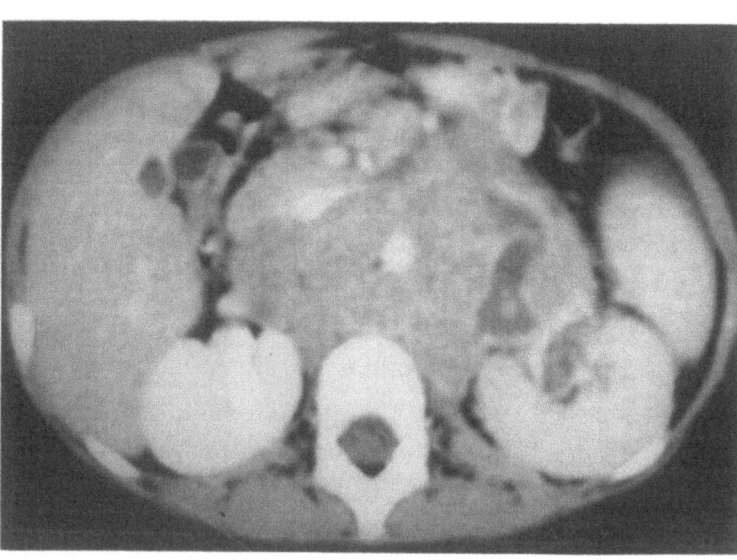

B

Figure 1.10. Partial renal obstruction. Prominent tracer retention by the left renal parenchyma and in the right pelvicalyceal system is identified on this posterior image obtained 4 hours following ⁹⁹ᵐTc-MDP administration (A). Computed tomography (B) performed immediately after intravenous administration of iodinated contrast reveals a large soft tissue mass encasing vessels and extending across the abdominal midline anterior to the spine. The right kidney shows a dense nephrogram and pelvicalyceal dilatation. There is relatively poor enhancement of the left kidney, indicating that the scintigraphic abnormality is analogous to the delayed nephrogram that can be present with renal obstruction on intravenous pyelography. The diagnosis in this case was neuroblastoma.

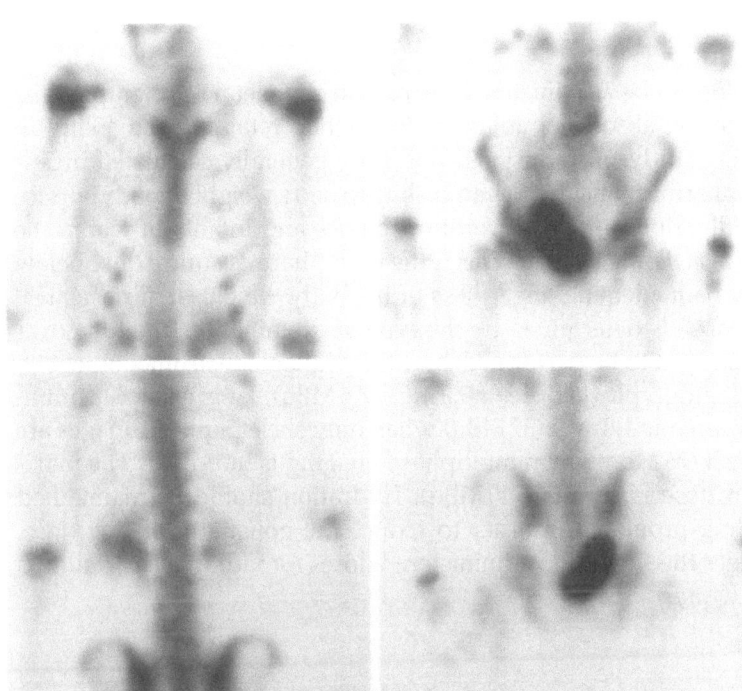

Figure 1.11. Urinary bladder displacement and hydronephrosis. Anterior (upper row) and posterior skeletal scintigrams are depicted (A). The urinary bladder is displaced to the right. The left ureter is deviated from its normal course and crosses anterior to L5 and the left renal pelvis is dilated.

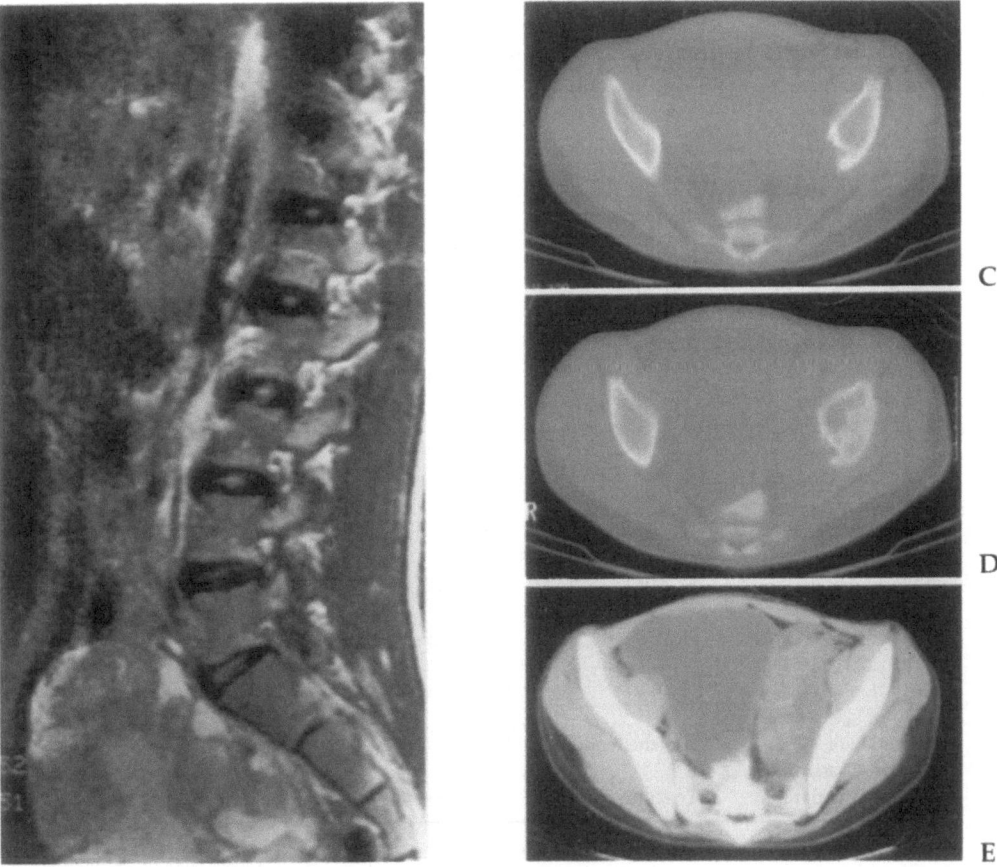

Figure 1.11 (*cont'd.*) A large pelvic soft tissue mass is identified anterior to the sacrum and L4 by magnetic resonance imaging (MRI) (B). Computed tomography shows lytic destruction of the left acetabulum and a soft tissue mass displacing the urinary bladder (C–E). This 17-year-old boy presented for MRI with a question of disk-related pain. The diagnosis was Ewing sarcoma.

Administered Dose

In estimating the dose to be administered for pediatric skeletal scintigraphy, the goal is to minimize the absorbed radiation dose while retaining the ability to obtain a high-quality study. Administered doses are generally calculated by adjusting adult radiopharmaceutical doses according to body weight or body surface area. Special consideration must be given to neonates and infants in whom the concept of *minimal total dose* is applied. This is the radiopharmaceutical dose below which a study will be inadequate regardless of the body weight or surface area. The minimal total dose is determined by the type of examination, the time over which the examination is to be performed, and the available instrumentation.

For ^{99m}Tc-MDP scintigraphy, a dose of 0.2 mCi (7.4 MBq)/kg is used. The minimum dose administered is 1.0 mCi (37 MBq) when only skeletal phase images are obtained and 2.0 mCi (74 MBq) when multiphase imaging is indicated. The maximum administered dose is 20 mCi (740 MBq). Hydration should be maintained and frequent voiding promoted in order to reduce the gonadal radiation dose. Table 1.1 summarizes the suggested administered doses for radiopharmaceuticals discussed in this chapter[39a].

Table 1.1. Radiopharmaceuticals used in assessing pediatric skeletal disorders.

Procedure	Radiopharmaceutical	Route of administration	Dose/kg		Minimal total dose		Dose/70 Kg	
			mCi	MBq	mCi	MBq	mCi	MBq
Skeletal scintigraphy	^{99m}Tc-methylene diphosphonate (MDP)	Intravenous	0.2	7.4	1.0	37	20	740
Localization of inflammation and infection, tumor assessment	^{67}Ga-citrate	Intravenous	0.04	1.48	0.25	9.25	6	222
Localization of inflammation, infection	^{99m}Tc-white blood cells	Intravenous	0.2	7.4	0.5	18.5	20	740
Localization of inflammation, infection	^{111}In-white blood cells	Intravenous	0.005	0.185	0.05	1.85	0.3	11.1
Detection of tumor	^{201}Tl as thallous chloride	Intravenous	0.03	1.11	0.5	18.5	2.0	74
Detection of tumor activity	^{99m}Tc-MIBI	Intravenous	0.4	14.8	2.0	74	20	740
Detection of neuroblastoma	^{131}I-MIBG	Intravenous	0.014	0.52	0.1	3.7	1.0	37
Detection of neuroblastoma	^{123}I-MIBG	Intravenous	0.2	7.4	1.0	37	10	370
Detection of neuroblastoma	^{111}In-pentetreotide	Intravenous	0.04	1.5	0.5	18.5	3.0	111
Marrow scintigraphy	^{99m}Tc-sulfur colloid	Intravenous	0.10	3.7	0.5	18.5	5.0	185

Modified from reference 39a, with permission.

Personnel

Pediatric nuclear medicine personnel must possess the necessary skills to reassure children and parents. Physicians, technologists, and receptionists must be trained to convey information and show patience, understanding, and compassion. An ability to reassure and a willingness to assist in distracting the pediatric patient during the course of an examination reduce the need for sedation.

The need for specific training in pediatric nuclear medicine as a prerequisite for all practitioners of the field cannot be emphasized too strongly. Pediatric nuclear medicine practitioners must have a sound knowledge of the fundamental principles of pediatrics and pediatric nuclear medicine. It is often necessary to tailor an examination according to the information required and the ability of the child to cooperate. Understanding the strengths and limitations inherent to various imaging techniques allows the examination to be adapted to the child rather than forcing the child to adapt to the examination. To do this whenever appropriate and possible, physicians and technologists must have detailed knowledge of a wide range of equipment capabilities including pinhole magnification, electronic zoom, collimators, and single photon emission computed tomography (SPECT). Since the most frequent route of radiopharmaceutical administration is intravenous, an effective technologist must be expert at obtaining and securing venous access.

Instrumentation

The basis of nuclear medicine imaging is the detection of photons, usually gamma rays, that are emitted during radionuclide decay. The principal detection instrument is the gamma camera. This consists of a collimator, one or more sodium iodide detectors, a photomultiplier tube array, electronic position logic circuits, and a pulse height analyzer.

Single-detector systems are the most versatile and commonly used in clinical practice. Dynamic scintigraphy (such as radionuclide angiography), whole body and multiple spot planar scintigraphy, pinhole magnification scintigraphy, and SPECT can be performed with a single-detector gamma camera. The configuration of single-detector systems provides easy access to the patient. Such access can be valuable when evaluating acutely ill children and enables a reassuring parent or technologist to calm an anxious child during image acquisition.

Multiple-detector systems allow more rapid completion of examinations than do single-detector systems. Dual-detector systems enable simultaneous acquisition of opposing planar projections while triple-detector systems allow simultaneous acquisition of planar images in degrees of obliquity. Compared with SPECT performed on a single-detector system, SPECT of an equal count density are obtained in approximately one half the time with dual-detector and approximately one third the time with triple-detector systems. The configuration required for dual- and particularly for triple-detector systems somewhat limits physical access to the patient. This potential disadvantage for imaging acutely ill children is offset by the ability to more rapidly complete an examination, however. Triple-detector systems are specially designed and optimized for SPECT. Pinhole imaging is not possible with some dual- and all currently available triple-detector systems.

An important consideration regarding gamma camera systems, particularly SPECT cameras, is that the failure of manufacturers to address peculiarities of pediatric imaging often requires modifications related to imaging table size, restraining devices, and autocontouring.

Patient Preparation, Immobilization, and Sedation

Prior to imaging, it is important to allay any fears a child has concerning the study and to determine if the child will be able to cooperate during the examination. As a child reflects the parents' attitudes, it is essential that parents be well informed and cooperative. Once a child's trust has been gained, continued cooperation is usually assured by relatively simple methods. The gentle hand of a trained technologist or aide is often the most effective means of achieving immobilization, especially for infants. Various other methods such as sheets wrapped around the body, sandbags, and/or special holding devices can be employed. Offering a bottle to a hungry infant, particularly if he or she has been sleep deprived or the examination is immediately before the usual nap time, is also effective. Entertainment in the form of television, videotapes, music, reading, and the proximity of favorite toys or blankets is helpful in calming and distracting older children. Parents should be encouraged to accompany their children during the course of a study and to provide needed emotional support.

Sedation is only rarely required for skeletal scintigraphy at our specialized institution, where a team of individuals with experience and expertise in imaging children has been assembled. Sedation is used when, on the basis of careful consideration, it is anticipated that the above methods will prove inadequate or when they prove unsuccessful. The goal of sedation is a minimally depressed level of consciousness in which a patient remains responsive to physical stimulation and verbal commands, while independently and continuously maintaining a patent airway and protective reflexes.[9] Only a rare extreme case requires the use of general anesthesia for a satisfactory examination.

Prior to sedation, assessment of the child's medical history and physical examination is necessary. Patient selection is based on the American Society of Anesthesiologists (ASA) physical status classification (Table 1.2). Generally, patients in

Table 1.2. American Society of Anesthesiologists physical status classification.

Class	Description
I	Healthy patient with no systemic disease
II	Patient with mild systemic disease but no functional impairment
III	Patient with severe systemic disease having definite functional impairment
IV	Patient with severe systemic disease that is a constant threat to life
V	Moribund patient who is not expected to survive

ASA categories I and II are considered eligible for sedation, while those in categories III and IV require further evaluation, preferably by an anesthesiologist. Informed consent should be obtained from a parent or guardian. During sedation, patient monitoring must be the primary responsibility of a designated health practitioner (often a nurse), who is trained in pediatric basic life support. After the procedure, the patient must be monitored in a suitably equipped area until established discharge criteria are met. Detailed instructions are reviewed with the parents or guardians before discharge. A 24-hour postprocedure telephone check is recommended to determine if any adverse effects, such as prolonged sedation or incoordination, vomiting, or hyperactivity, have occurred.[1,3,41]

Specific sedation protocols, particularly regarding the recommended medications and their dosages, vary from institution to institution. These protocols are continuously being reevaluated and are frequently customized according to the medical needs of an individual patient. Commonly used medications include chloral hydrate, pentobarbital, and fentanyl citrate. The availability of appropriate monitoring and resuscitative equipment, personnel trained in pediatric advanced life support, and an active quality assurance program are essential components of any sedation program.

Imaging Techniques

Skeletal scintigraphy may include radionuclide angiography, tissue phase imaging, and skeletal phase imaging. When all three phases are obtained, the study is referred to as a three-phase bone scan (Fig. 1.12). The need to include all three phases depends on the clinical question being asked and the patient's condition. Three-phase imaging is routinely performed in children with suspected musculoskeletal infection and may be of value in evaluating benign and malignant bone tumors, and stress injuries of the lower extremities. A four-phase study, which is rarely required in children, includes an additional set of skeletal phase images between 6 and 24 hours following tracer administration.

For radionuclide angiography, a gamma camera equipped with a high-resolution collimator is used. The patient is positioned so that the region of interest is within the field of view. Recording begins immediately after the administration of the radiopharmaceutical as a rapid bolus. Images are recorded at one frame per second for 60 seconds on a 128×128 matrix. The radionuclide angiogram is best evaluated on cinematic mode. It can also be printed on film or paper (Fig. 1.12A).

Immediately following the radionuclide angiogram, a tissue phase image is obtained (300,000–500,000 counts) of the region of interest (256×256 matrix). Tissue phase images can be obtained in various projections for the same number of counts or time if desired. Tissue phase images depict tracer in the blood pool,

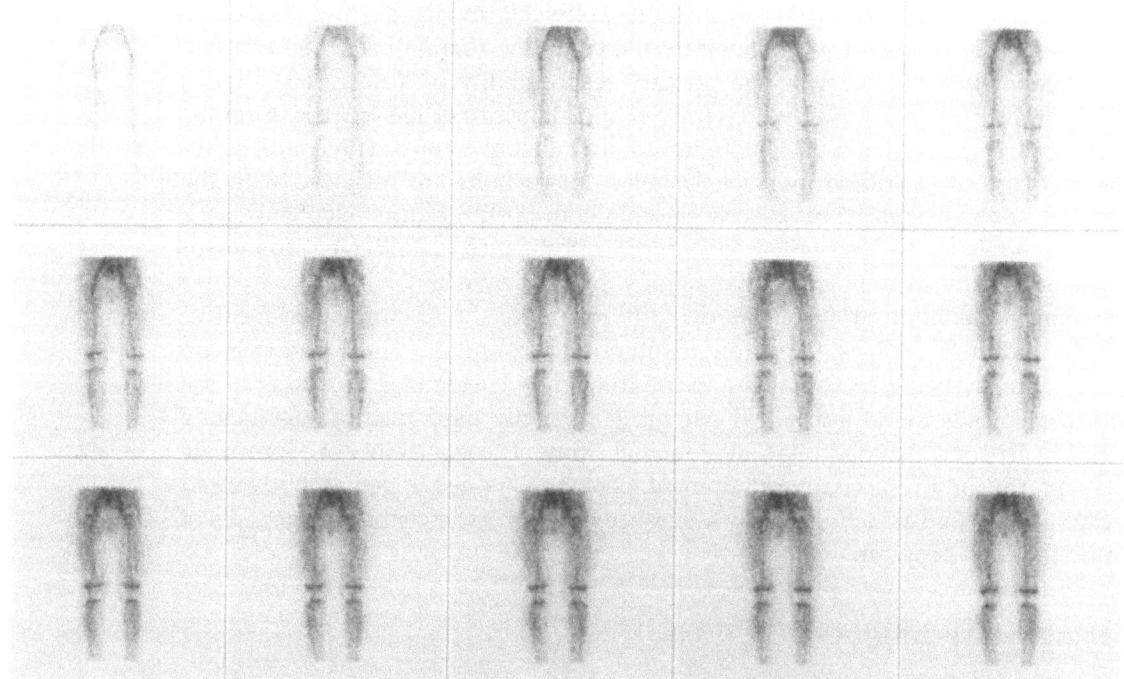

A

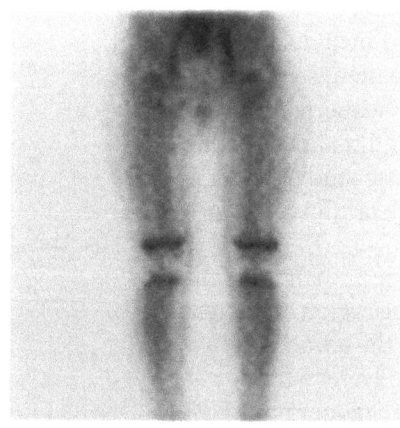

B

Figure 1.12. Three-phase skeletal scintigraphy. Radionuclide angiography (anterior projection) shows symmetric blood flow to the hips, knees and visualized portions of the lower extremities (A). Tissue phase imaging shows tracer within the soft tissues and bone (B).

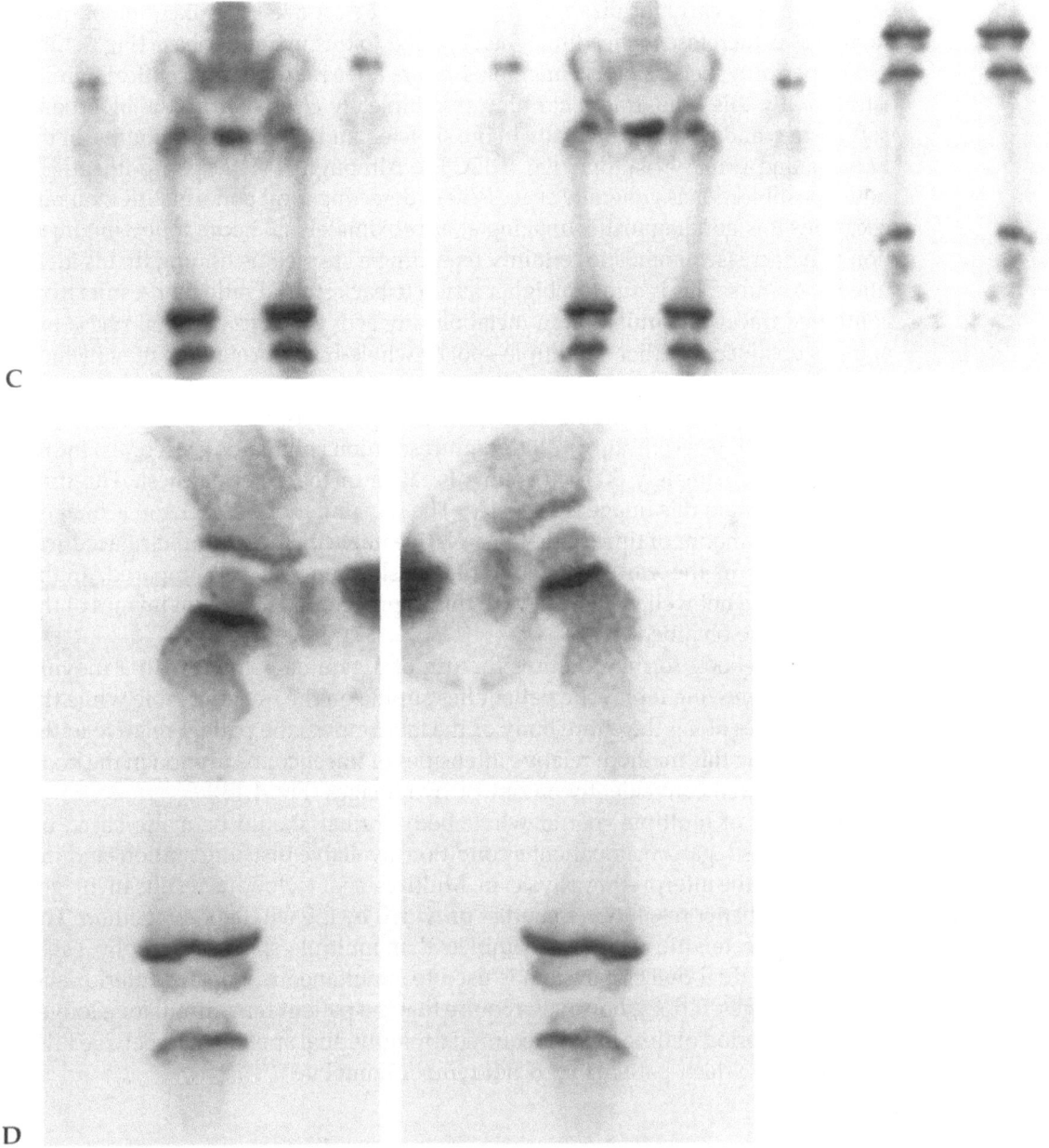

Figure 1.12 (cont'd.) Skeletal phase imaging, performed with a high-resolution collimator, reveals normal symmetric tracer distribution [C: posterior and anterior projections of the pelvis and femurs, anterior projection of the distal lower extremities]. Note that the patellae and naviculars are not visualized as they have not begun ossification in this 2-year-old girl. Pinhole magnification images confirm the symmetry of tracer localization in the hips and knees (D). Note the clarity with which details are depicted and the absence of ^{99m}Tc-MDP localization in the unossified ischiopubic synchondroses, trochanters, and patellae.

soft tissue, and early localization in the bone. The oft-used moniker "blood pool imaging" is therefore misleading when applied to this imaging phase (Fig. 1.12b).

We perform skeletal phase imaging 4 hours after radiopharmaceutical administration. By this time, tracer has almost completely cleared from the blood and soft tissues, and is seen principally in the skeleton and, in variable amounts, in the kidneys and urinary bladder (Fig. 1.12C,D). Although skeletal phase imaging 4 hours postinjection is generally successful in detecting focal abnormalities, on rare occasions it is nondiagnostic. Imaging at approximately 24 hours following injection may increase diagnostic certainty regarding a suspicious finding that is identified at 4 hours. This is due to a higher lesion to background ratio that results from continued tracer accumulation in metabolically active lesions. Skeletal phase imaging is obtained in either a multiple-spot or whole-body format and may include magnification and/or SPECT.

With multiple-spot imaging (Fig. 1.3), a large field-of-view gamma camera fitted with a high-resolution or ultra–high-resolution collimator is used. An initial image of approximately 500,000 counts is taken of the anterior chest. The time required to obtain this image is recorded. The remainder of the skeleton is imaged for the same amount of time so that the relative intensities of radiopharmaceutical concentration in the various regions of the skeleton can be compared. If the extremities are not well visualized with this approach, 300,000 count images of the extremities are obtained.

The whole-body format requires the use of a gamma camera with a moving detector or a moving table. The patient lies supine on the imaging table while the detector moves along the entire body or the table moves the patient relative to the detector. Using this method, relative intensities of tracer concentration in the body can be compared conveniently on one or two images (Fig. 1.13).

The choice of multiple-spot or whole-body format should be made based on considerations regarding a patient's condition, available instrumentation, and the preference of the interpreting physician. Multiple-spot technique results in images with slightly better resolution than that provided by the whole-body method. The whole-body technique is faster to complete than multiple-spot scintigraphy, especially when a dual-detector system is used to simultaneously obtain anterior and posterior images. It does, however, require that the patient remain still for a longer continuous period of time than is required for individual spot images, between the acquisition of which patients need not remain immobile.

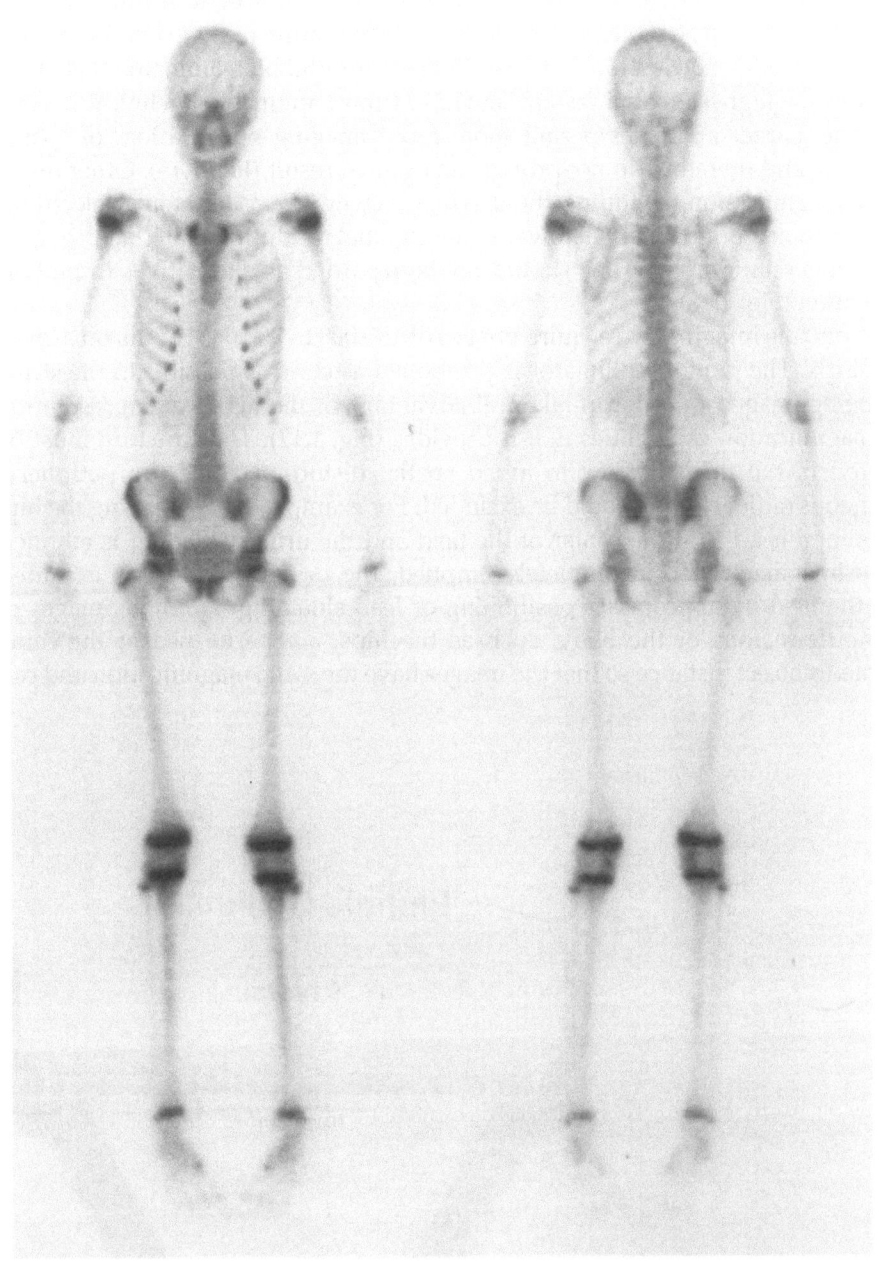

Figure 1.13. Whole-body skeletal scintigraphy. These anterior (left panel) and posterior images of a 13-year-old girl were obtained with a moving detector system.

Magnification is required in some cases to assess small structures such as the femoral capital epiphysis and the bones of the hands and feet, to further evaluate bone adjacent to growth centers, or to localize the nidus of an osteoid osteoma. Optical magnification with a 2- to 3-mm aperture pinhole collimator (Fig. 1.14) provides the highest spatial resolution (1.5–2.0 mm) attainable in clinical nuclear medicine. Larger apertures permit more rapid imaging but at a loss of spatial resolution and therefore do not provide an optimal result (Fig. 1.15). Other methods of magnification, including the use of a converging collimator or electronic magnification (zoom), result in lower system spatial resolution than that provided by pinhole scintigraphy. They should not be regarded as alternatives to pinhole collimation (Fig. 1.16).[12,36]

For pinhole imaging, we acquire images of 150,000 to 300,000 counts on a 256 × 256 matrix. The pinhole collimator is positioned as close as possible to the structure being imaged in order to take full advantage of the high system resolution and magnification capabilities that it provides (Fig. 1.17). The structure must be centered in the field of view to avoid spatial distortion along the periphery. Extraneous radioactivity should be excluded. For example, when imaging the hip, the femoral head is in the center of the field and the urinary bladder is emptied before imaging. When incompletely emptied, the urinary bladder is excluded from the field by appropriate positioning or lead shielding.[10] Pinhole images of symmetric regions of the body, such as the hips, are performed at the same pinhole-to-object distance so that the images have the same magnification and can

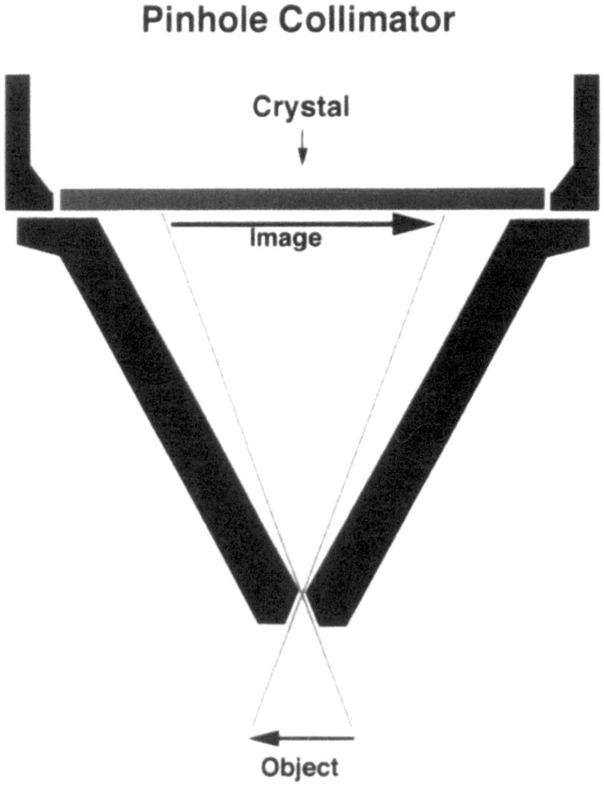

Figure 1.14. Pinhole collimator. A pinhole collimator projects an inverted magnified image of the object on the detector crystal as long as the object is closer to the aperture than the aperture is to the crystal. The magnification factor equals the crystal to aperture distance divided by the aperture to object distance.

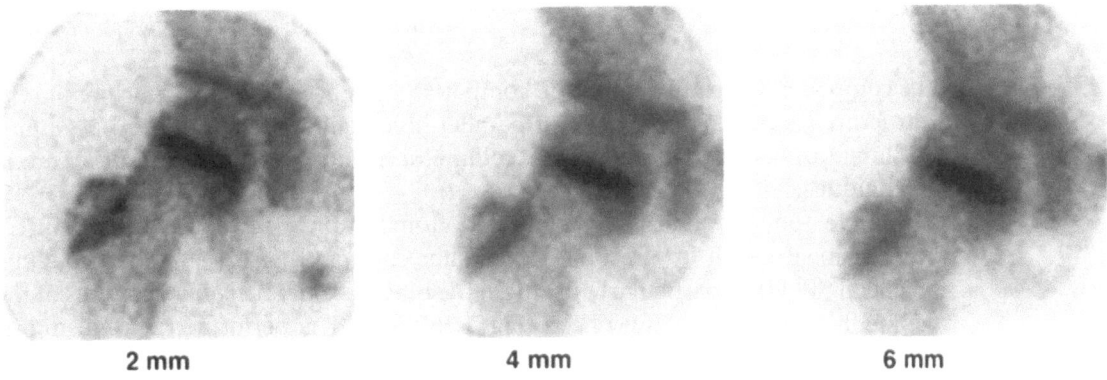

| 2 mm | 4 mm | 6 mm |

Figure 1.15. Effect of aperture size. The smaller the pinhole aperture, the better the resolution. This relationship is governed by the equation: $R = d(a + b)/a$, where R = resolution, d = diameter of aperture, a = crystal to aperture distance, and b = aperture to object distance. (Reprinted from Davis et al,[12] with permission.)

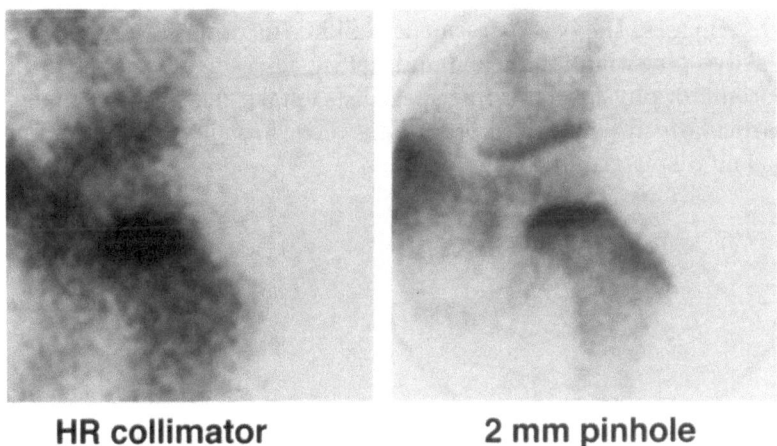

HR collimator   **2 mm pinhole**

Figure 1.16. Electronic vs. optical magnification. Skeletal detail, particularly the femoral capital epiphysis is better depicted with the pinhole image than the electronically magnified high-resolution image. (Reprinted from Davis et al,[12] with permission.)

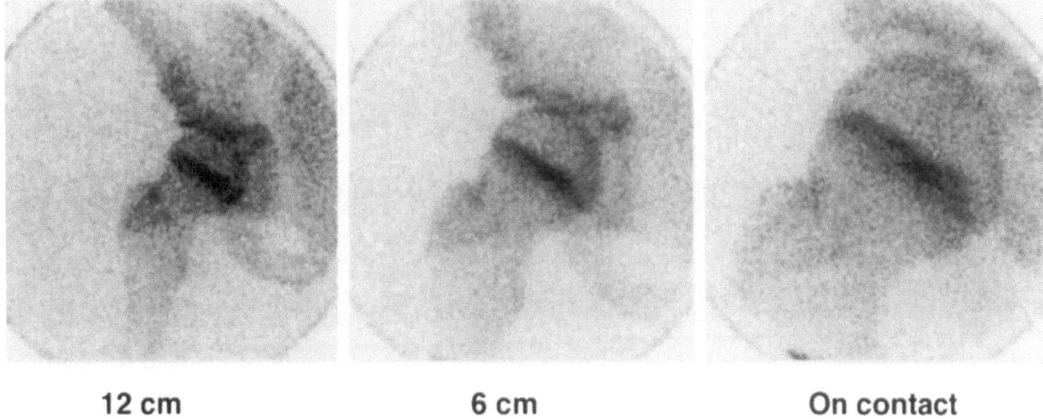

| 12 cm | 6 cm | On contact |

Figure 1.17. Effect of pinhole to object distance. The closer the object is to the pinhole aperture, the higher the magnification factor and the better the resolution. The field of view becomes progressively smaller, however. Distances noted are from the skin surface. (Reprinted from Davis et al,[12] with permission.)

be compared. Generally, however, comparison of tracer distribution in symmetric structures is better made using a parallel hole collimator rather than a pinhole collimator, as slight variations in collimator positioning occur despite careful technique.

Single photon emission computed tomography provides better three-dimensional lesion localization and greater contrast than does planar imaging. Skeletal SPECT is particularly useful in the diagnosis of focal abnormalities of the spine, hips, feet, knees, and head (Fig. 1.18). SPECT is performed with a single-, dual-, or triple-detector gamma camera system.[16] Although similar spatial resolution is obtainable with these systems, a triple-detector system offers advantages discussed previously. When undergoing SPECT, the child lies on the imaging table while the detector(s) rotates around the body. Typically, 120 images are obtained on a 128×128 matrix using an ultra–high-resolution collimator. We employ a noncircular 360° orbit. With this standard technique, imaging times are in the range of 20 to 30 minutes per examination and the total number of counts recorded are in the range of 3.6 to 10.0 million. Studies are evaluated using multiple slices in the coronal, transverse, and sagittal planes, as well as rotating volume rendered images. The best assessment of SPECT is done at the computer monitor with active physician interaction and not by assessment of printed images. It is important for physician imaging specialists to take an active role in data processing, particularly in choosing appropriate reconstruction filtering, gray-scale intensity, and display contrast (Fig. 1.19).

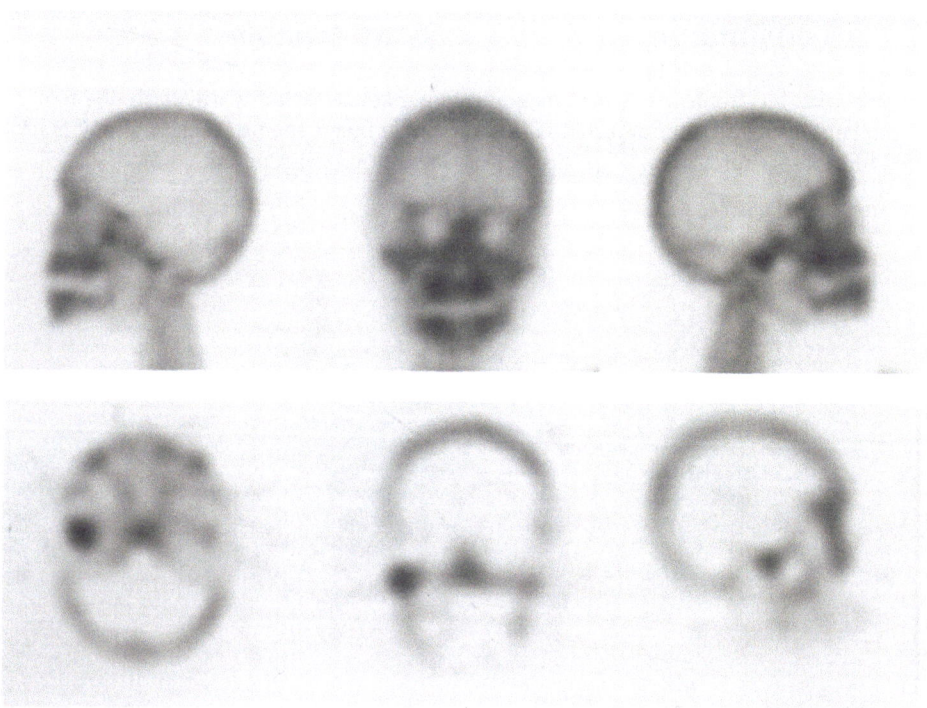

Figure 1.18. Single photon emission computed tomography. Planar imaging (upper row) and SPECT (lower row) shows intense tracer localization in the right temporomandibular region. Anatomic positioning of this finding to the right mandibular condyle is better achieved with SPECT in the transverse, coronal, and sagittal planes (left to right). This individual had significant facial asymmetry with the condylar localization reflecting continuing asymmetric mandibular growth.

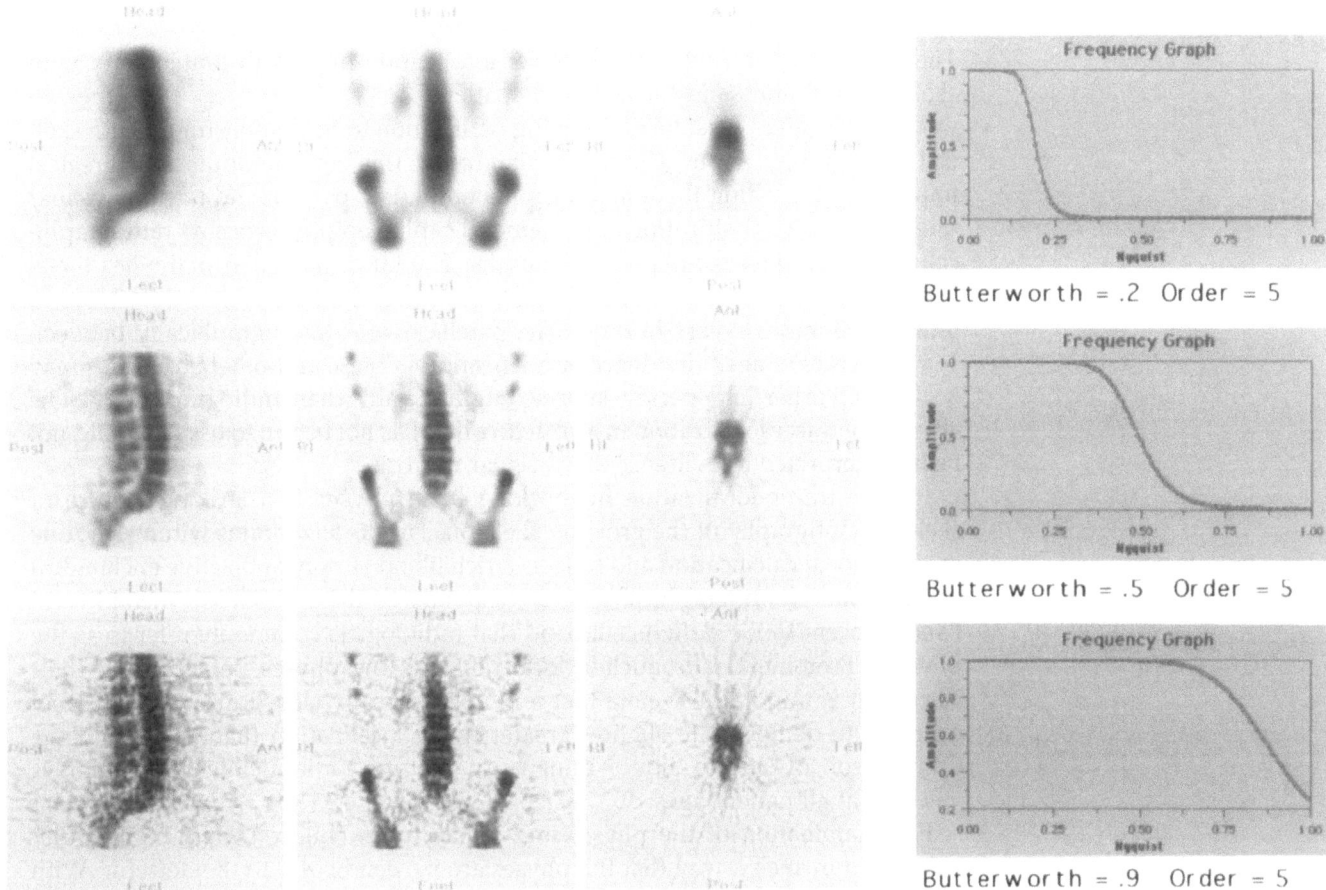

Figure 1.19. SPECT filter selection. Reconstructions corresponding to different filter shapes for a Butterworth filter are depicted. Anatomic structures are poorly defined when the images are too smooth (top row) or too sharp (bottom row). With appropriate filter selection (middle row), excellent anatomic detail is provided by SPECT.

The Normal Study and Potential Pitfalls in Interpretation

The appearance and intensity of tracer localization in growth centers vary with skeletal maturation and the age of the patient.

Growth centers must be undergoing ossification to be demonstrated with skeletal scintigraphy. From a practical standpoint this consideration is of greatest importance regarding the femoral capital epiphysis, patella, and tarsal navicular (Figs. 1.20–1.22). Ossification of the femoral capital epiphysis occurs radiographically between the ages of 2 and 7 months. The tarsal navicular is the last tarsal bone to ossify radiographically, doing so between the ages of 1 and $3\frac{1}{2}$ years in girls and 3 and $5\frac{1}{2}$ years in boys. The patella ossifies radiographically between $1\frac{1}{2}$ and 6 years of age.[28] Evidence of ossification in these and other structures may be visible earlier and persist later scintigraphically than radiographically. The absence of tracer localization in a structure that has not begun to ossify should not be misinterpreted as evidence of avascular necrosis.

Intense tracer localization in the long bone physes is a striking feature of skeletal scintigraphy of the growing skeleton. This localization is within the zone of provisional calcification and reflects a rich blood supply and active enchondral ossification.[7,8] Radiographically, it corresponds to the radiodense metaphyseal band adjacent to the radiolucent band that radiologists commonly refer to as the physis.[17] Prominent radionuclide localization at the physes persists until their closure. It is important to note that a radiographically closed growth plate may continue to demonstrate slightly greater tracer localization than adjacent bone. Comparison of side to side symmetry of physeal radionuclide localization is valuable at all patient ages.

For examination of the physes and metaphyses, children must be carefully positioned in such a way that the physes are perpendicular to the detector. With this orientation, physes appear as clearly defined transverse bands of prominent tracer localization.[38] Improper positioning results in apparent blurring of physeal margins. Infants deserve special mention as they tend to lie with their legs abducted and externally rotated. Imaging an infant in this position results in blurring of all lower extremity physes. Adduction of the feet is necessary to clearly delineate the distal tibial and fibular physes and adjacent bone.

Tracer localization is also prominent at apophyses and synchondroses. Tracer localization at certain of these ossification centers could be misinterpreted as representing a pathologic state. A brief review of some of the more common sources of such error is warranted.

Figure 1.22. Unossified naviculars. Absence of tracer localization in the naviculars is due to their not having begun to ossify in a 2-year-old boy (A). The right navicular of a 3-year-old girl has begun ossification; the left has not (B). Note also that internal rotation of the feet allows for separation of the tibial from the fibular physes for both cases.

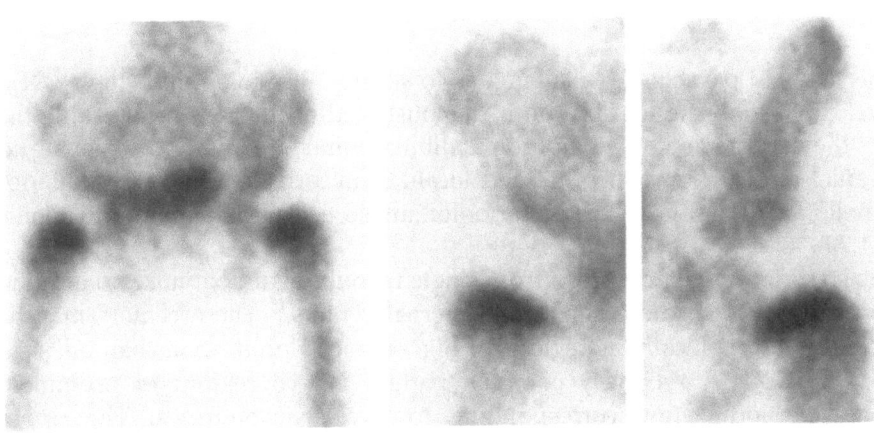

Figure 1.20. Unossified femoral capital epiphysis. The femoral capital epiphyses have not begun ossification in the 2-month-old infant whose images are depicted here.

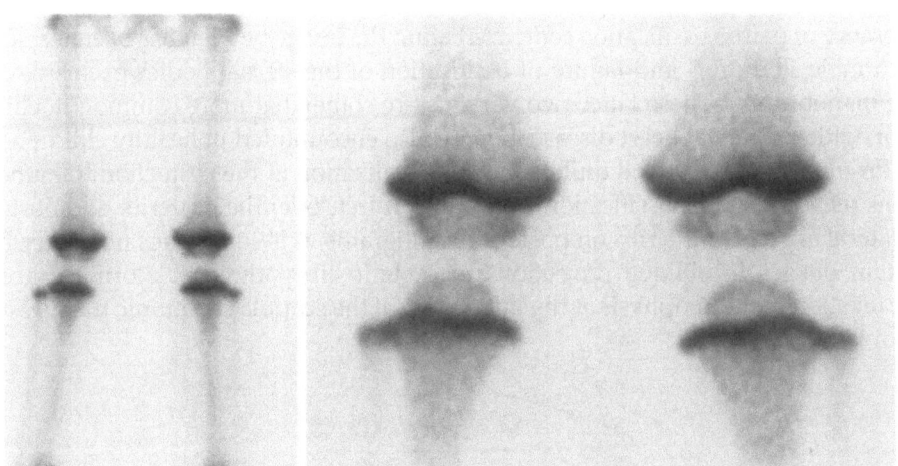

Figure 1.21. Unossified patellae. The patellae are not visualized with either high-resolution planar imaging or pinhole imaging in a 2-year-old girl.

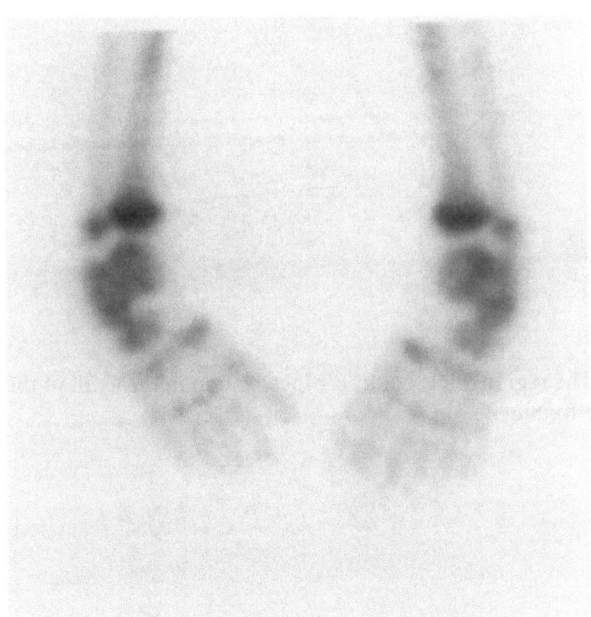

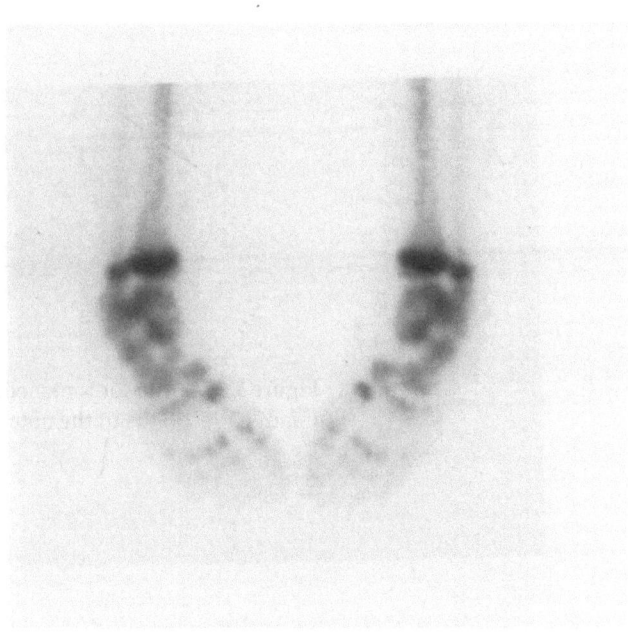

A

B

The skull is particularly challenging to assess. Physiologically high ^{99m}Tc-labeled diphosphonate localization is demonstrated at the base of the skull, the orbits, the nasal region, the temporomandibular joints, the mastoid regions, and the cranial sutures. Low to absent tracer localization corresponding to the anterior fontanelle, and occasionally the posterior fontanelle, are normal findings in infants (Fig. 1.23).

The sternum usually develops from single manubrial and xiphoid ossification centers and three separate single mesosternal centers.[26] These centers may be depicted scintigraphically as regions of higher tracer localization than adjacent bone (Fig. 1.24). A relatively common pattern is two regions of prominent radionuclide localization corresponding to two synchondroses. The upper synchondrosis is identified in adults as the manubriosternal joint. The caudal synchondrosis, which normally ossifies between 16 and 25 years of age, is identified as a transverse line of prominent radionuclide localization in many children. Persistent sternal segmentation, the multipartite sternum, is occasionally observed in the adult.[2] Other patterns that are rarely observed in children include the presence of paired ossification centers creating the image of what has been termed a "double sternum," and failure of ossification of the sternal bodies exclusive of the manubrium.[24] These latter two variants are somewhat more common in children with congenital heart disease, but are also encountered in healthy children.[37]

Prominent ^{99m}Tc-labeled diphosphonate localization at the costochondral junctions reflects ongoing ossification. Since this projects over the posterior and posterolateral aspects of the ribs on posterior scintigrams, it is sometimes necessary to obtain images in oblique projections to exclude rib pathology. Normal tracer localization in the apophysis at the inferior tip of the scapula can mimic fracture or neoplasm (Fig. 1.25).

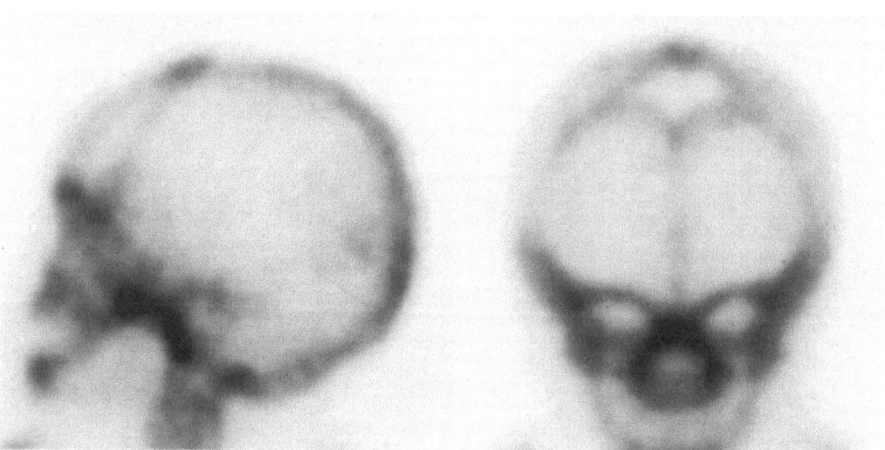

Figure 1.23. Anterior fontanelle. The region of absent tracer localization in the skull of this infant corresponds to the anterior fontanelle.

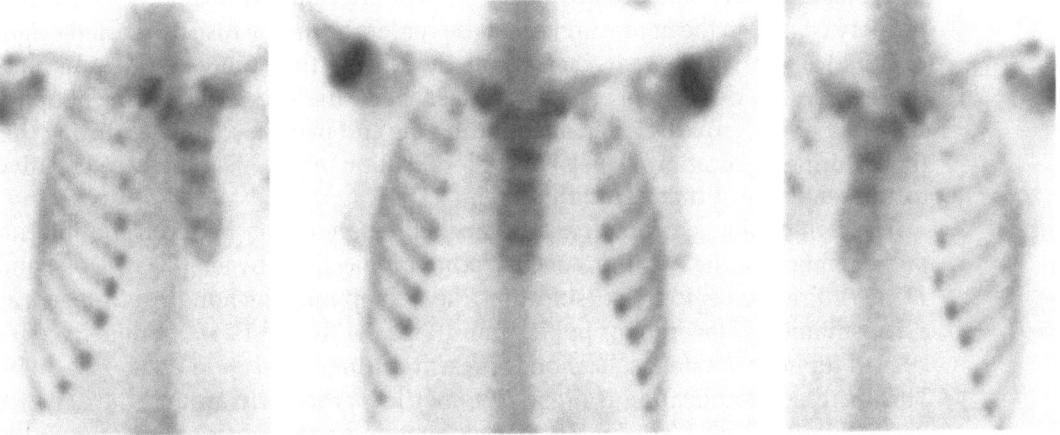

Figure 1.24. Sternal ossification centers. Three bands of high tracer localization corresponding to sternal growth centers are identified in this 18-year-old male.

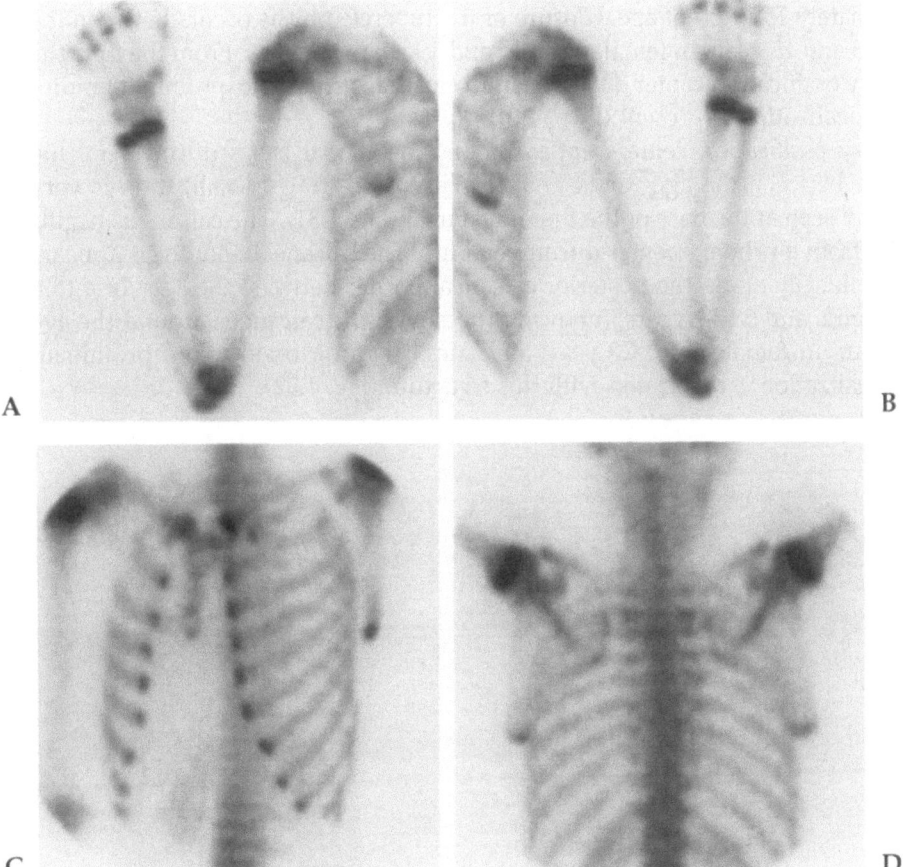

A

B

C

D

Figure 1.25. Scapular apophyses. Higher tracer localization is present at the apophyses of the inferior scapular tips than in adjacent bone. This overlies ribs on the posterior projections (A,B). Oblique imaging (C) and posterior imaging with the arms raised (D) assist in delineating this finding.

Vertebral ossification occurs at a single primary center in the body and at two primary centers in the neural arches. These centers normally fuse between the ages of 3 and 6 years. Secondary centers at the tips of the spinous and transverse processes ossify during puberty and the teenage years. The vertebral ring apophysis, a secondary growth center surrounding the end plate, also ossifies during this time. During ossification, skeletal tracer localization may appear increased relative to adjacent bone at these growth centers.[23]

The ischiopubic synchondrosis, a cartilaginous junction between the inferior pubic ramus and the ischium, ossifies radiographically between the ages of 4 and 12 years. Prior to beginning ossification, the ischiopubic synchondrosis appears as a discontinuity of the inferior pubic ramus (Figs. 1.12D and 1.26). Prominent ^{99m}Tc-labeled diphosphonate localization is present during ossification (Figs. 1.27–1.29). This increased localization is often asymmetric, particularly around the age of 8 years (Figs. 1.28 and 1.29). An asymmetric anatomic appearance to the ischiopubic synchondroses is also common radiographically.[4] Some imaging specialists experience difficulty in confidently excluding osteomyelitis when symptoms are referable to the ischiopubic region. With awareness of the normal pattern of tracer localization, this should rarely pose a significant problem, however. Increased radionuclide localization in adjacent bone, poor definition of the synchondrosis margins, tracer localization exceeding that related to the triradiate cartilage, and increased localization on the radionuclide angiogram are signs of osteomyelitis or trauma.[6,19]

The tibial tubercle, which originates as an inferior extension of the proximal tibial chondroepiphysis, develops a secondary center of ossification by 7 to 9 years of age. The epiphyseal tubercle center fuses with the main proximal tibial center at approximately 15 years of age. Closure of the tubercle physis occurs between the ages of 13 and 15 years in females and 15 and 19 years in males. From the time the secondary ossification center develops until closure is complete, prominent radionuclide localization is present (Fig. 1.30).

Primary ossification centers appear at the metatarsal bases during fetal life and close between the ages of 14 and 21 years. High tracer localization is very commonly seen at the base of the first metatarsal (Fig. 1.31). The calcaneus begins to ossify from a primary center during fetal life. The calcaneal apophysis appears radiographically along the posterior calcaneal border between the ages of 4 to 6 years in girls and 5 to 9 years in boys. It fuses with the calcaneus around the age of 16 years in females and 20 years in males.[39] During ossification, prominent tracer localization is associated with this structure (Fig. 1.32).

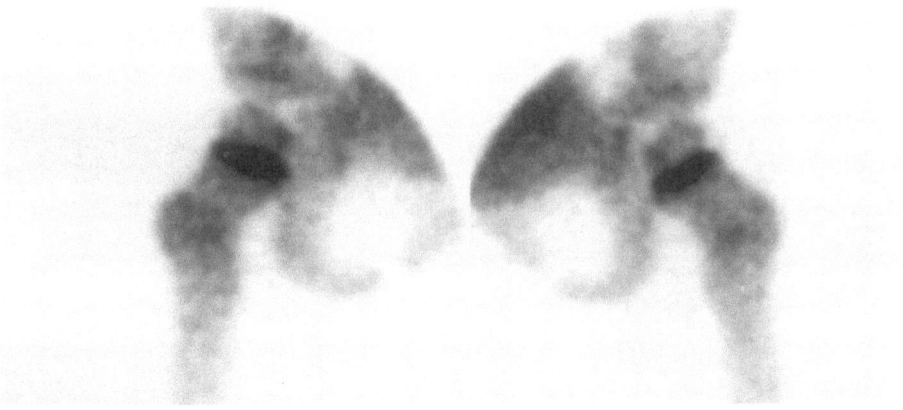

Figure 1.26. Ischiopubic synchondroses. Both synchondroses are devoid of tracer localization in this 5-year-old girl as shown by pinhole imaging.

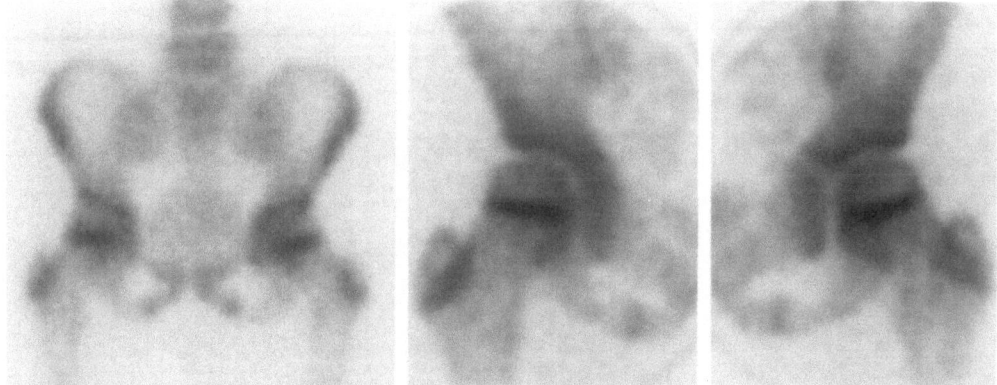

Figure 1.27. Ischiopubic synchondroses. High tracer localization is present symmetrically at both ischiopubic synchondroses of a 9-year-old girl (high-resolution planar and pinhole images).

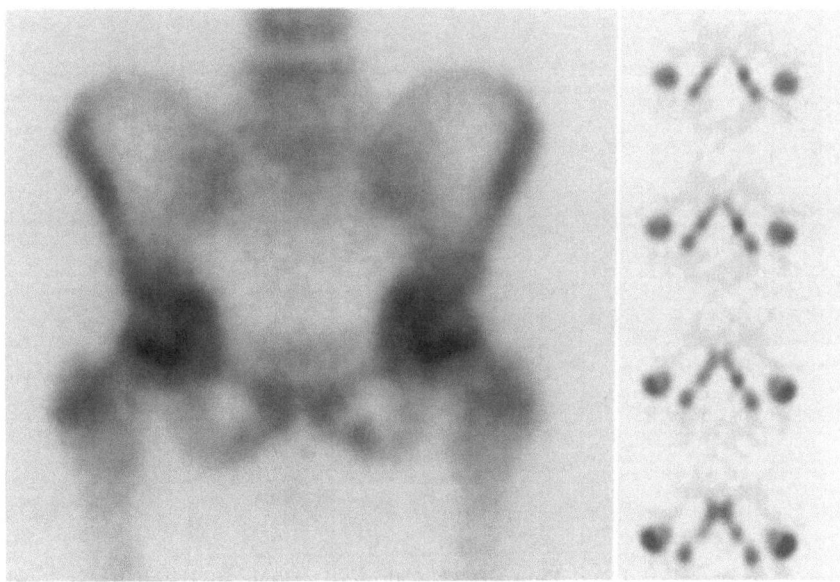

Figure 1.28. Ischiopubic synchondroses. Localization of ^{99m}Tc-MDP in the ischiopubic synchondroses of an 8-year-old girl is asymmetric as depicted by high-resolution planar scintigraphy (left image) and transverse SPECT images.

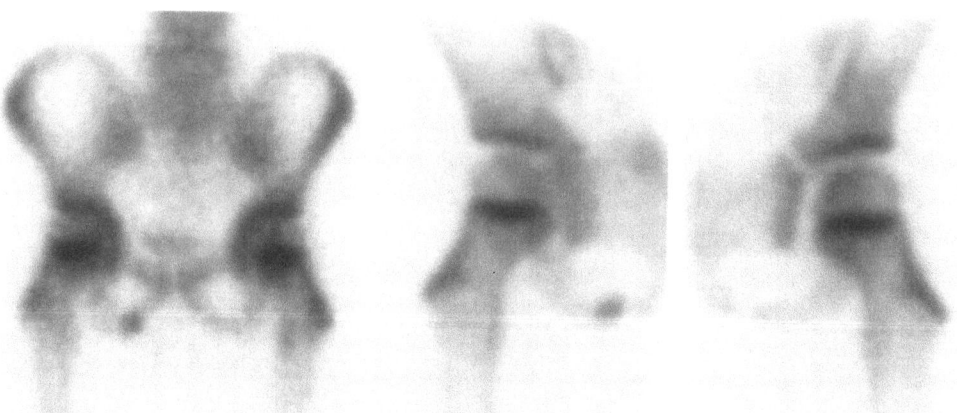

Figure 1.29. Ischiopubic synchondroses. The right ischiopubic synchondrosis intensely localizes ^{99m}Tc-MDP while the left ischiopubic synchondrosis shows an absence of tracer localization in an 8-year-old boy. Note also that the greater trochanters have not begun ossification.

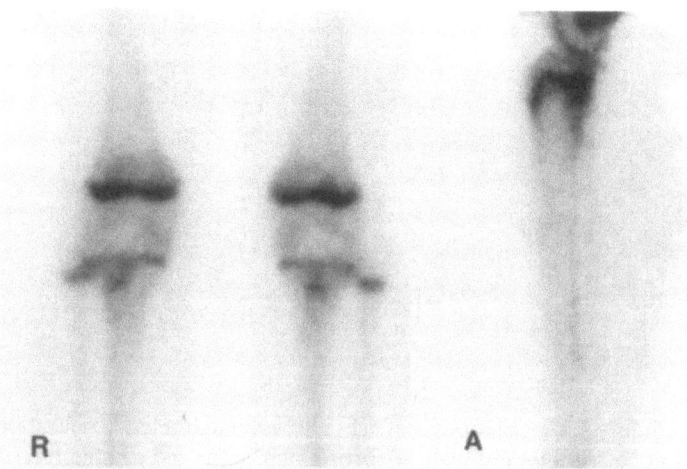

Figure 1.30. Tibial tubercle. Prominent tracer localization is frequently identified at the tibial tubercles (R, right; A; anterior).

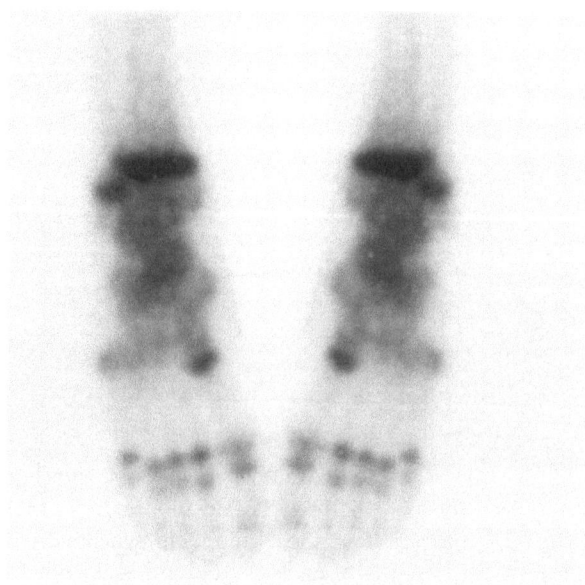

Figure 1.31. Metatarsal growth centers. Metatarsal and phalangeal growth centers demonstrate high ^{99m}Tc-MDP localization.

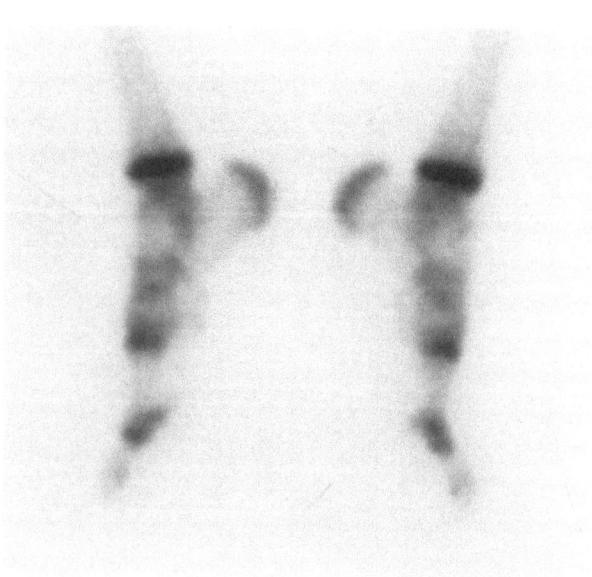

Figure 1.32. Calcaneal apophysis. High tracer localization along the calcaneus posteriorly corresponds to the calcaneal apophysis.

Other Radiotracers Used in Evaluating the Pediatric Skeleton

Radiotracers that localize to sites of infection, tumors, and the bone marrow are useful in evaluating pathologic conditions affecting the pediatric skeleton. The mechanism of localization and the imaging characteristics of these tracers are reviewed below. Suggested administered doses for radiopharmaceuticals discussed in this section are summarized in Table 1.1.

Gallium-67

Gallium-67 (^{67}Ga) citrate is used in the assessment of suspected infection and various neoplasms, most notably lymphoma. This cyclotron-produced radiopharmaceutical has a physical half-life of 78.1 hours. Photons used in imaging are emitted at 93 keV, 184 keV, 296 keV, and 388 keV. The energy of these photons requires appropriate collimation.

Gallium-67 is a group III transition metal that acts as a ferric ion analogue when administered in trace amounts. Accumulation of ^{67}Ga in sites of infection and inflammation is multifactorial. It is related to direct uptake into leukocytes and bacteria, as well as binding to lactoferrin, which accumulates with leukocyte breakdown, and siderophores, compounds that facilitate iron uptake by microorganisms.[40] The mechanism of ^{67}Ga localization in tumors varies with tumor type. With lymphoma, transferrin binding and alterations in cellular plasma membranes are most likely involved.[13]

The suggested administered doses for ^{67}Ga scintigraphy are 0.04 mCi (1.48 MBq)/kg (minimum 0.25 mCi [9.25 MBq], maximum 6.0 mCi [222 MBq]). Imaging is performed 24 or more hours following administration.

The normal distribution of ^{67}Ga includes bone and bone marrow, the nasopharynx, lacrimal and salivary glands, liver, spleen, and bowel (Fig. 1.33). The normal passage of ^{67}Ga into the bowel often necessitates serial imaging over 3 days to 14 days when abdominal pathology is questioned. The kidneys may be demonstrated during the initial 48 hours following tracer administration due to normal renal excretion. Breast uptake is frequently observed during menarche, with pregnancy and lactation and in association with oral contraceptives. In children, the thymus often accumulates ^{67}Ga. Localization of ^{67}Ga in reactive and reparative bone somewhat limits its use in evaluating suspected skeletal infection and significantly limits its use in assessing the response of skeletal malignancies to therapy.

Labeled Leukocytes

Scintigraphy with radiolabeled leukocytes provides a means for identifying sites of infection and inflammation. Labeling is accomplished with either indium-111 (^{111}In), using ^{111}In oxine, or ^{99m}Tc, using ^{99m}Tc-hexamethylpropylene amine oxime (HMPAO). Although there is a larger body of published experience with ^{111}In-labeled leukocytes, the superior imaging characteristics of ^{99m}Tc, the more favorable radiation dosimetry of ^{99m}Tc-labeled leukocytes, and the greater convenience of labeling with ^{99m}Tc render the use of ^{99m}Tc-labeled leukocytes the preferred technique for use in children.

The suggested administered dose of ^{99m}Tc-labeled leukocytes is 0.2 mCi (7.4 MBq)/kg (minimum 0.5 mCi [18.5 MBq], maximum 20.0 mCi [740 MBq]). Im-

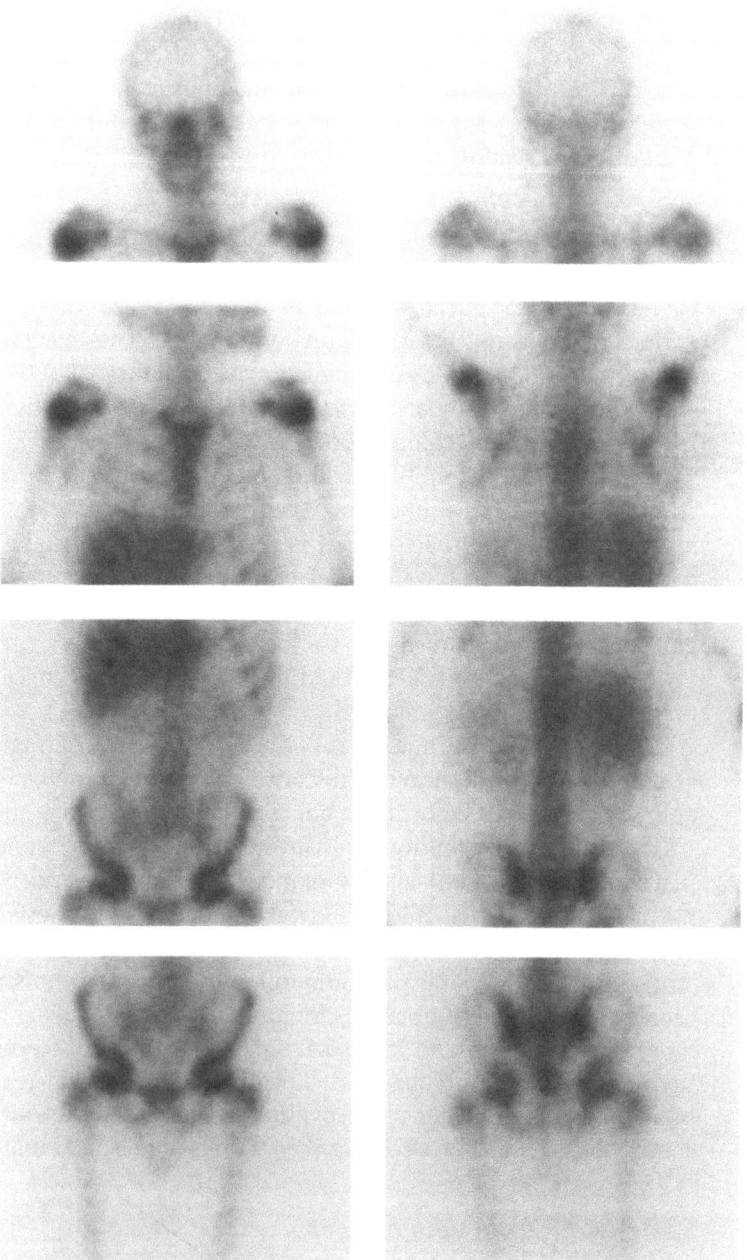

Figure 1.33. Normal gallium-67 study. The lacrimal glands, the nasopharynx, salivary glands, liver, spleen, and bone are visualized. Bowel excretion is minimal in this patient (anterior images: left panels; posterior images: right panels).

aging is performed 1 and 4 hours following administration. Images obtained in the first hour normally demonstrate the spleen, in which localization is intense, liver, lungs, and bone marrow. The urinary bladder and, frequently, the kidneys are visualized due to excreted ^{99m}Tc, probably as pertechnetate. The gallbladder is seen in some patients, due to excretion of ^{99m}Tc-HMPAO or a secondary metabolite. Images obtained 4 or more hours after ^{99m}Tc-labeled leukocyte administration show more prominent bone marrow localization and less prominent pulmonary localization. Bowel may be visualized due to hepatic excretion. Radionuclide distribution is otherwise unchanged (Fig. 1.34).[33]

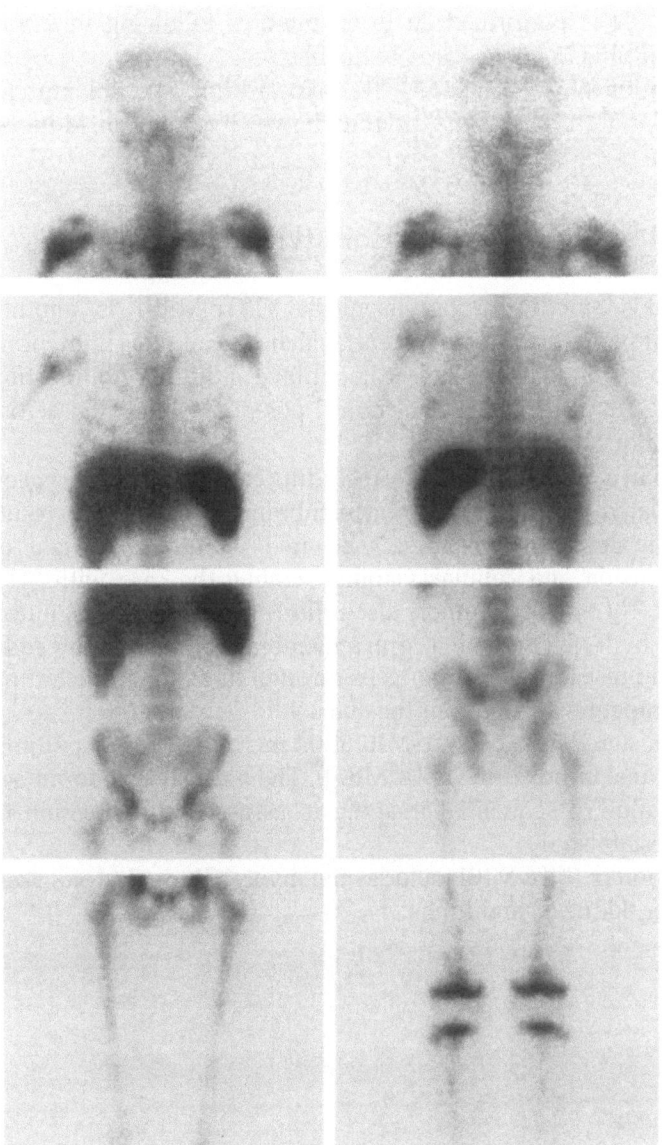

Figure 1.34. Normal ^{99m}Tc-labeled leukocyte examination. Anterior (left panels) and posterior (right panels) images of the head, neck, thorax, abdomen, and pelvis, and anterior images of the lower extremities (lowermost panels) show the most intense accumulation of radiotracer to be in the spleen. Note that the peripheral appendicular skeleton is visualized secondary to the presence of red marrow. Images were obtained 4 hours following tracer administration.

Thallium-201 Chloride

Thallium-201 (^{201}Tl) chloride is a cyclotron-produced radiopharmaceutical that is widely used for myocardial perfusion scintigraphy. The half-life of ^{201}Tl is 73 hours. Mercury x-rays of 69 to 83 keV, emitted during the decay of ^{201}Tl, are used for imaging.

This potassium analogue is distributed in the myocardium in proportion to blood flow with its entry into myocytes dependent on an intact adenosine triphosphatase (ATPase)-mediated sodium-potassium transport system. Owing to its similarity to potassium, ^{201}Tl is also concentrated in various tumors, most notably osteosarcoma. The uptake of ^{201}Tl by bone malignancies is influenced by blood flow, cellular viability, malignancy grade, and density of viable tumor cells (Fig. 1.35).[21]

The suggested administered doses for ^{201}Tl chloride scintigraphy are 0.03 mCi (1.11 MBq)/kg (minimum 0.5 mCi [18.5 MBq], maximum 2.0 mCi [74 MBq]). Tumor imaging with ^{201}Tl is performed 20 to 60 minutes following injection. High-quality planar and SPECT images are obtainable.

The normal distribution of ^{201}Tl includes the myocardium, skeletal muscle, lacrimal and salivary glands, nasopharynx, thyroid, bowel, liver, spleen, kidneys, and genitalia (Fig. 1.36).

Technetium-99m Hexakis-2-Methoxyisobutylisonitrile

Technetium-99m hexakis-2-methoxyisobutylisonitrile (^{99m}Tc-MIBI) is another widely used myocardial perfusion imaging agent, which concentrates in myocardium according to regional blood flow. Myocardial uptake of this lipophilic cation occurs by passive diffusion in response to electrical potentials generated across sarcolemmal and mitochondrial membranes.

Uptake of ^{99m}Tc-MIBI in a number of tumors, including osteosarcoma,[5] has been reported. This is postulated to reflect high transmembrane potentials that result from the high metabolic demand of tumors.[31] As with ^{201}Tl, tumoral uptake of ^{99m}Tc-MIBI reflects perfusion and cellular viability. Unlike the case with ^{201}Tl, uptake and retention of ^{99m}Tc-MIBI in tumors also reflects this agent's recognition as a transport substrate by P-glycoprotein (Pgp), a membrane protein involved in the development of drug resistance in tumor cells through its action in excluding a number of chemotherapeutic agents from the cytosol.[18,30]

The suggested administered dose of ^{99m}Tc-MIBI is 0.4 mCi (14.8 MBq)/kg (minimum 2.0 mCi [74 MBq], maximum 20 mCi [740 MBq]). The optimal time for imaging and the possible value of sequential imaging to assess Pgp expression in tumors have not been established.

The normal distribution of ^{99m}Tc-MIBI includes the myocardium, thyroid, skeletal muscle, bowel, liver, kidneys, and lungs.

Figure 1.36. Normal thallium-201 study. Anterior images depict the normal distribution of ^{201}Tl in the lacrimal glands, nasopharynx, salivary glands, thyroid, heart, liver, spleen, kidneys, bowel, genitalia, and muscle.

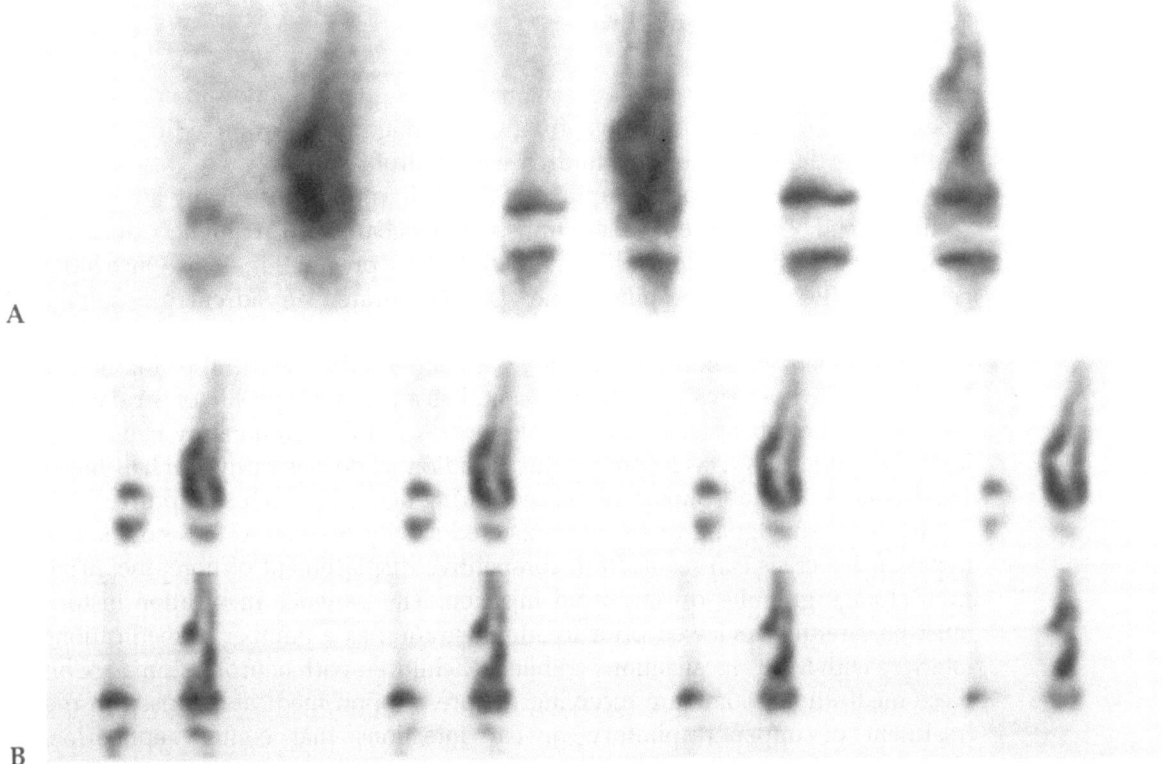

A

B

Figure 1.35. Thallium-201 in osteosarcoma. The distribution of ^{201}Tl in a right femoral osteosarcoma (A, left panel) is similar, but not identical, to that of ^{99m}Tc-MDP during tissue phase imaging (A, middle panel). The skeletal phase ^{99m}Tc-MDP image shows a markedly different distribution of ^{99m}Tc-MDP relative to that of ^{201}Tl (A, right panel). Differing distribution of the two tracers is well demonstrated with coronal SPECT (B, upper row: ^{201}Tl; lower row: ^{99m}Tc-MDP skeletal phase). Thallium-201 localization in osteosarcoma reflects perfusion and cellularity. Technetium-99m MDP distribution reflects perfusion, particularly on radionuclide angiography and tissue phase imaging, and either reactive or malignant bone formation. Additional images of this patient are presented in Figure 5.3.

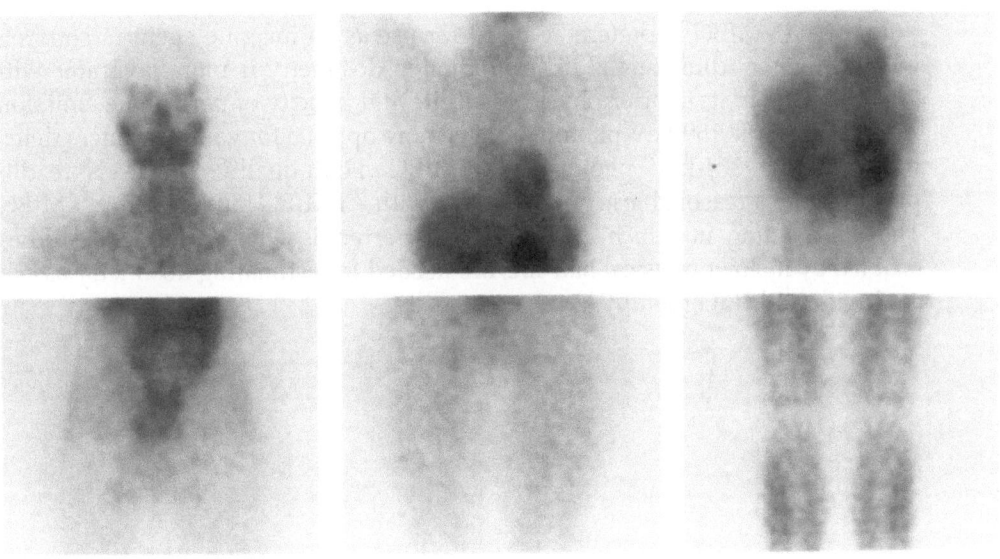

Metaiodobenzylguanidine

Metaiodobenzylguanidine (MIBG), an analogue of guanethidine and norepinephrine (Fig. 1.37), localizes in various tumors. The major application of this tracer in
pediatrics is the assessment of children with neuroblastoma.

At doses used for imaging, uptake of MIBG into the cytosol is by a neuronal
sodium- and energy-dependent transport mechanism. At higher doses, a
nonneuronal sodium-independent mechanism may prevail (Fig. 1.38). Once intra-
cellular, MIBG, like norepinephrine, is concentrated in adrenergic storage
vesicles.[14]

Metaiodobenzylguanidine is labeled with either iodine-131 (^{131}I) or iodine-123
(^{123}I). Iodine-131, a reactor-produced agent, has a physical half-life of 8.1 days. It
decays with both beta and gamma emissions. A 364-keV gamma ray is used for
imaging. Iodine-123, a cyclotron-produced radionuclide, has a physical half-life of
13.3 hours. A 159-keV photon is emitted during decay by electron capture.

Metaiodobenzylguanidine is administered slowly over 20 to 30 seconds as a
hypertensive crisis can result from competitive displacement of norepinephrine
from storage granules during rapid injection. The patient's medication history
must be carefully reviewed prior to administration as a number of medications
interfere with MIBG localization.[35] While few children with neuroblastoma are on
these medications, some are receiving nonprescription medications used in the
treatment of upper respiratory or ear infections that contain ephedrine,
phenylephridine, or other potentially interfering agents.

The suggested administered dose of ^{131}I-MIBG is 0.014 mCi (0.52 MBq)/kg
(minimum 0.1 mCi [3.7 MBq], maximum 1.0 mCi [37 MBq]). To limit thyroidal
irradiation, we recommend that 1 drop of supersaturated potassium iodide (SSKI)
solution be administered three times daily beginning 1 day before and continuing
for 5 days following ^{131}I-MIBG administration. Imaging is performed 2 or more
days following administration (Fig. 1.39). The suggested dose of ^{123}I-MIBG is
0.2 mCi (7.4 MBq)/kg (minimum 1.0 mCi [37 MBq], maximum 10.0 mCi [370 MBq]).
SSKI is administered in a dose of one drop three times daily beginning the day
before and continuing for 3 days after ^{123}I-MIBG administration. Imaging is performed 24 hours and, if deemed necessary, 48 hours following administration (Fig.
1.40).

Normal tracer distribution is to the heart, liver, thyroid, salivary and lacrimal
glands, kidneys, urine, adrenals, bowel, and muscle. Pulmonary localization occasionally occurs. Uptake of MIBG does not occur in normal bone and bone
marrow.[14,15,29]

Iodine-123 MIBG is preferable to ^{123}I for use as an imaging agent in children.
Even in higher administered doses, radiation dosimetry is more favorable with
^{123}I-MIBG due to its shorter physical half-life and paucity of particulate emission.
Additionally, the 159-keV photon of ^{123}I is more optimal for gamma camera detection than the 364-keV photon of ^{131}I-MIBG. High-quality SPECT is readily
performed in a reasonable acquisition time with ^{123}I-MIBG but not with ^{131}I-MIBG.
The only setting in which ^{131}I-MIBG is preferred is when prolonged studies,
enabled by its long physical half-life, are needed for estimating dosimetry associated with ^{131}I-MIBG therapy.

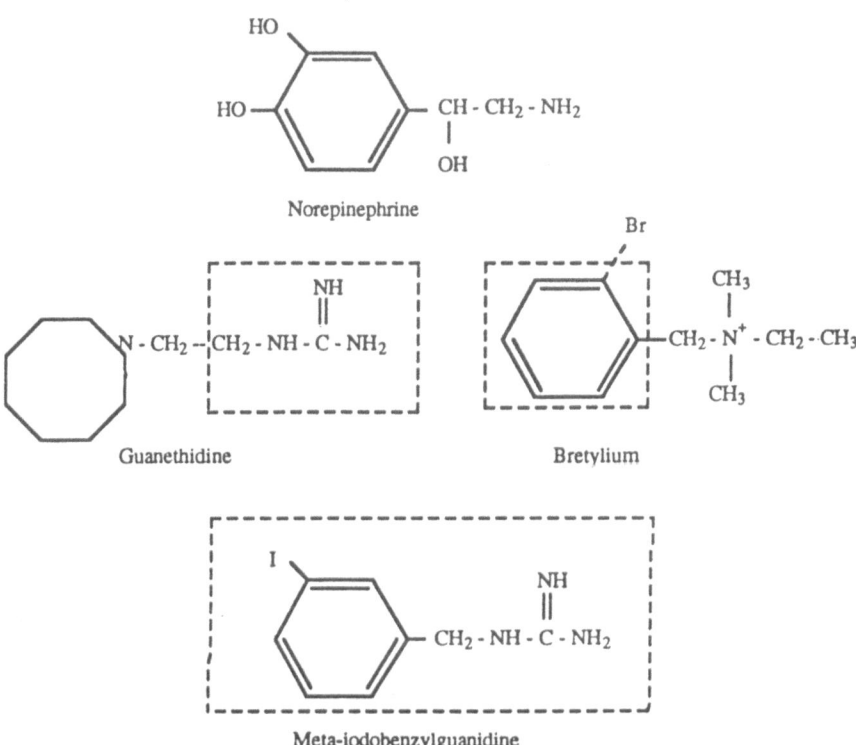

Figure 1.37. Chemical structures of norepinephrine, guanethidine, bretylium, and MIBG. The guanidine group of guanethidine is combined with the benzyl group of bretylium to synthesize MIBG. (Reprinted from Farahati et al,[14] with permission.)

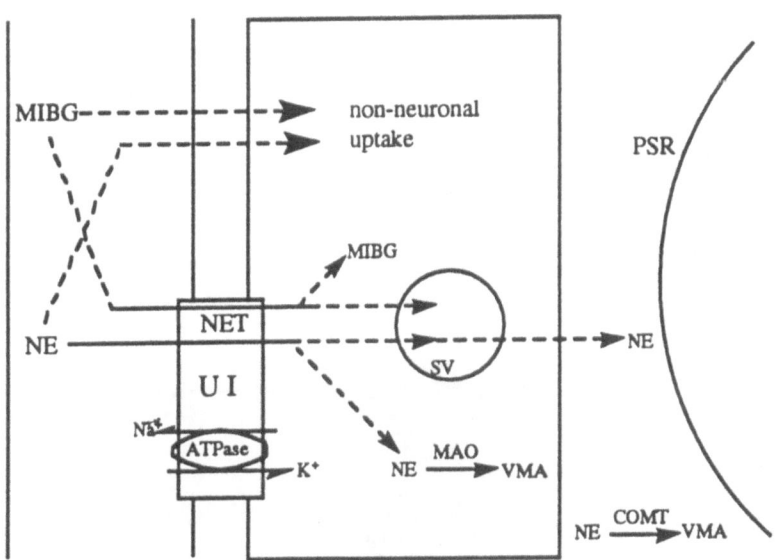

Figure 1.38. Norepinephrine and MIBG uptake mechanism. UI, sodium- and energy-dependent transport mechanism uptake; NE, norepinephrine; NET, norepinephrine transporter; SV, synaptic vesicle; MAO, monoamine oxidase; COMT, catechol-o-methyl-transferase; VMA, vanillylmandelic acid; PSR, postsynaptic receptor. (Reprinted from Farahati et al,[14] with permission.)

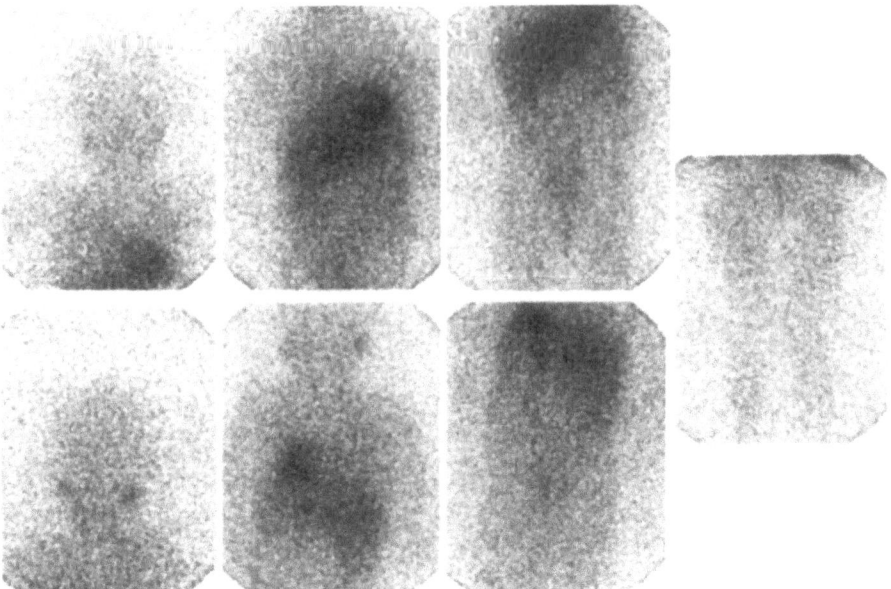

Figure 1.39. Iodine-131 metaiodobenzylguanidine imaging. The salivary glands, heart, liver, urinary bladder, and skeletal muscle are identified on these images obtained 2 days following ^{131}I-MIBG administration. Upper row: anterior projections; lower row: posterior projections, anterior lower extremity image.

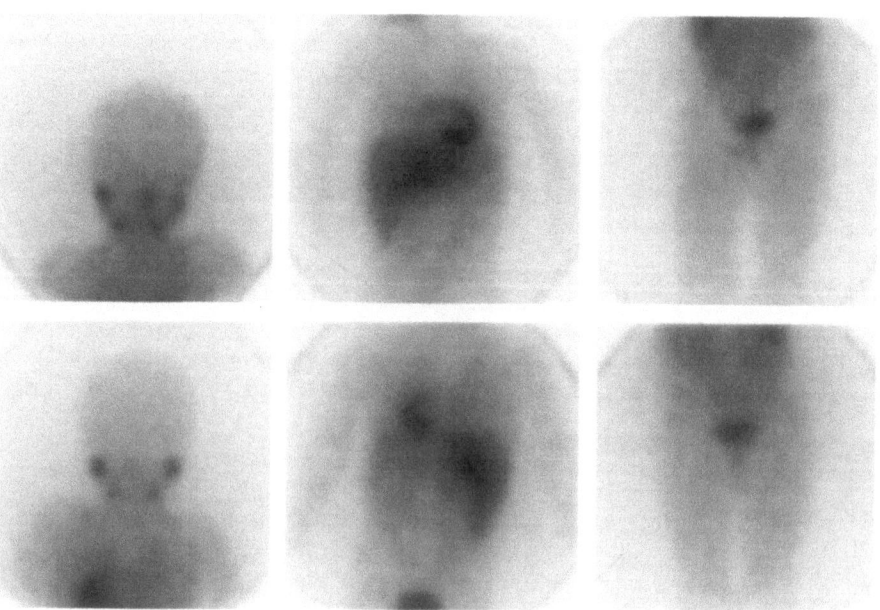

Figure 1.40. Iodine-123 metaiodobenzylguanidine imaging. Tracer is seen in salivary glands, heart, liver, urinary bladder, and skeletal muscle on these images obtained 24 hours following administration of ^{123}I-MIBG (upper row: anterior projections; lower row: posterior projections). Definition is clearer than with ^{131}I-MIBG imaging.

Indium-111 Pentetreotide

Pentetreotide is formed by conjugation of diethylenetriamine pentaacetic acid to the somatostatin analogue octreotide. This agent has potential applications in a number of tumors that possess somatostatin receptors. These include neuroblastoma. Radiolabeling is with [111]In. From the recommended adult dose of 3.0 mCi (111 MBq), a pediatric dose of 0.04 mCi/kg (1.5 MBq/kg) is estimated. Imaging is performed from 4 to 48 hours following tracer administration. Tracer accumulation is seen in the pituitary, spleen, liver, kidneys, urine, gallbladder, bowel, breasts, thyroid, nasal region, and lung hili.[20,25]

Technetium-99m Sulfur Colloid

Radiolabeled colloids allow scintigraphic visualization of the reticuloendothelial system, where colloidal particles undergo phagocytosis. The most commonly used agent in the United States is ^{99m}Tc-sulfur colloid. This radiopharmaceutical is formed in particle sizes ranging from 0.1 to 2 μm during heating of an acid mixture of ^{99m}Tc pertechnetate and sodium thiosulfate.

The suggested administered dose of ^{99m}Tc-sulfur colloid is 0.10 mCi/kg (3.7 MBq/kg) (minimum 0.50 mCi [18.5 MBq], maximum 5.0 mCi [185 MBq]).

Tc-99m–sulfur colloid most avidly localizes in the reticuoendothelial cells of the liver and spleen. Approximately 5% of administered dose localizes in the bone marrow. Except for portions of the thoracic and lumbar spine that are obscured by tracer uptake in the liver and spleen, this degree of uptake is adequate to image most of the bone marrow. The normal pattern of ^{99m}Tc-sulfur colloid uptake in the marrow differs with age, reflecting the distribution of active marrow. In children older than 10 years of age, the uptake pattern is similar to that seen in adults. In younger children, there is more extensive uptake in the extremities. Through 2 years of age, the entire femur and tibia may be demonstrated. From ages 2 to 10, extremity uptake decreases, initially in the distal tibia and later in the femur. Peripheral marrow expansion following chemotherapy may alter this appearance.[27,34]

Other marrow imaging agents include smaller size colloids, such as ^{99m}Tc-nanocolloid and ^{99m}Tc-antimony sulfide colloid. Indium-111 chloride may also be used. Bone marrow localization of this ^{111}In-chloride is due to either phagocytosis of an indium colloid that forms in vivo after injection or indium acting as a mimic of iron in hematopoiesis.

References

1. American Academy of Pediatrics Committee on Drugs. Guidelines for monitoring and management of pediatric patients during and after sedation for diagnostic and therapeutic procedures. *Pediatrics* 1992;89:1110–1115.
2. Baas J, Eijsvogel M, Dijkstra P. Persistent sternum synchondroses on bone scintigraphy. *Eur J Nucl Med* 1988;13:572–573.
3. Burrows PE. Pediatric sedation for nuclear medicine procedures. In: Treves ST, ed. *Pediatric Nuclear Medicine*. 2nd ed. New York: Springer-Verlag; 1995:12–16.
4. Caffey J, Ross SE. The ischiopubic synchondrosis in healthy children: some normal roentgenologic findings. *AJR* 1956;76:488–494.
5. Caner B, Kitapci M, Aras T, et al. Increased accumulation of hexakis (2-methoxyisobutylisonitrile) technetium (I) [Tc-MIBI] in osteosarcoma and its metastatic lymph nodes. *J Nucl Med* 1991;32:1977–1978.
6. Cawley KA, Dvorak AD, Wilmot MD. Normal anatomic variant: scintigraphy of the ischiopubic synchondrosis. *J Nucl Med* 1983;24:14–16.

7. Christensen SB, Krogsgaard OW. Localization of Tc-99m MDP in epiphyseal growth plates of rats. *J Nucl Med* 1981:22:237–245.

8. Comar CL, Lotz WE, Boyd GA. Autoradiographic studies of calcium, phosphorus, and strontium distribution in the bones of the growing pig. *Am J Anat* 1952;90:113–129.

9. Committee on Drugs Section on Anesthesiology. Guidelines for the elective use of conscious sedation, deep sedation and general anesthesia in pediatric patients. *Pediatrics* 1985;76:317–321.

10. Conway JJ. Scintigraphic classification of Legg-Calvé-Perthes disease. *Semin Nucl Med* 1993;23:274–295.

11. Datz FL. *Gamuts in Nuclear Medicine*. Norwalk: Appleton and Lange; 1987.

12. Davis RT, Zimmerman RE, Treves ST. Magnification in pediatric nuclear medicine. In: Treves ST, ed. *Pediatric Nuclear Medicine*. 2nd ed. New York: Springer-Verlag; 1995:24–32.

13. Dillehay GL, Papatheofanis FJ. Gallium imaging of tumors. In: Henkin RE, Boles MA, Dillehay GL, et al, eds. *Nuclear Medicine*. Philadelphia: Mosby Year Book; 1996:1463–1492.

14. Farahati J, Mueller SP, Coennen HH, et al. Scintigraphy of neuroblastoma with radioiodinated m-iodobenzylguanidine. In: Treves ST, ed. *Pediatric Nuclear Medicine*. 2nd ed. New York: Springer-Verlag; 1995:528–545.

14a. Fischer KC, Shapiro S, Treves ST. Visualization of the spleen with a bone-seeking radionuclide in a child with sickle cell anemia. Radiology 1977;122:398.

15. Gelfand MJ. Meta-iodobenzylguanidine in children. *Semin Nucl Med* 1993;23:231–242.

16. Groch MW, Erwin WD, Bieszk JA. Single photon emission computed tomography. In: Treves ST, ed. *Pediatric Nuclear Medicine*. 2nd ed. New York: Springer-Verlag; 1995:33–87.

17. Harcke HT, Mandell GA. Scintigraphic evaluation of the growth plate. *Semin Nucl Med* 1993;23:266–273.

18. Kartner N, Riordan JR, Ling V. Cell surface P-glycoprotein associated with multidrug resistance in mammalian cell lines. *Science* 1983;221:1285–1288.

19. Kloiber R, Udjus K, McIntyre W, et al. The scintigraphic and radiographic appearance of the ischiopubic synchondroses in normal children and in osteomyelitis. *Pediatr Radiol* 1988;18:57–61.

20. Krenning EP, Kwekkeboom DJ, Bakker WH, et al. Somatostatin receptor scintigraphy with [In-111-DTPA-D-Phe1] and [123I-Tyr3]-octreotide: the Rotterdam experience with more than 1,000 patients. *Eur J Nucl Med* 1993;20:716–731.

21. Lepanto PB, Rosenstock J, Littman P, et al. Gallium-67 scans in children with solid tumors. *AJR* 1976;126:179–186.

22. Lutrin CL, McDougall IR, Goris ML. Intense concentration of technetium-99m pyrophosphate in the kidneys of children treated with chemotherapeutic drugs for malignant disease. *Radiology* 1978;128:165–167.

23. Mandell GA, Harcke HT. Scintigraphy of persistent vertebral process epiphysis. *Clin Nucl Med* 1987;12:359–362.

24. Mandell GA, Heyman S. Absent sternum on bone scan. *Clin Nucl Med* 1983;8:327.

25. Manil L, Edeline V, Lumbroso J, et al. Indium-111-pentetreotide scintigraphy in children with neuroblast-derived tumors. *J Nucl Med* 1996;37:893–896.

26. Ogden JA, Conlogue GJ, Bronson ML, et al. Radiology of postnatal skeletal development: II. The manubrium and sternum. *Skeletal Radiol* 1979;4:189–195.

27. Oseas RS, Siddiqui AR, Wellman HN, et al. Usefulness of bone marrow imaging in childhood malignancies. *J Pediatr* 1982;101:206–209.

28. Ozonoff MB. *Pediatric Orthopedic Radiology*. 2nd ed. Philadelphia: W.B. Saunders; 1992.

29. Paltiel HJ, Gelfand MJ, Elgazzar AH, et al. Neural crest tumors: [123]I MIBG imaging in children. *Radiology* 1994;190:117–121.

30. Piwnica-Worms D, Chiu ML, Budding M, et al. Functional imaging of multidrug-resistant P-glycoprotein with an organotechnium complex. *Cancer Res* 1993;53:977–984.

31. Piwnica-Worms D, Holman BL. Noncardiac applications of hexakis (alkylisonitrile) technetium-99m complexes (editorial). *J Nucl Med* 1990;31:1166–1167.

32. Roack PJ, Itrato D, Treves ST. Bowel visualization on bone scan because of protein losing enteropathy. *Clin Nucl Med* 1994;19:1114–1116.

33. Roddie ME, Peters Am, Danpure HJ, et al. Inflammation: imaging with Tc-99m HMPAO-labeled leukocytes. *Radiology* 1988;166:767–772.

34. Siddiqui AR, Oseas RS, Wellman HN, et al. Evaluation of bone marrow scanning with technetium-99m sulfur colloid in pediatric oncology. *J Nucl Med* 1979;20:379–386.

35. Solanki KK, Bomanji J, Moyes J, et al. A pharmacological guide to medicines which interfere with the biodistribution of radiolabelled meta-iodobenzylguanidine (MIBG). *Nucl Med Commun* 1992;13:513–521.

36. Sorenson JA, Phelps ME. *Physics in Nuclear Medicine.* 2nd ed. Philadelphia: W.B. Saunders; 1987.

37. Steiner RM, Kricun ME, Shapiro J. Absent mesosternum in congenital heart disease. *AJR* 1976;127:923–925.

38. Sty JR, Wells RG, Starshak RJ, Gregg D. The musculoskeletal system. In: Sty J, Wells R, Starshak R, Gregg D, eds. *Diagnostic Imaging of Infants and Children.* Vol. 3. Gaithesburg: Aspen; 1992:233–405.

39. Tachdjian MO. *The Child's Foot.* Philadelphia: W.B Saunders; 1985.

39a. Treves ST, Introduction. In: Treves ST, Pediatric Nuclear Medicine, New York: Springer-Verlag 1995:1–8.

40. Tsan M. Mechanisms of gallium-67 accumulation in inflammatory lesions. *J Nucl Med* 1985;26:88–92.

41. Weiss S. Sedation of pediatric patients for nuclear medicine procedures. *Semin Nucl Med* 1993;23:190–198.

2
Skeletal Infection

Suspected skeletal infection is one of the most common indications for skeletal scintigraphy in children. This chapter reviews infections of the pediatric skeleton and the role of skeletal scintigraphy in their diagnosis. The imaging strategy that we employ in assessing suspected acute osteomyelitis is described.

Acute Osteomyelitis

Clinical Considerations

Acute osteomyelitis is a common pediatric problem that occurs at any age. Children younger than 5 years of age are most frequently affected.

During childhood, acute osteomyelitis is usually the result of hematogenous spread of infection related to transient and often asymptomatic bacteremia. Acute osteomyelitis usually involves a single bone but can be multifocal, particularly in neonates. Thirty percent of patients have a history of upper respiratory infection, otitis media, or other infection that presumably serves as the source of bacteremia.[56] A history of recent trauma to the affected bone is elicited in one third of cases. This suggests that traumatized bone is at increased risk for osteomyelitis.[37] Direct puncture wounds and spread of infection from contiguous structures such as the skin or paranasal sinuses account for a small percentage of cases.

The long tubular bones are involved in approximately 75% of cases. Acute osteomyelitis of the long bones predominantly affects the metaphysis (Figs. 2.1 and 2.2). Blood-borne organisms become lodged in the metaphyses due to high vascularity and physiologic slowing of flow in looping arterial and venous sinusoidal vessels. Organisms concentrated in the metaphyseal microcirculation incite an exudative response. This produces a local increase in intraosseous pressure and slows blood flow. The most rapidly growing and largest metaphyses are preferentially affected. In decreasing order of frequency, the distal femur, proximal femur, proximal tibia, distal tibia, proximal humerus, distal humerus, fibula, and other long bones are involved.[46] The epiphysis is commonly involved in infants and children younger than 18 months of age as transphyseal vessels allow infection to spread from metaphysis to epiphysis. After these vessels are obliterated at around 15 to 18 months of age, the relatively avascular physis serves as a natural barrier to spread of infection in most cases. Only occasionally is the epiphysis involved primarily (Fig. 2.3). Extension directly across the physis and spread from septic arthritis or intraarticular osteomyelitis are other mechanisms by which osteomyelitis develops in an epiphysis of a child older than 18 months of age. Primary diaphyseal involvement with acute hematogenous osteomyelitis is unusual, but loose attachment of the periosteum to the cortex permits subperiosteal spread of metaphyseal infection into and along the diaphysis.

The flat and irregular bones are involved in approximately 25% of cases (Fig. 2.4). Acute osteomyelitis of the flat and irregular bones characteristically develops in bone adjacent to cartilage. These regions, termed metaphyseal equivalents, have a similar vascular anatomy to that of the long bone metaphyses. The most common sites of involvement, in decreasing order of frequency, are the ilium, vertebrae, calcaneus, ischium, scapula, talus, pubis, patella, tarsal navicular, and sternum.[46]

Staphylococcus aureus is the infective organism in approximately 70% of cases.[16,20] One third of neonatal cases are caused by group B β-hemolytic streptococcus.[6] Less frequent causative organisms include salmonella species, mycobacterium, fungi, and viral agents. *Pseudomonas aeruginosa* is associated with acute osteomyelitis secondary to penetrating foot wounds.

Early diagnosis of acute osteomyelitis is necessary to prevent significant complications such as sepsis, chronic infection, growth arrest, and deforming bone damage. Unfortunately, the clinical diagnosis of acute osteomyelitis is frequently difficult in young children, who frequently present with only limping or refusal to bear weight. Pain is often not well localized and swelling and tenderness are often absent. Older children are better able to report localized symptoms and signs such as pain aggravated by motion, limitation in use of the affected extremity, and muscular spasm. Fever may accompany other signs, may be the only sign, or may be absent in children of any age with acute osteomyelitis.

The single most consistently abnormal hematologic parameter is an elevated erythrocyte sedimentation rate (ESR). This is noted in 90% of cases. Only about one third of affected children have leukocytosis. Bacteriologic cultures often provide important information, but are frequently negative. The infective organism is identified by blood and/or bone culture in 50% to 70% of cases.[20,44,65]

Acute osteomyelitis is treated with intravenous followed, in children who are likely to be compliant, with oral antibiotics. Intravenous cephalosporins are useful for initial empiric therapy, while culture results are awaited. There is no consensus regarding the time to change from intravenous to oral antibiotics. Improvement in local symptoms and a return to normal temperature and pulse should be achieved prior to this therapeutic change. The median duration of intravenous antibiotic therapy ranges from 5 to 15 days in different reports.[45,71] The total duration of antibiotic therapy is typically 4 to 6 weeks in uncomplicated cases.

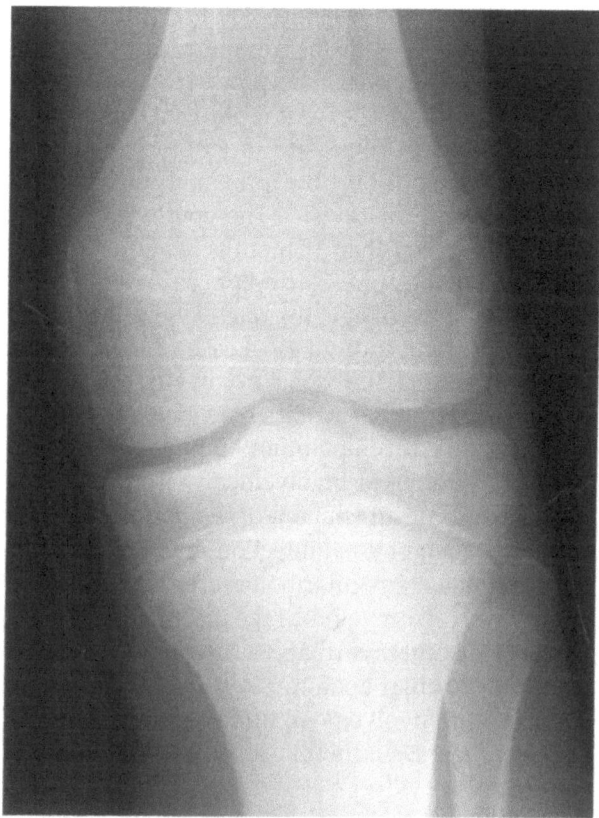

Figure 2.1. Acute osteomyelitis. The left knee appears normal radiographically (A).

A

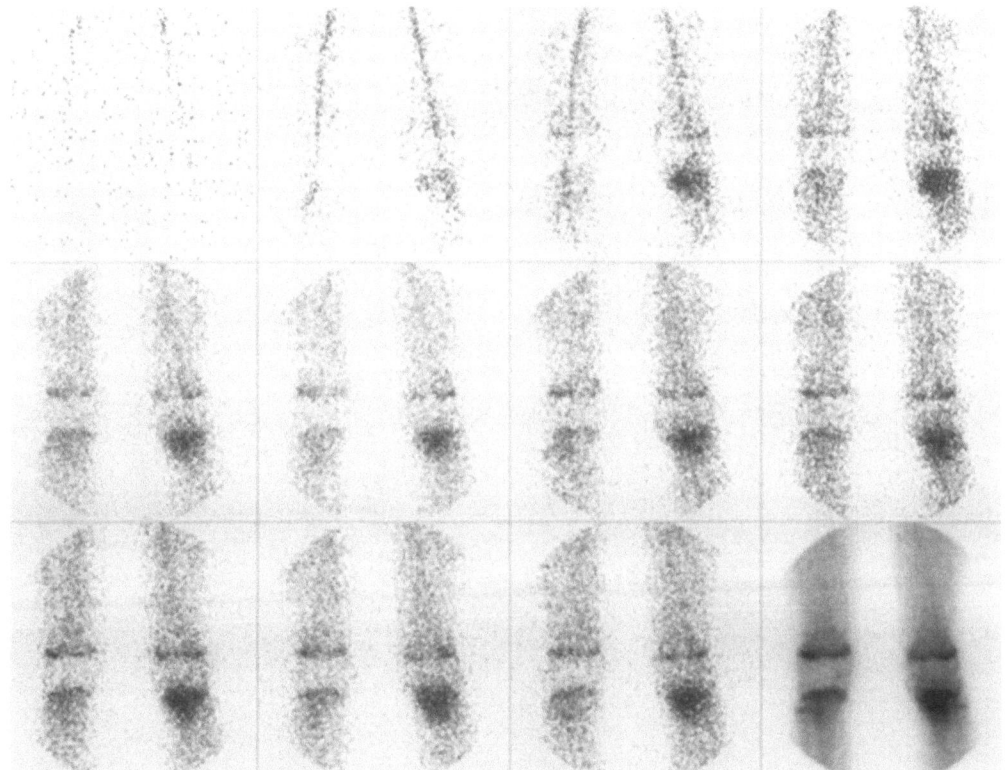

B

Figure 2.1 (*cont'd.*) Anterior radionuclide angiography and a tissue phase image (lower right panel) reveal increased tracer delivery to, and early localization in, the left proximal tibial metaphysis (B).

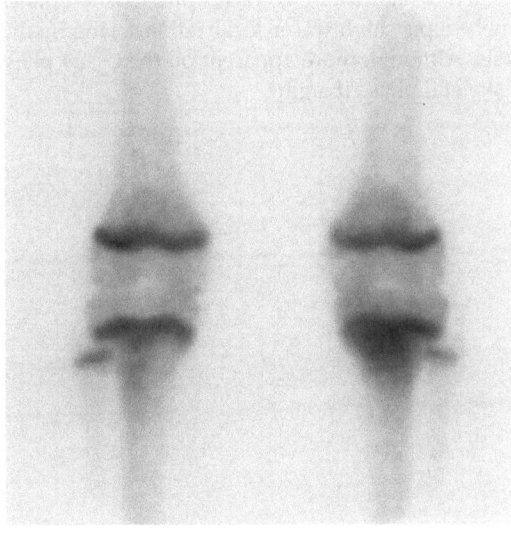

C

Figure 2.1 (*cont'd.*) This persists as a focal abnormality on skeletal phase imaging (C).

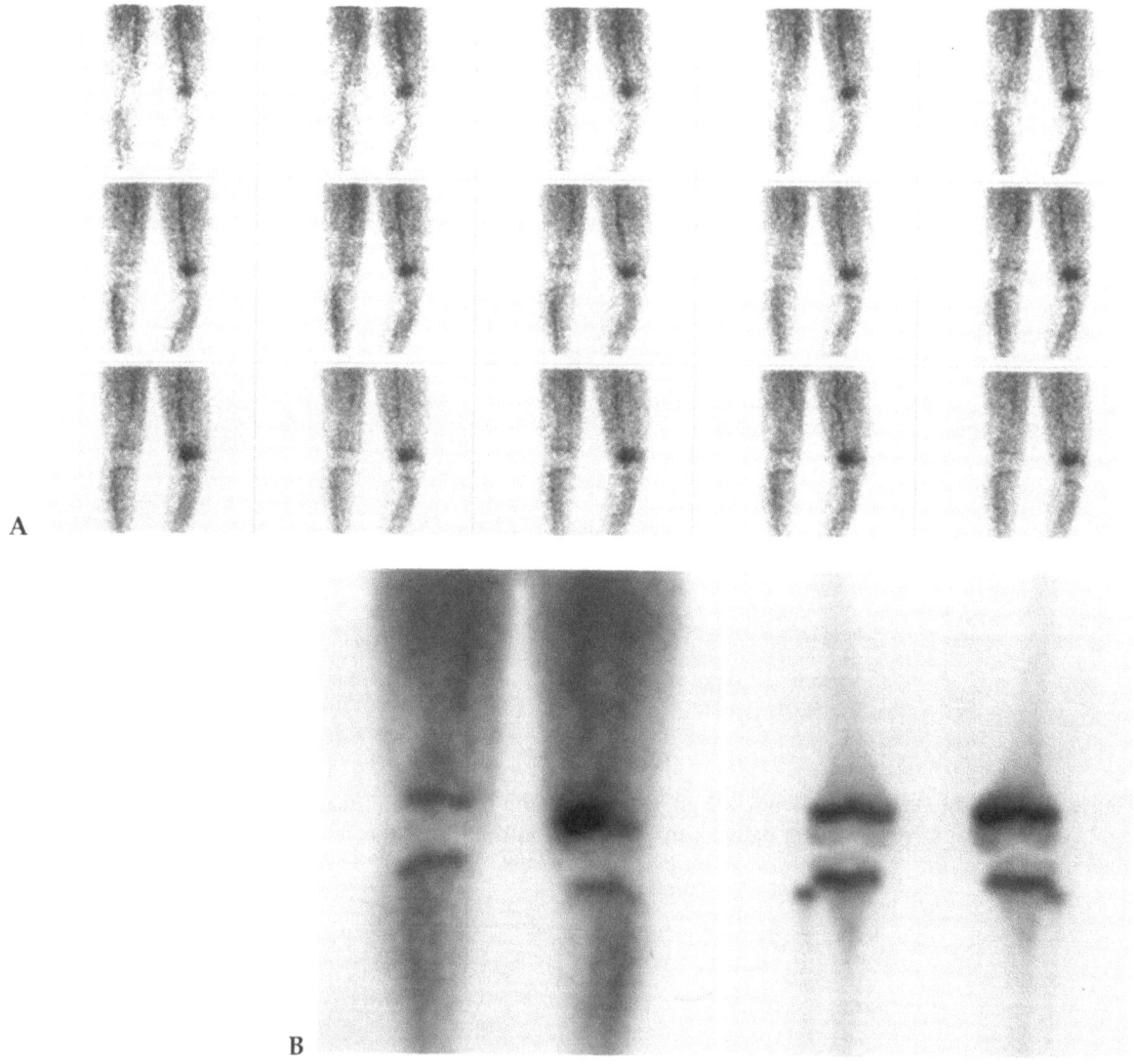

Figure 2.2. Acute osteomyelitis. Radionuclide angiography (anterior projection) demonstrates increased ^{99m}Tc-MDP delivery to the left distal femur (A). Tissue phase (B, left panel) and skeletal phase imaging (B, right panel) depict high tracer localization in the medial aspect of the left distal femoral metaphysis. Although more apparent on the tissue phase image, the focal abnormality persists on skeletal phase imaging.

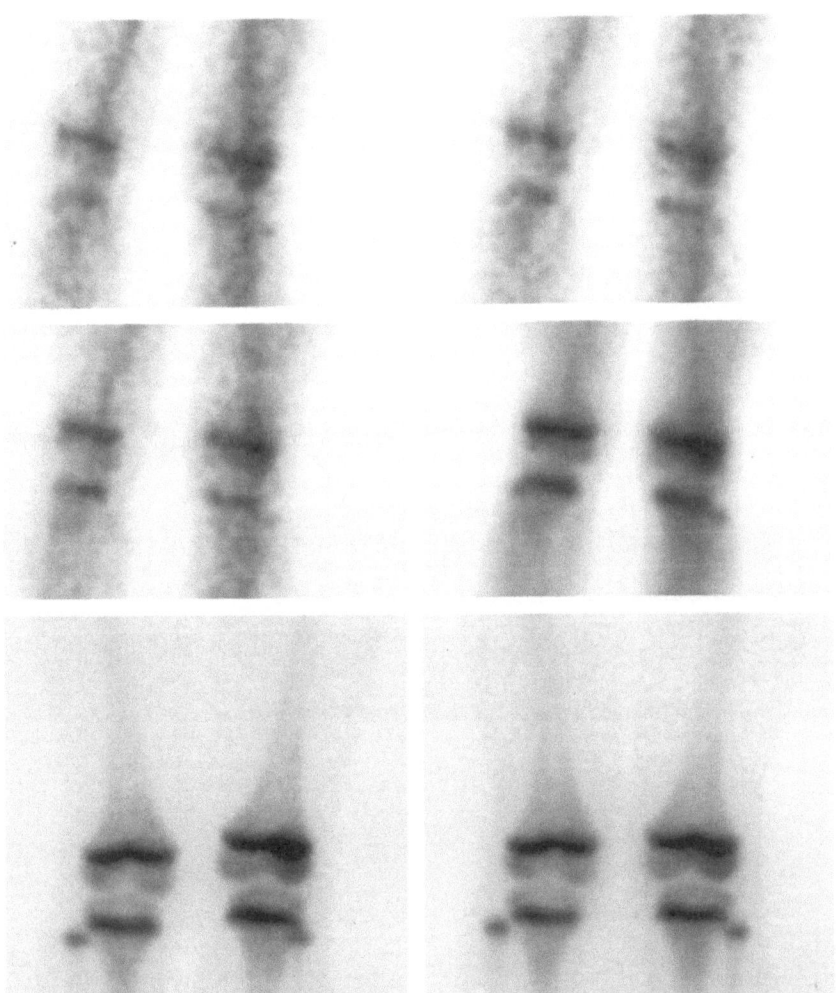

Figure 2.3. Epiphyseal osteomyelitis. Radionuclide angiography and tissue phase imaging (anterior projection) demonstrate prominent tracer delivery and early localization to the region of the distal left femur. Skeletal phase imaging in the anterior (lower left panel) and posterior (lower right panel) projections shows focally increased tracer localization in the distal left femoral epiphysis laterally.

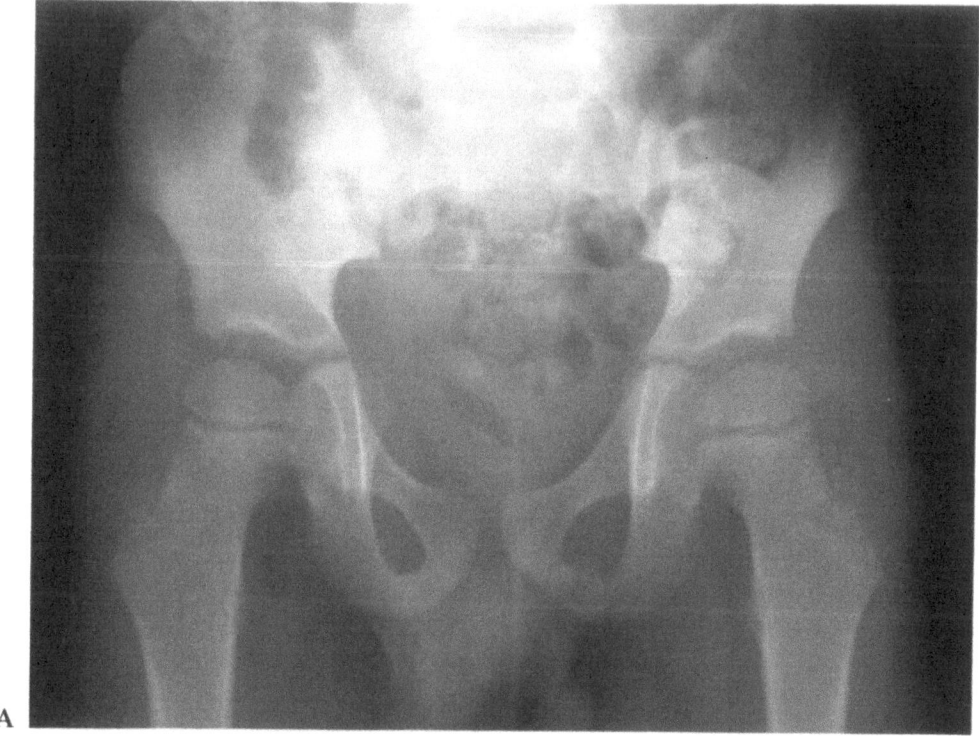

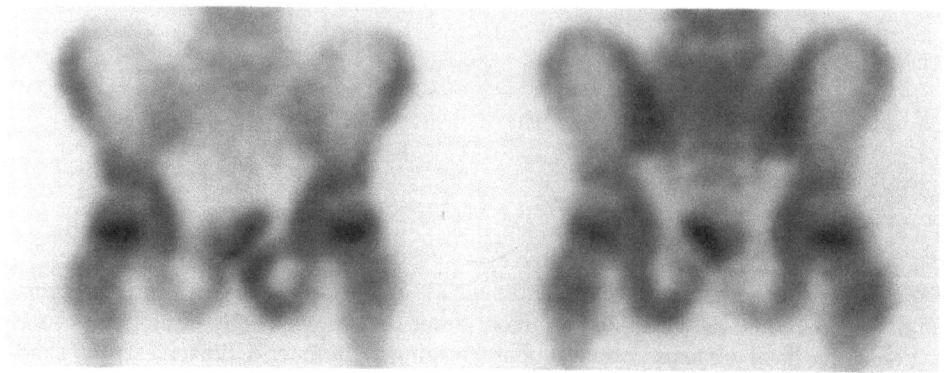

Figure 2.4. Acute osteomyelitis. A pelvic radiograph of a 7-year-old boy with left hip pain demonstrates an asymmetric appearance to the ischiopubic synchodroses (A). This can be seen in normals. Skeletal phase imaging (B) shows increased tracer localization extending from the left ischiopubic synchondrosis along the symphysis pubis and into the superior pubic ramus (left image: anterior projection; right image: posterior projection).

Imaging

Radiography

The imaging evaluation of children with suspected acute osteomyelitis usually begins with radiographs.

Radiographic diagnosis of acute osteomyelitis in its early stages is difficult as the earliest radiographic manifestations of acute osteomyelitis are neither consistently observed nor specific. These findings include deep soft tissue swelling, obliteration of soft tissue planes, and subcutaneous edema. They are present as early as 48 hours following the onset of infection in some cases but are often not observed. Osseous manifestations of focal or confluent radiolucencies and periosteal new bone are not visualized until 7 to 10 days after the onset of infection. This reflects an insensitivity of radiographs to loss of less than 30% of bone matrix.[20,37] In cases where symptom duration is less than 7 days, radiographs are most valuable in helping to exclude other pathologic conditions, including fracture and tumor, that may resemble acute osteomyelitis clinically. An important consideration regarding radiographic diagnosis is that, in some cases, the site of infection may not be included on the radiographs due to poorly localized symptoms.

Further imaging is generally required to assist in evaluating cases of suspected acute osteomyelitis. The modalities most frequently employed for this purpose are skeletal scintigraphy, magnetic resonance imaging (MRI), and ultrasonography.

Skeletal Scintigraphy

Based on multiple reported series, the sensitivity and specificity of skeletal scintigraphy for the diagnosis of acute osteomyelitis are approximately 95%.[54] Skeletal scintigraphy is typically abnormal within 24 to 72 hours of symptom onset.[69]

Skeletal scintigraphy is useful in all pediatric age groups when a diagnosis of acute osteomyelitis is considered (Fig. 2.5). Early reports detailing poor results for skeletal scintigraphy in the diagnosis of neonatal osteomyelitis[5,38,42,63] are refuted

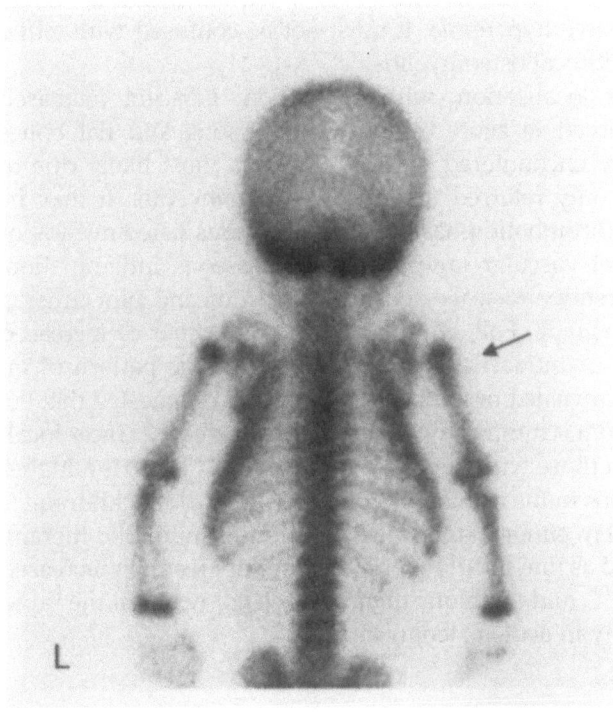

Figure 2.5. Neonatal osteomyelitis. Increased tracer localization affects the right proximal humeral metaphysis (posterior projection). (Reprinted from Treves et al,[68] with permission.)

by later experience showing skeletal scintigraphy to be reliable in detecting osteomyelitis during the first 6 weeks of life.[13] This apparent discrepancy is due to technical and interpretation-related factors. The use of modern imaging equipment, high-resolution collimation, pinhole magnification, and meticulous care in patient positioning are especially important when assessing the neonate. Due to difficulties in performing and interpreting studies in neonates, the value of skeletal scintigraphy in the diagnosis of neonatal osteomyelitis is greatly reduced when the imaging team is not well versed in performing and interpreting scintigrams in this pediatric group.

Multiphase skeletal scintigraphy is useful in distinguishing acute osteomyelitis from cellulitis. A radionuclide angiogram and tissue phase image of the region of highest clinical suspicion and high- or ultra–high-resolution skeletal phase images of the entire skeleton are obtained in children with suspected acute osteomyelitis. The occurrence of multifocal bone involvement, particularly in neonates (22% incidence of multifocality[6]) and occasionally in older children, and the frequent absence of localizing signs in young children renders a whole-body survey essential. Whole-body imaging is also valuable in cases where diseases such as metastatic neuroblastoma[3] and leukemia[17] clinically mimic acute osteomyelitis. Pinhole imaging is used to more convincingly demonstrate or more accurately delineate an abnormality that is visible on planar skeletal phase images (Fig. 2.6). Due to the typical metaphyseal location of acute osteomyelitis, pinhole imaging is also useful for confirming the absence of focal abnormalities adjacent to the intensely tracer avid physis. When pelvic osteomyelitis is suspected, single photon emission computed tomography (SPECT) is often valuable for these purposes (Figs. 2.7, 2.8, 2.9).

Radionuclide angiographic and tissue phase images of acute osteomyelitis typically reveal regionally increased tracer delivery and localization to the infected bone and adjacent soft tissues. Cellulitis may have a similar appearance. A focal osseous abnormality is demonstrated on tissue phase imaging in many cases of acute osteomyelitis but not cellulitis. Skeletal phase images demonstrate focally increased tracer localization in an infected bone. Skeletal phase imaging of cellulitis shows less intense tracer localization than is demonstrated on the first two phases. Focally increased skeletal localization does not occur with cellulitis. An extended pattern of increased localization involving the adjacent physis and bones distal or proximal to an involved metaphysis may be observed with acute osteomyelitis of a long bone (Fig. 2.10). This pattern reflects increased tracer delivery resulting from reactive hyperemia. It must not be confused with either physeal involvement or multifocal osteomyelitis.

Focally decreased tracer localization, with or without adjacent increased localization, has been observed in acute osteomyelitis of long and flat bones (Fig. 2.11).[13,31,42,66] This rarely encountered pattern, which is most likely due to regional ischemia, is commonly referred to as "cold" osteomyelitis. It may be demonstrated in the early thrombotic phase of hematogenous osteomyelitis or later when there is regional vascular tamponade. Intraosseous inflammation, edema, or abscess, as well as subperiosteal extension of infection and joint effusion are possible causes of tamponade. Following aspiration and relief of increased intraosseous, subperiosteal, or intraarticular pressure, the classic pattern of increased tracer localization is revealed in some cases. It has been suggested that the prognosis of children in whom scintigraphy demonstrates decreased tracer localization is poorer than that in those with increased localization.[62] There is a higher incidence of cold osteomyelitis in the neonate as compared with older children.[13,42]

Clinicians should not delay either diagnostic aspiration or antibiotic therapy until scintigraphy is obtained as fine-needle aspiration does not result in increased skeletal tracer localization[15,40,67] and antibiotic therapy does not result in the rapid normalization of scintigraphy in acute osteomyelitis.

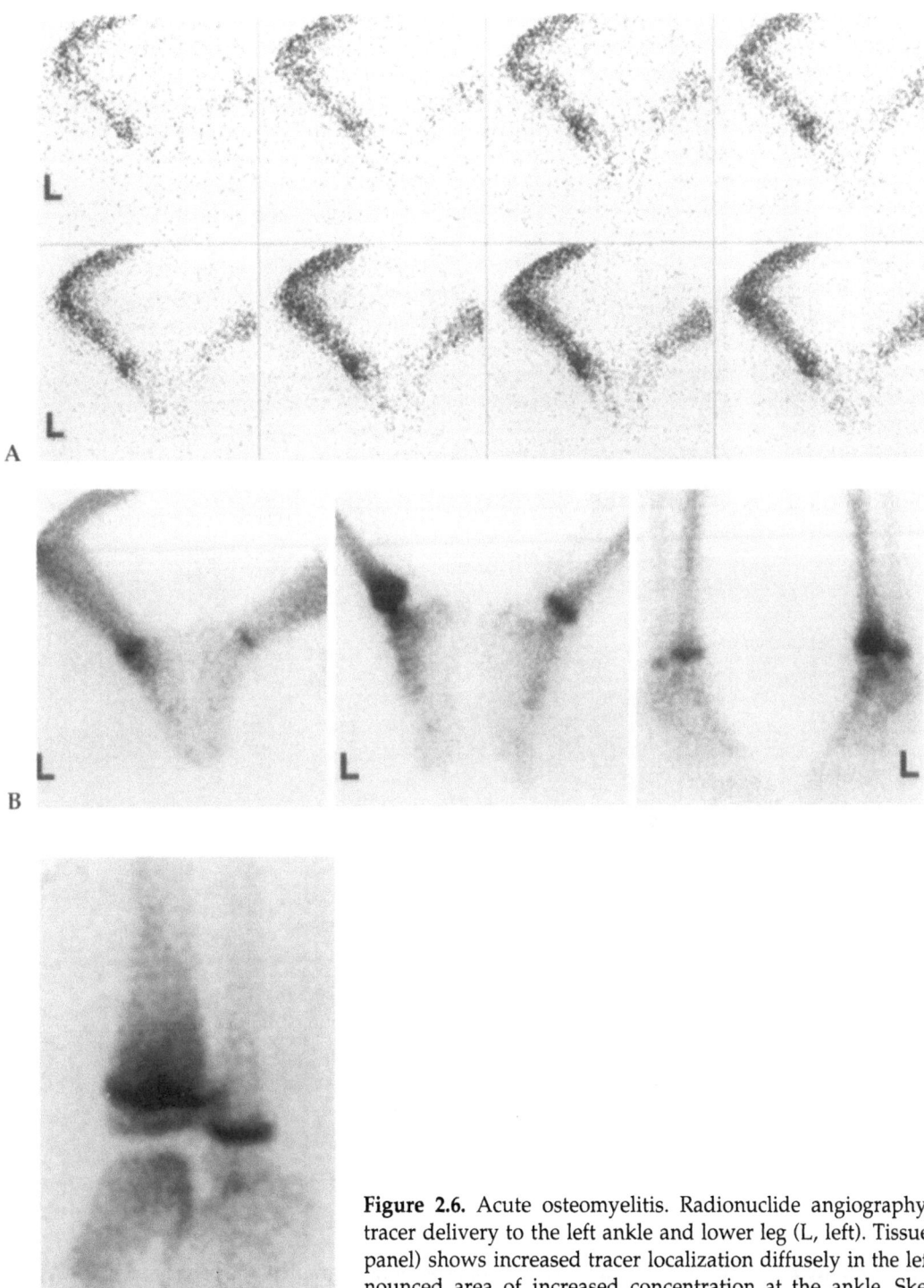

Figure 2.6. Acute osteomyelitis. Radionuclide angiography (A) reveals increased tracer delivery to the left ankle and lower leg (L, left). Tissue phase imaging (B, left panel) shows increased tracer localization diffusely in the left lower leg with a pronounced area of increased concentration at the ankle. Skeletal phase images (B, middle and right panels) demonstrate focally intense tracer accumulation in the distal left tibial metaphysis. This is more optimally depicted by pinhole magnification (C).

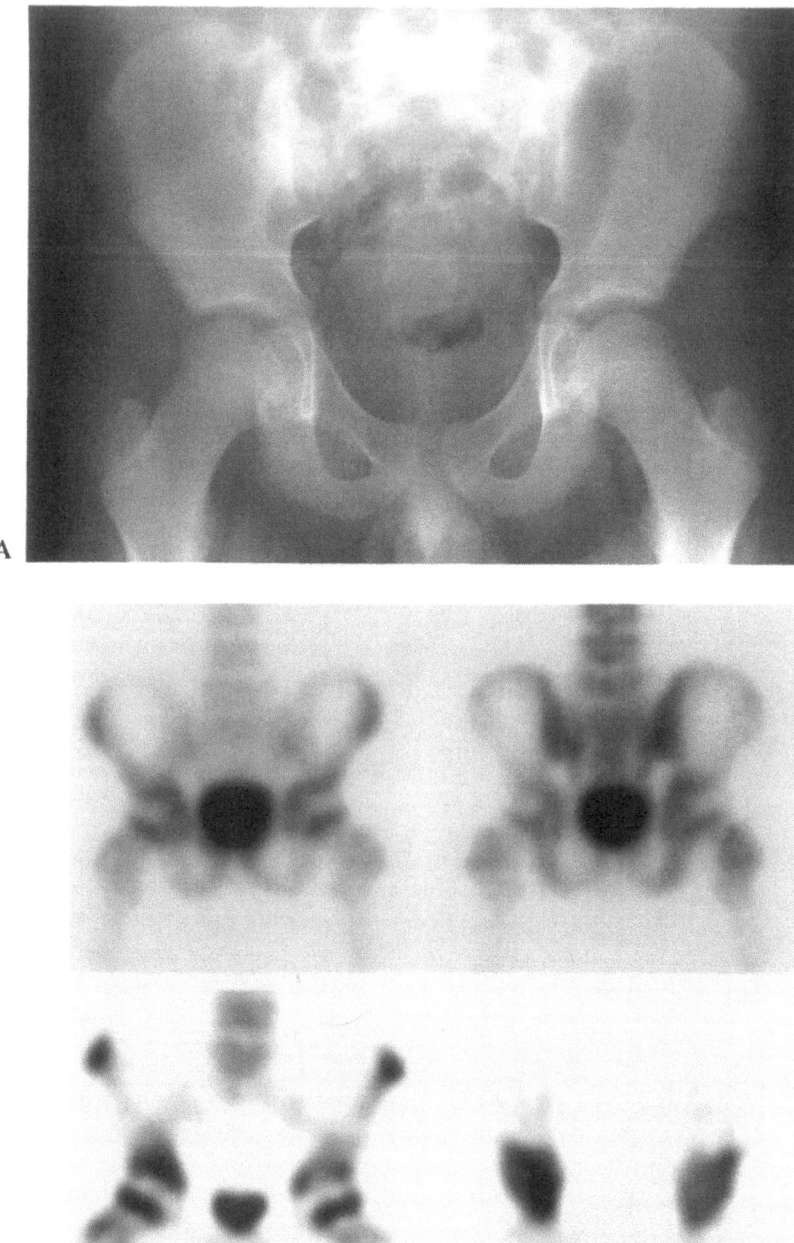

Figure 2.7. Acute osteomyelitis. An anteroposterior radiograph of the pelvis is normal (A). Skeletal phase images (B, upper row) in anterior and posterior projections reveal slightly greater ^{99m}Tc-MDP localization in the right than left acetabulum. This is confirmed and more convincingly shown with SPECT (B, lower row, coronal and transverse images).

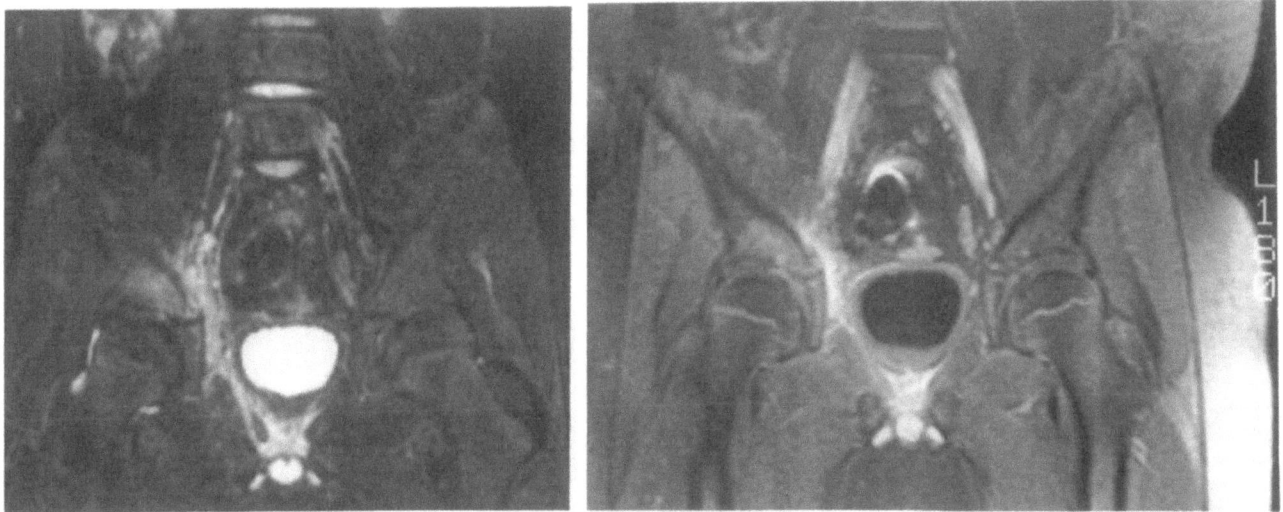

C   D

Figure 2.7 (*cont'd.*) Increased signal is demonstrated in the right acetabulum on a coronal T2-weighted image (C). Increased signal extends into the right obturator internus muscle and surrounding soft tissues. A small right hip effusion is present. The majority of the area that demonstrates abnormal T2 signal also demonstrates enhancement on a T1-postgadolinium image (D). A fluid collection amenable to drainage is not identified.

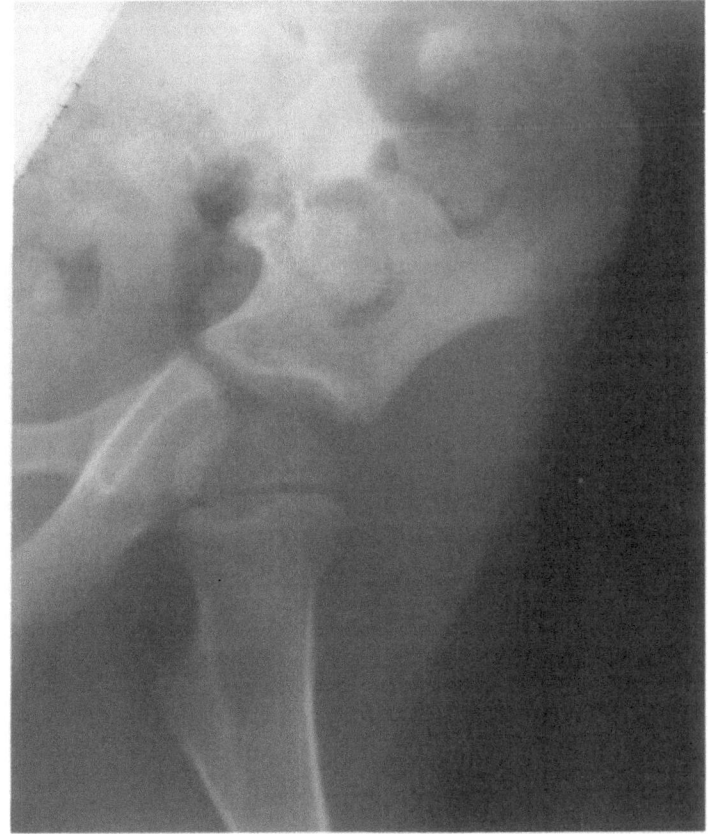

Figure 2.8. Acute osteomyelitis. Images of an 11-year-old with left hip pain. A left hip radiograph reveals no osseous abnormality (A).

A

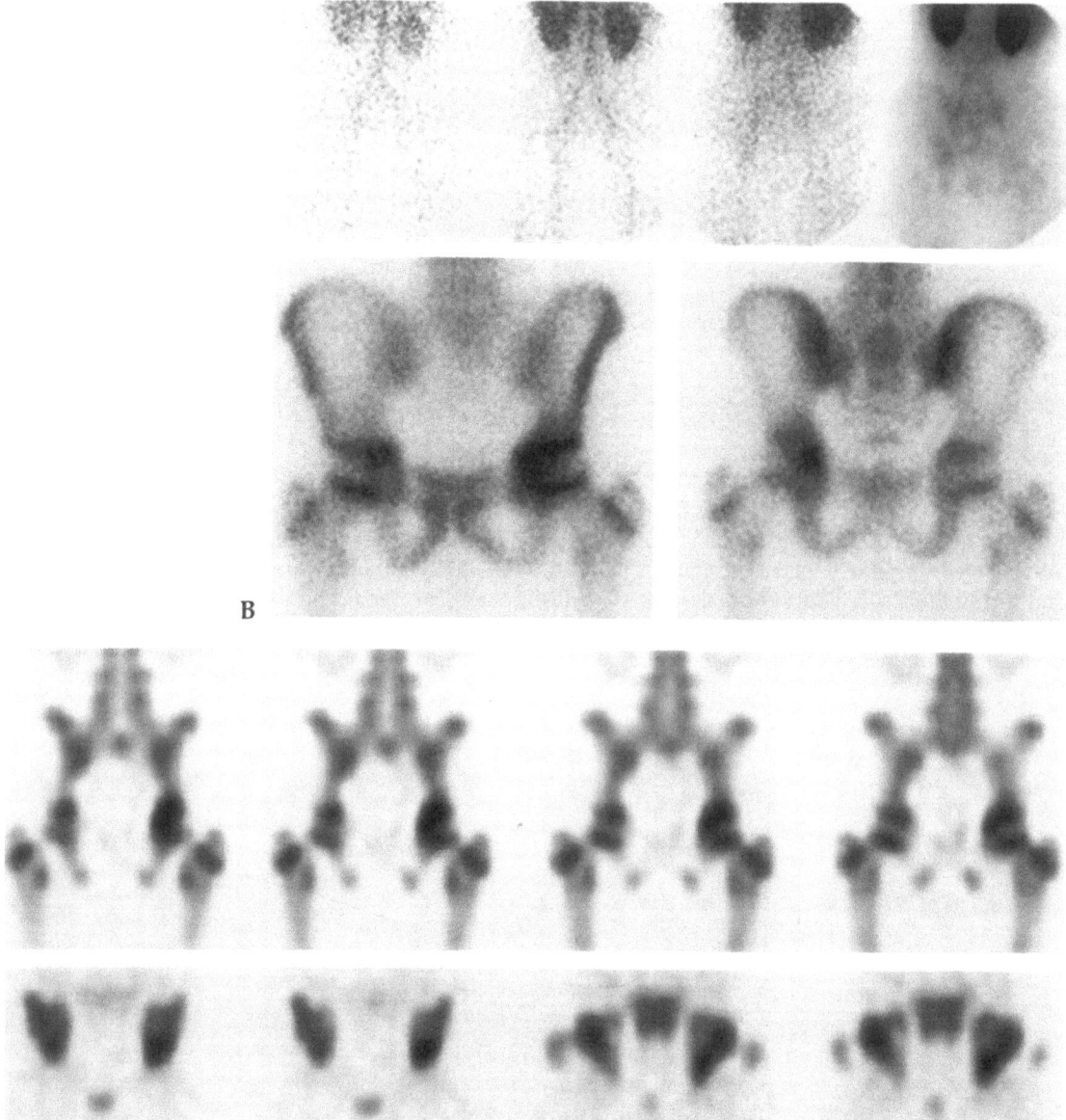

Figure 2.8 (_cont'd._) There is mildly increased blood flow to the left hip region depicted with three selected posterior images from radionuclide angiography (B, upper row left). Increased tracer localization in the left acetabulum is depicted on the posterior tissue phase image (upper right) and skeletal phase images (lower left: anterior projection; lower right: posterior projection). This is confirmed with coronal (upper row) and transverse (lower row) SPECT (C).

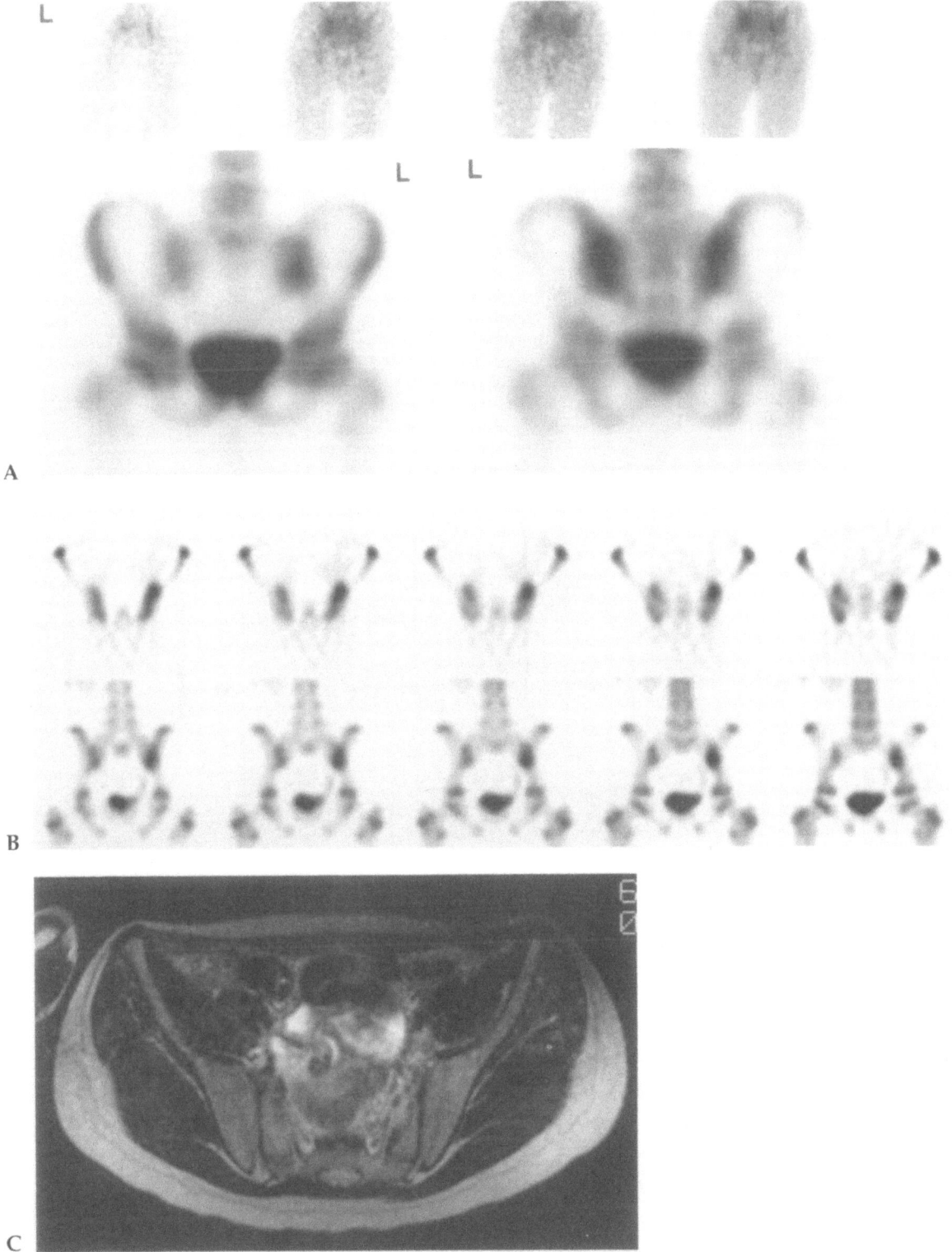

Figure 2.9. Acute osteomyelitis. Posterior radionuclide angiography and tissue phase imaging (A, upper row) reveal increased blood flow to, and early tracer localization in, the region of the left sacroiliac joint. Skeletal phase images (A, lower row) and SPECT (B) depict increased tracer localization in the left ilium. Fast multiplanar inversion recovery (FMPIR) imaging reveals only a very slight increase in signal intensity in the left ilium with a small amount of fluid tracking anteriorly along the left iliac wing (C).

Figure 2.10. Acute osteomyelitis: extended pattern. In addition to focally intense tracer localization in the proximal left tibial metaphysis, there is prominent tracer localization involving the diaphysis (left panel: anterior projection; right panel: posterior projection).

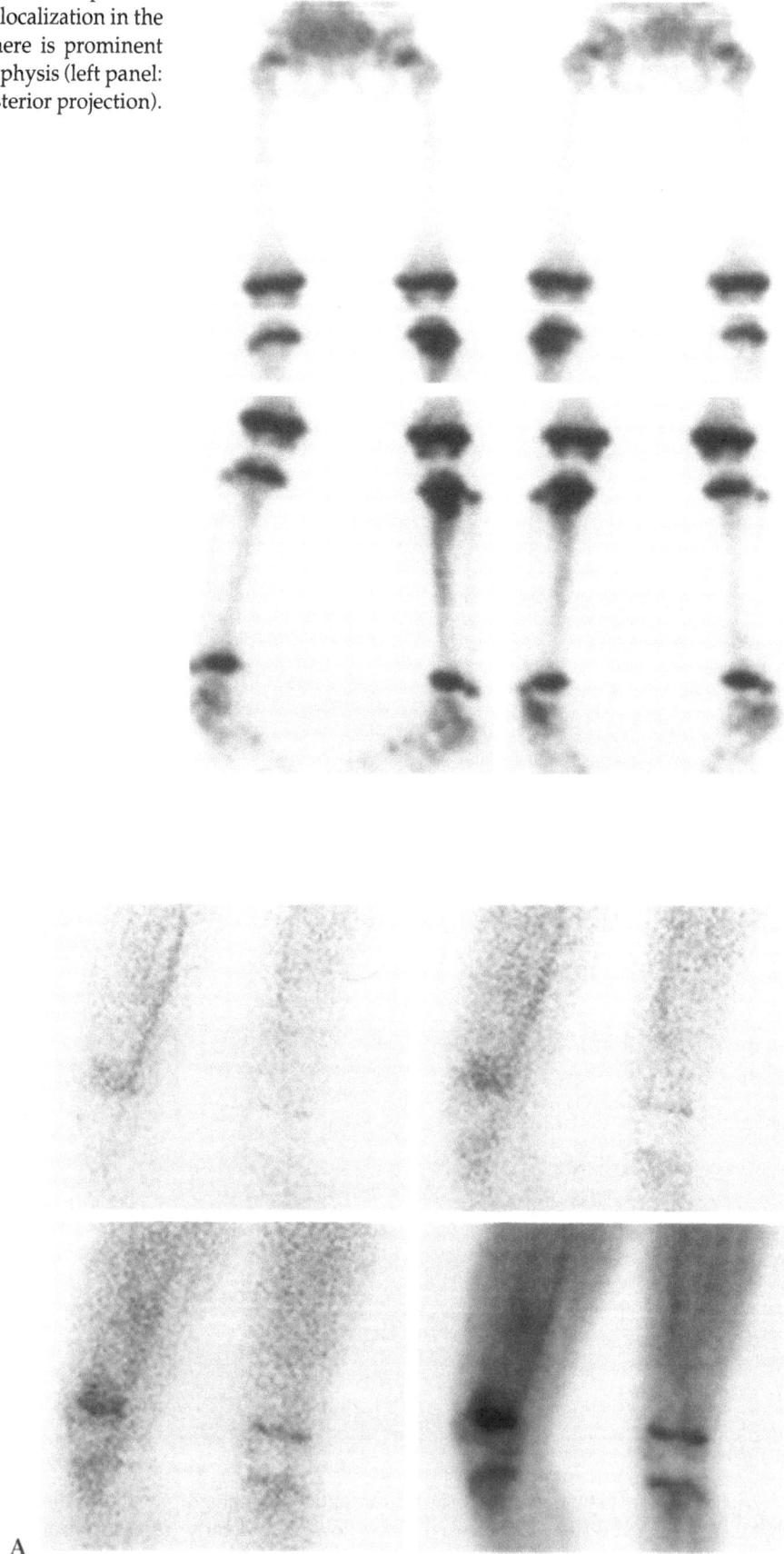

A

Figure 2.11. Acute osteomyelitis: cold osteomyelitis. Selected anterior images from the radionuclide angiogram and the tissue phase image of a 13-year-old boy reveal increased perfusion to, and ^{99m}Tc-MDP localization in, the distal right femoral metaphysis and less prominently superior to this in the midthigh or femur (A).

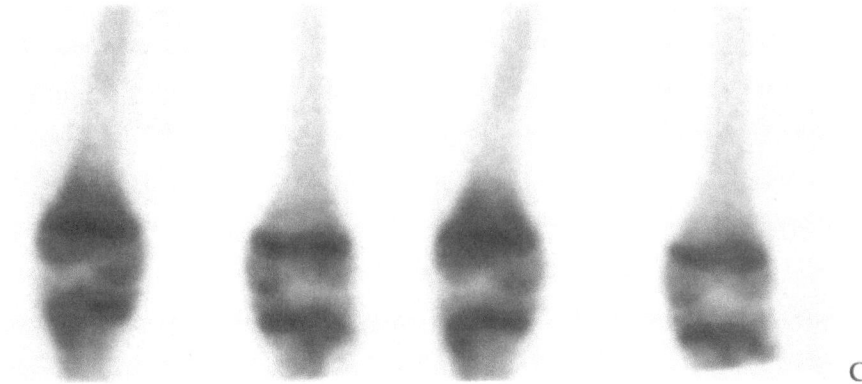

B   C

Figure 2.11 (*cont'd.*) Skeletal phase images in the anterior (B) and posterior (C) projections show increased right femoral metaphyseal ^{99m}Tc-MDP localization, with a region of decreased localization in the adjacent diaphysis. A large amount of subperiosteal pus was drained surgically.

Magnetic Resonance Imaging

Changes in signal intensity resulting from increased fluid in the bone marrow and soft tissues allow the detection of acute osteomyelitis by MRI within 24 to 48 hours following symptom onset. Marrow edema appears as decreased signal intensity on T1-weighted and increased signal intensity on T2-weighted images. Abnormal perfusion patterns indicative of ischemia, necrosis, or intraosseous abscess, can be demonstrated with gadolinium-enhanced MRI.[37] Magnetic resonance imaging is especially valuable in cases of acute osteomyelitis of the spine and pelvis, where extension to the epidural space or pelvic soft tissues may be the main cause of morbidity (Fig. 2.12). MRI is also useful in identifying extension of infection into the physis, in which case MRI assists with surgical treatment aimed at decreasing the risk of growth arrest.

The sensitivity of MRI relative to that of scintigraphy has not been conclusively established.[27] Based on the experience at our institution and published series, MRI and scintigraphy appear to be equally sensitive for the early diagnosis of acute osteomyelitis providing that symptoms are sufficiently localized to direct MRI.[18,39]

Ultrasonography

The primary role of ultrasonography in pediatric skeletal infections is detecting and guiding aspiration of fluid from the hip joint (Fig. 2.13). The main limitation of this modality is its inability to detect osseous disease. Ultrasonography may, however, reveal periosteal elevation, subperiosteal fluid, increased echogenicity in the deep soft tissues corresponding to early deep soft tissue swelling,[1,51] and soft tissue abscess or phlegmon (Fig. 2.14). Although potentially helpful, ultrasonography should not be used in place of skeletal scintigraphy or MRI.[27]

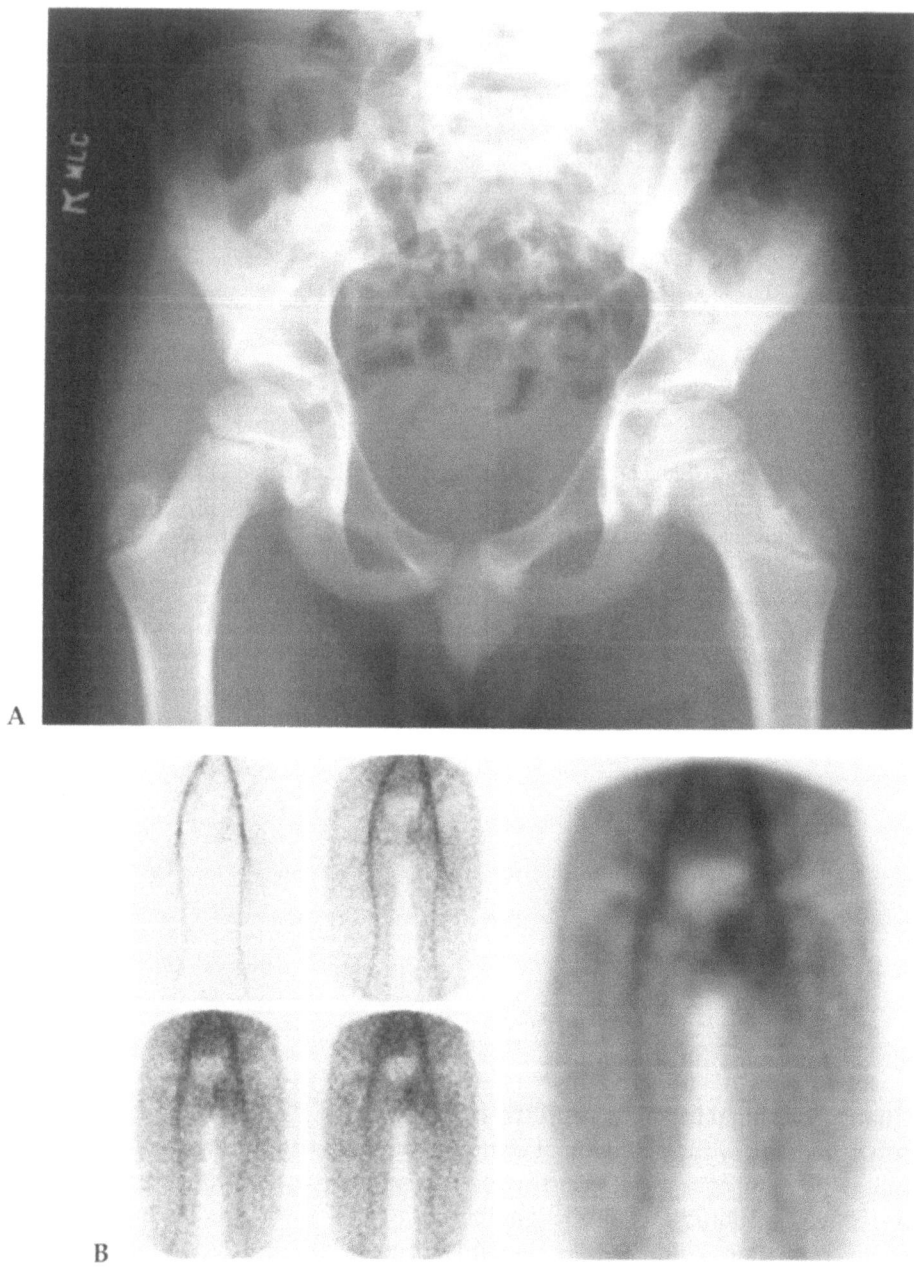

Figure 2.12. Acute osteomyelitis. An anteroposterior radiograph of the pelvis shows asymmetry of the ischiopubic synchondroses (A). Radiolucency extending from the left synchondrosis and displacement of the obturator internus fat pad medially suggest osteomyelitis with soft tissue abscess. Selected anterior images from a radionuclide angiogram (B) demonstrate increased blood flow to the left inguinal region. The tissue phase image (B) shows a corresponding increase in tracer localization.

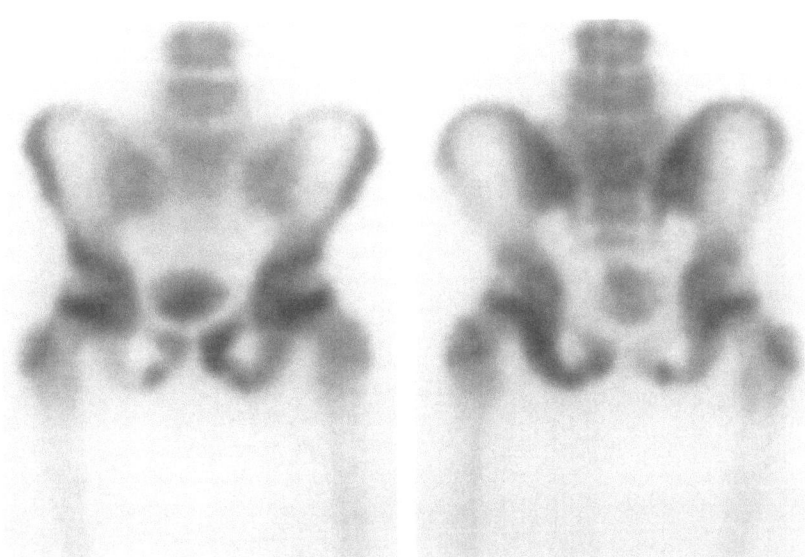

Figure 2.12 (*cont'd.*) Anterior (left) and posterior skeletal phase images depict increased tracer localization in the left ischium and pubis (C). Tracer localization in the right ischiopubic synchondrosis is within normal limits.

C

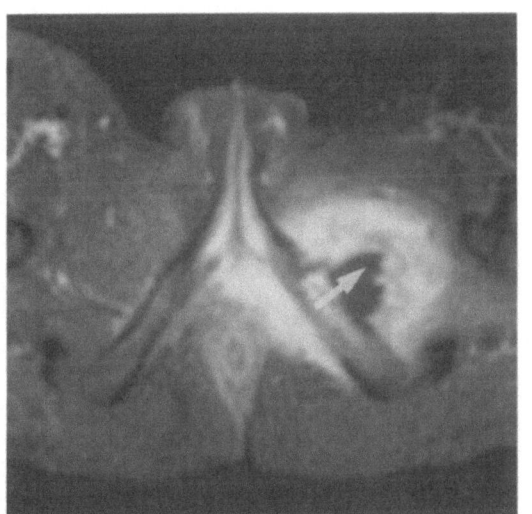

D

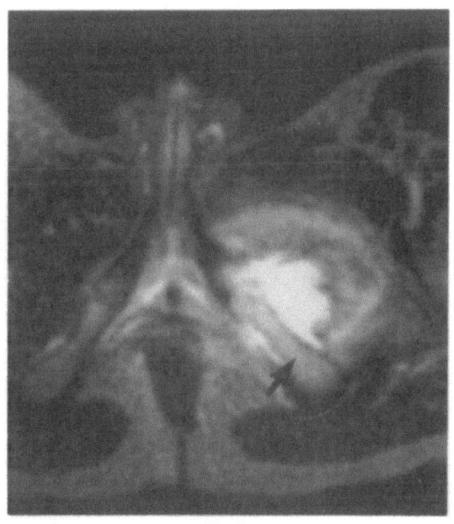

E

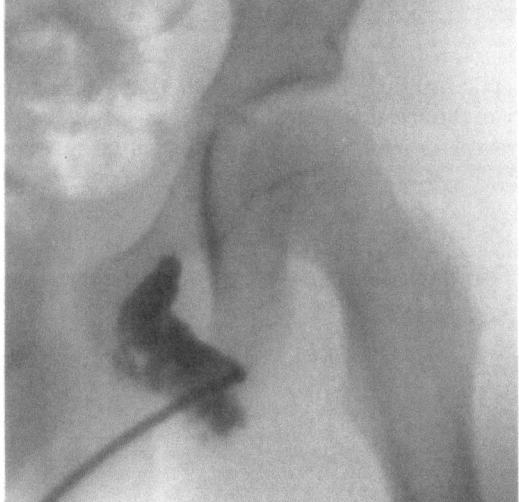

F

Figure 2.12 (*cont'd.*) A large abscess centered about the left ischiopubic synchondrosis is depicted with MRI (D,E). The bulk of the lesion shows moderate to marked enhancement with gadolinium, with an area of central liquefaction (D, arrow). The left ischium shows increased T2 signal, with no central signal change suggesting sequestrum (E, arrow). Radiographic contrast instilled following percutaneous abscess drainage delineates the abscess cavity (F).

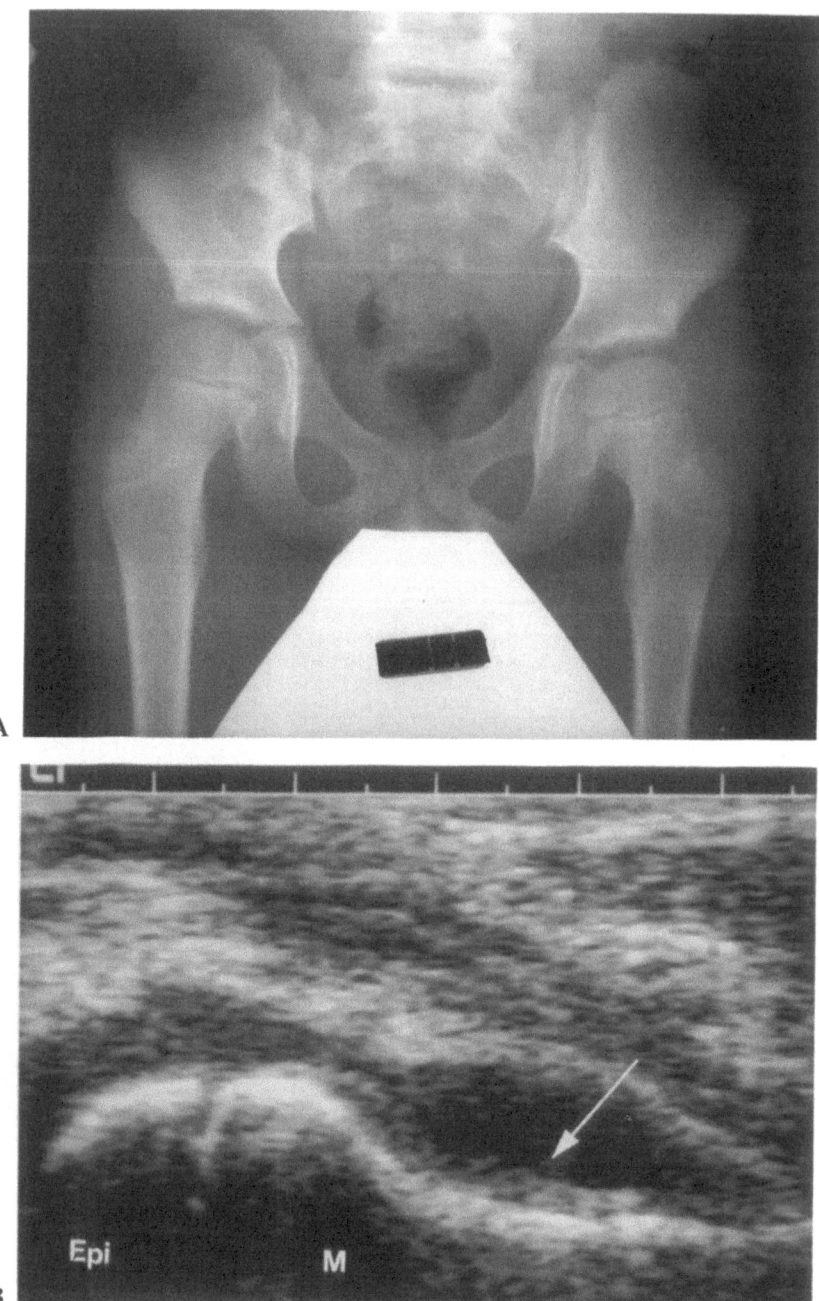

A

B

Figure 2.13. Acute osteomyelitis and septic arthritis. The bones of the left hip appear normal radiographically (A). Asymmetry of the acetabular "teardrop" distance suggests a left hip effusion. Ultrasonography (B) reveals a moderate left hip effusion (arrow; epi, femoral capital epiphysis; m, metaphysis).

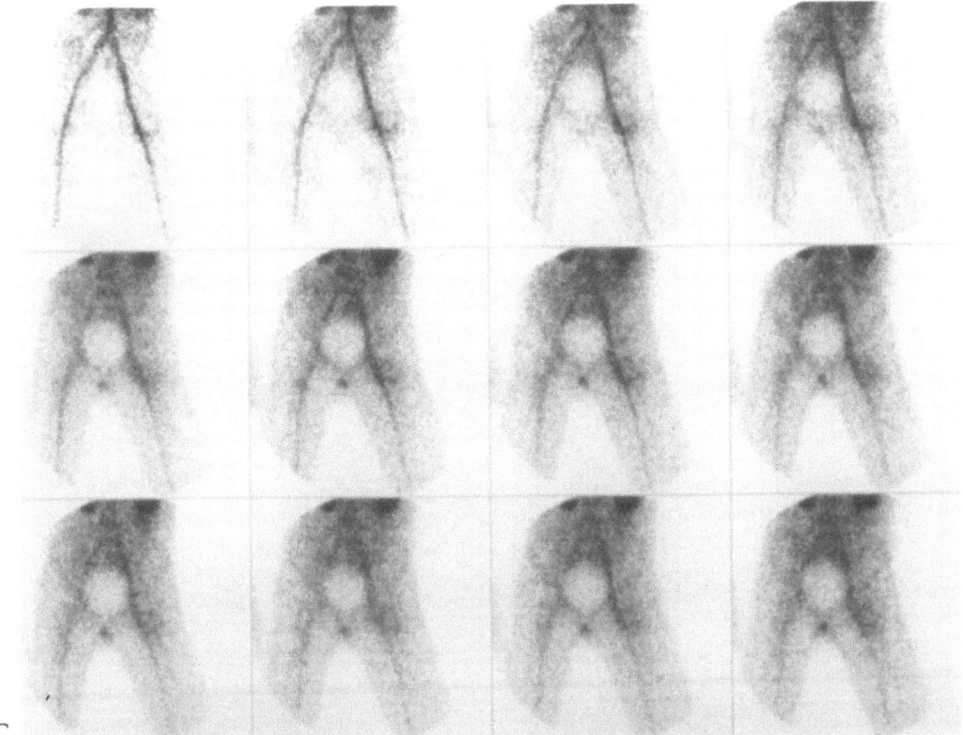

C

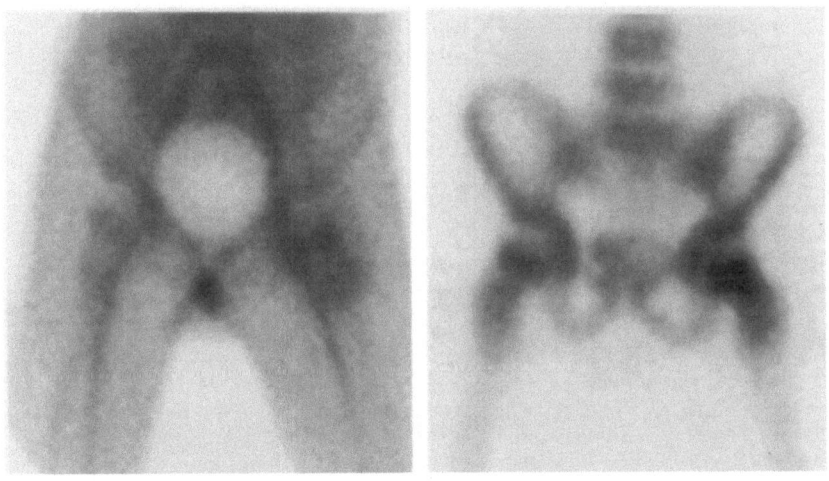

D

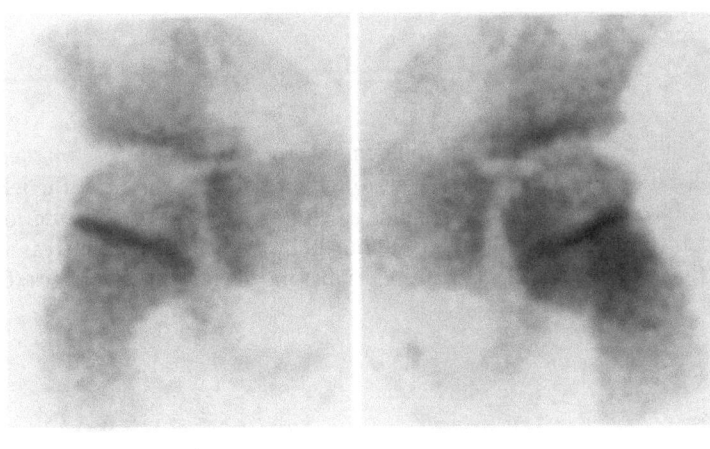

E

Figure 2.13 (*cont'd.*) Radionuclide angiography (anterior projection) depicts increased perfusion to the left hip region (C). Diffusely increased tracer localization at the time of tissue phase imaging (D, left panel) appears focal in the left proximal femoral metaphysis on the skeletal phase image (D, right panel). This is better depicted with pinhole magnification (E).

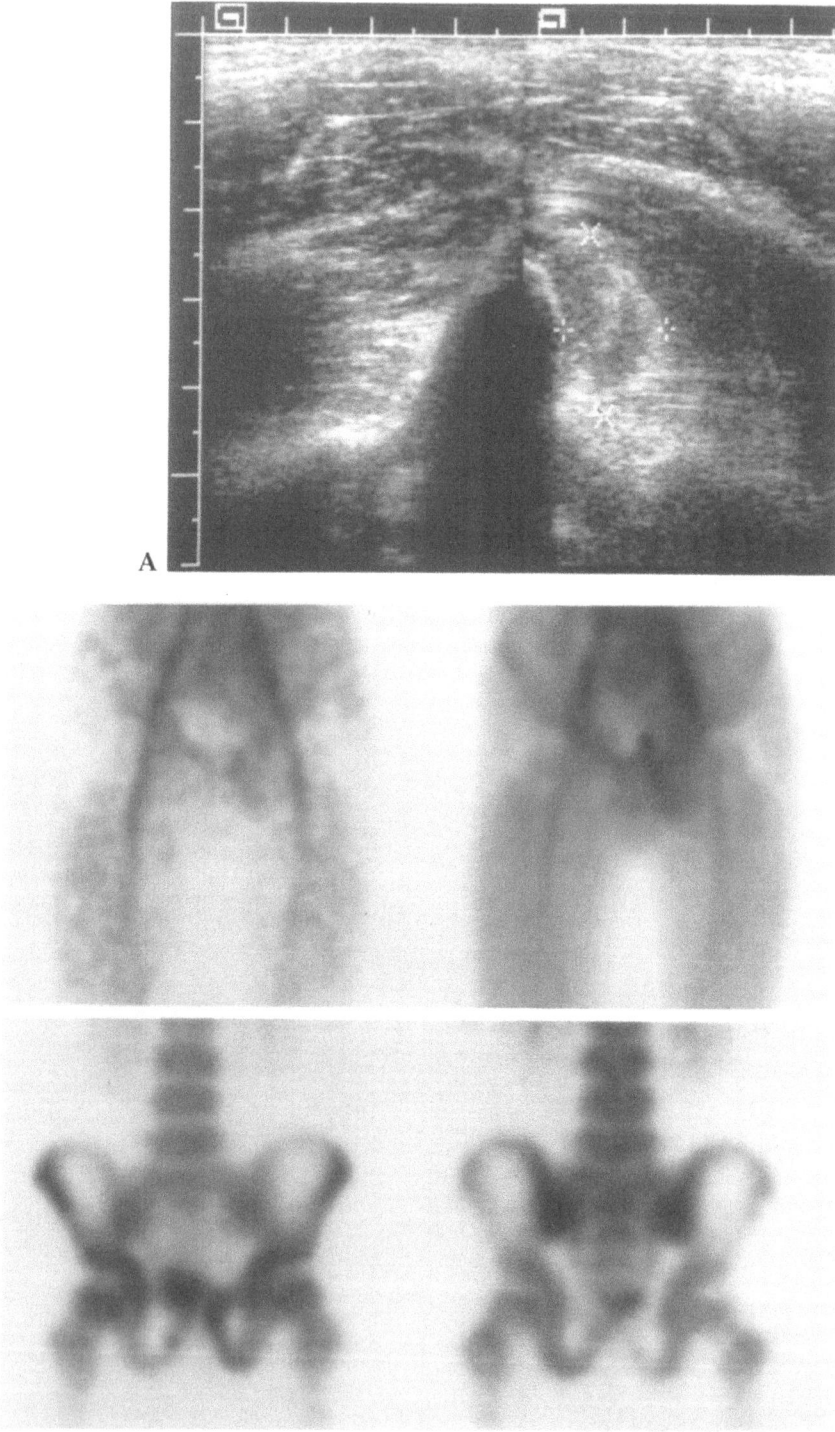

Figure 2.14. Osteomyelitis with inflammatory phlegmon. An echogenic mass (marked with cursors) is visualized sonographically adjacent to the inferolateral aspect of the left ischium (A). Increased blood flow to the left inguinal region is depicted on the anterior radionuclide angiogram (B, upper left). The left inferior pubic ramus exhibits increased tracer localization on the tissue phase image (B, upper right) and skeletal phase images (B, lower panels).

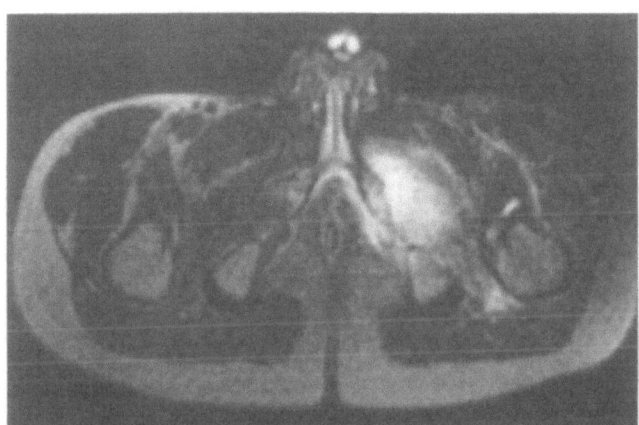
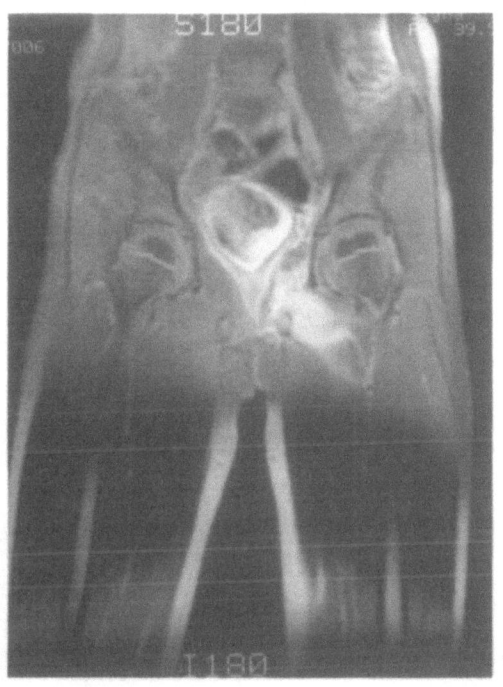

C   D

Figure 2.14 (*cont'd.*) MRI demonstrates increased T2 signal (C) and gadolinium enhancement (D) in the left inferior pubic ramus near the synchondrosis. Similar MR signal is seen in the adjacent muscles, mainly in the left obturator internus and externus, as well as the left adductor muscles. A drainable fluid collection is not identified. A small amount of fluid is present in the left hip joint.

Septic Arthritis and Transient Synovitis

Septic arthritis is usually caused by pyogenic organisms. The knee or hip is involved in approximately 70% of cases. Children younger than 3 years of age account for 50% of all cases of septic arthritis.[47] *S. aureus* and group A streptococci are the most common infective organisms in all age groups.[8,73]

Organisms enter a joint by three mechanisms. First, the synovium, which is vascular, may be infected during bacteremia. Second, infection may spread to a joint from intraarticular bone. This most commonly occurs in neonates and infants, in whom infection spreads from metaphysis to epiphysis through transphyseal blood vessels. It may also result from acute osteomyelitis of an intraarticular metaphysis or metaphyseal equivalent (Fig. 2.13). The relatively common occurrence of acute osteomyelitis in the proximal femoral metaphysis, which is partially intraarticular, and in metaphyseal equivalent bone adjacent to the triradiate cartilage makes the hip particularly susceptible to septic arthritis as a complication of osteomyelitis. Third, penetrating trauma may introduce organisms into a joint.

Within a joint, pathogenic organisms find an environment consisting of transudative joint fluid and avascular cartilage that is hospitable for their proliferation. Defense mechanisms are overwhelmed with pathogenic bacteria, such as *S. aureus*. Lytic enzymes, including proteases, collagenases, and peptidases in purulent articular fluid destroy articular and epiphyseal cartilages. Epiphyseal ischemia secondary to increased intracapsular pressure may progress to infarction. This is a particular concern at the hip, as the blood supply to the femoral capital epiphysis follows an intraarticular course (see Fig. 4.37). The

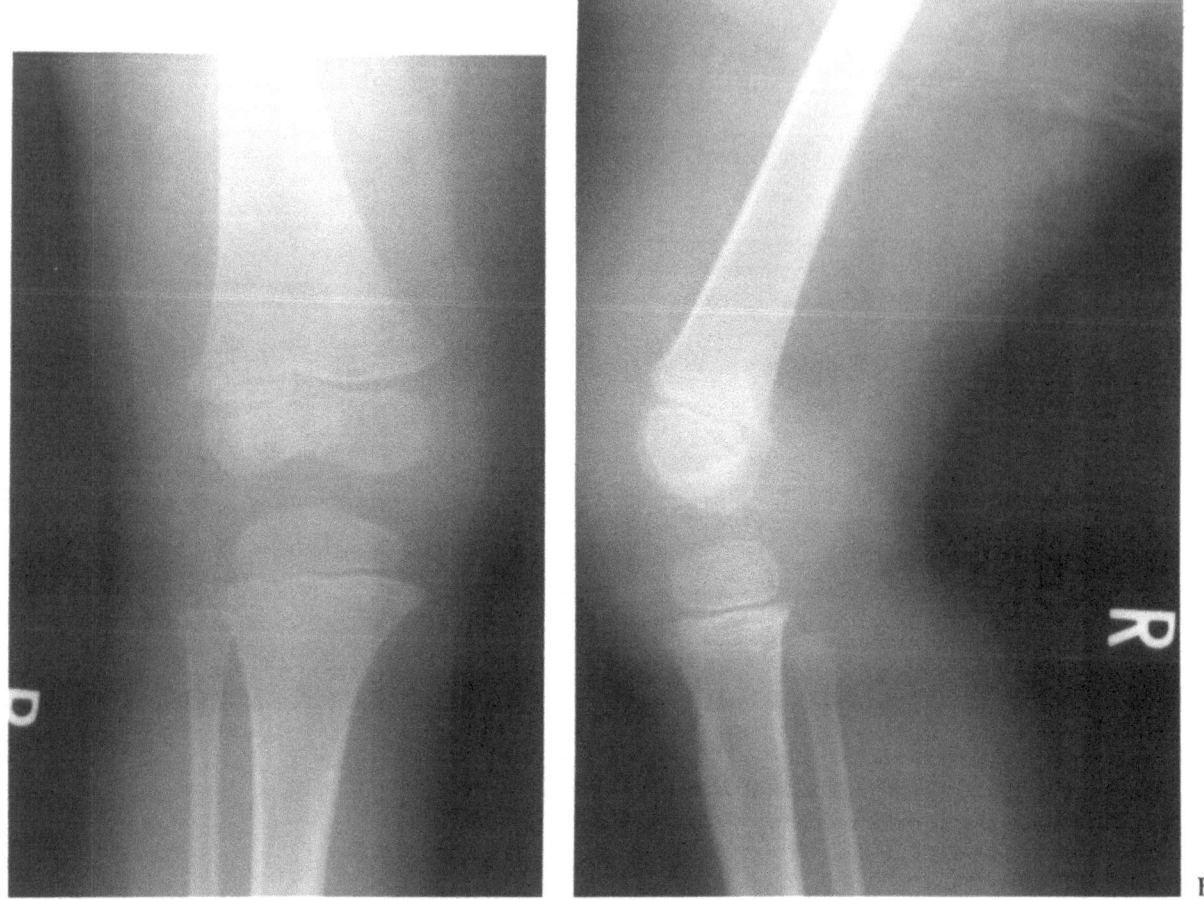

Figure 2.15. Transient synovitis. Anteroposterior (A) and lateral (B) radiographs of a 3-year-old girl with painful swelling of the right knee reveal a joint effusion but no osseous abnormality.

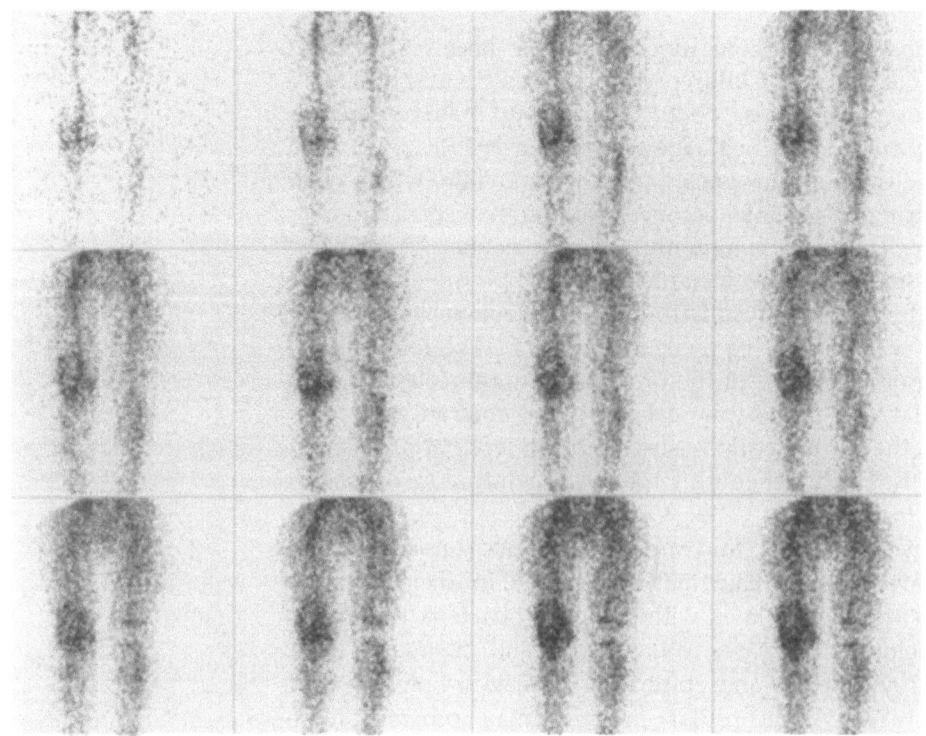

Figure 2.15 (*cont'd.*) Radionuclide angiography demonstrates increased ^{99m}Tc-MDP delivery to the right knee (C).

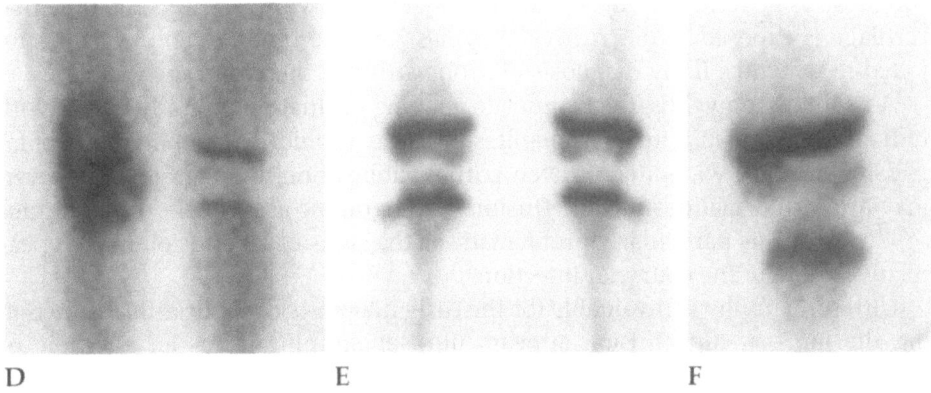

D   E   F

Figure 2.15 (*cont'd.*) Increased tracer localization on the tissue phase image (D) outlines the suprapatellar bursa. Skeletal phase images (E: planar; F: pinhole, right knee) reveal minimally increased tracer localization affecting the articulating surfaces of the right distal femur and proximal tibia.

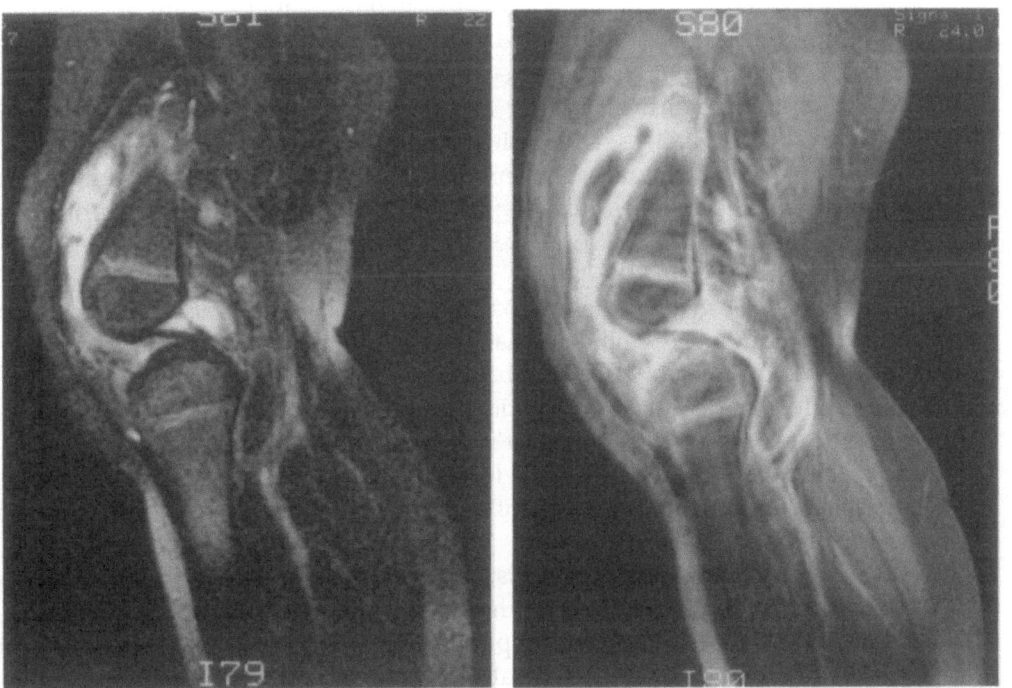

G   H

Figure 2.15 (*cont'd.*) Sagittal T2-weighted MRI of the right knee reveals a joint effusion (G). Enhancement of thickened synovium is seen on T1-weighted image following gadolinium (H).

prognosis is governed by the duration of symptoms, which reflects the time that cartilage is exposed to destructive enzymes, and the time the epiphysis is subjected to ischemia. Early diagnosis of septic arthritis, therefore, is imperative.

As with osteomyelitis, the diagnostic imaging evaluation typically begins with radiographs. A joint effusion is manifested radiographically by obliteration of fat pads, joint space widening, or even partial subluxation. Radiographs, however, may appear normal despite an effusion. Radiographic assessment of the hip for septic arthritis is particularly problematic as the signs of an effusion may appear relatively late in the course of infection.[72]

Ultrasonography is invaluable for the early diagnosis of septic arthritis involving the hip.[78] A hip effusion appears ultrasonographically as an anechoic or hypoechoic area separating the proximal femoral metaphysis from the joint capsule. Echogenic material within an effusion increases the examiner's concern for septic arthritis,[79] but the absence of such material does not assure the sterile nature of an effusion. Absence of fluid by ultrasonography greatly lessens the likelihood of septic arthritis.[78] A completely echogenic effusion, however, may be difficult to detect.

An effusion is not specific for septic arthritis. Examination of joint fluid is the most reliable means for differentiating septic arthritis from other causes of a joint effusion. Ultrasonography facilitates hip aspirations[30] but is generally not required for aspiration of other joints. Fluid aspirated from a septic joint characteristically has a marked leukocyte concentration. Leukocyte counts of infected articular fluid characteristically exceed 80,000/mL but may be less than 25,000/mL.[22] This and the fact that other inflammatory conditions may produce concentrations of leukocytes within joint fluid similar to those seen with septic arthritis prevent a definitive diagnosis from being made solely on this parameter.[7] Gram staining is useful for early guidance of therapy but is positive in only about one third of cases.[20,22,56] The positive yield of joint cultures ranges from 36% to 80%.[20,48,77]

Skeletal scintigraphy of joints affected with septic arthritis may be normal or reveal increased periarticular tracer localization on angiographic, tissue phase, and skeletal phase images. Diminished or apparently absent tracer localization may be noted in the femoral capital epiphysis and proximal femoral physis due to tamponade of the intracapsular epiphyseal vessels. This generally normalizes following arthrocentesis. A focal area of increased tracer localization indicates osteomyelitis.[35,41,61,62]

Magnetic resonance imaging may reveal prominent synovial enhancement on T1-weighted MR images following gadolinium administration. The MRI findings of osteomyelitis indicate associated bone infection.

The differential diagnosis of septic arthritis includes a number of conditions such as acute osteomyelitis, transient synovitis, Legg-Calvé-Perthes disease, juvenile rheumatoid arthritis, rheumatic fever, Kawasaki disease, and Lyme disease. Transient synovitis, the most frequent cause of hip pain in childhood,[36,58] warrants special consideration.

Transient synovitis (toxic synovitis, observation hip, irritable hip) is a nonspecific clinical condition associated with an acute history of hip or knee pain, limp, and spasm. Affected children are typically 5 to 10 years of age. There is a slight male predominance. Symptoms usually subside following a short period of rest. The etiology is unknown. Bacterial, viral, and allergic causes have not been found.[47] Transient synovitis is a diagnosis of exclusion.

Transient synovitis and septic arthritis are not differentiated with radiography, skeletal scintigraphy, or MRI (Fig. 2.15). Ultrasonography usually demonstrates a joint effusion. An effusion is not required for diagnosis, however.[9] Tracer localization in the femoral capital epiphysis may be decreased (Fig. 2.16). This is generally not severe in degree and typically returns to normal spontaneously or following arthrocentesis.[28] Joint aspiration is useful for decreasing intraarticular pressure, particularly in cases involving the hip, and essential for excluding septic arthritis.[37]

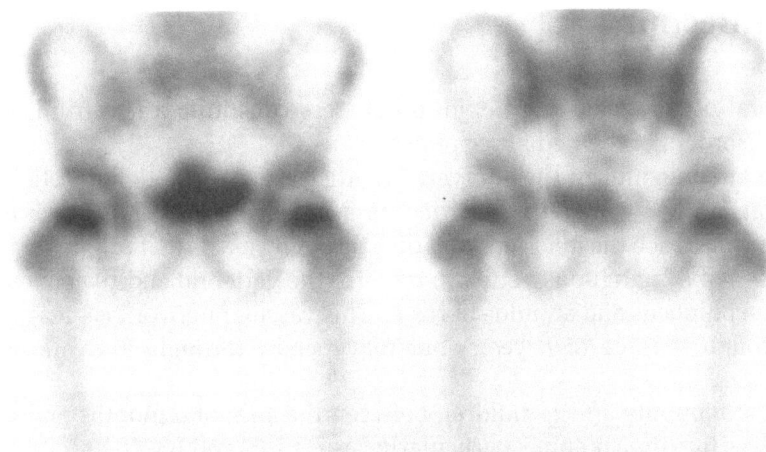

A

Figure 2.16. Septic arthritis with hip effusion. Anterior (left) and posterior skeletal phase images reveal slightly decreased tracer localization in the left femoral capital epiphysis (A). Pinhole imaging confirms this finding and shows that epiphyseal tracer localization, while decreased, is not absent (B). Echogenic material (arrow) layers posteriorly within the effusion (*) shown sonographically (C).

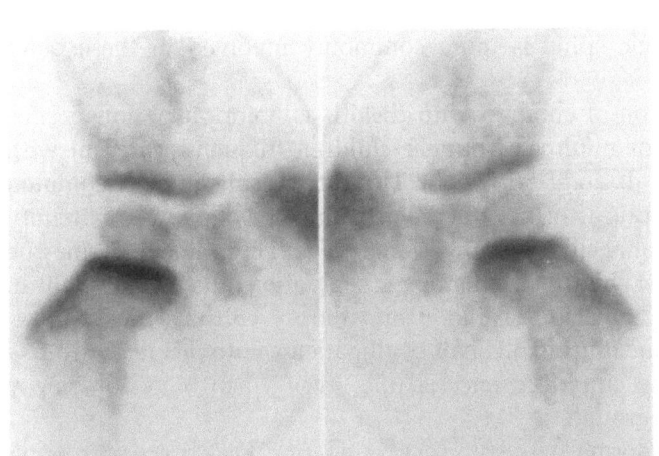

B

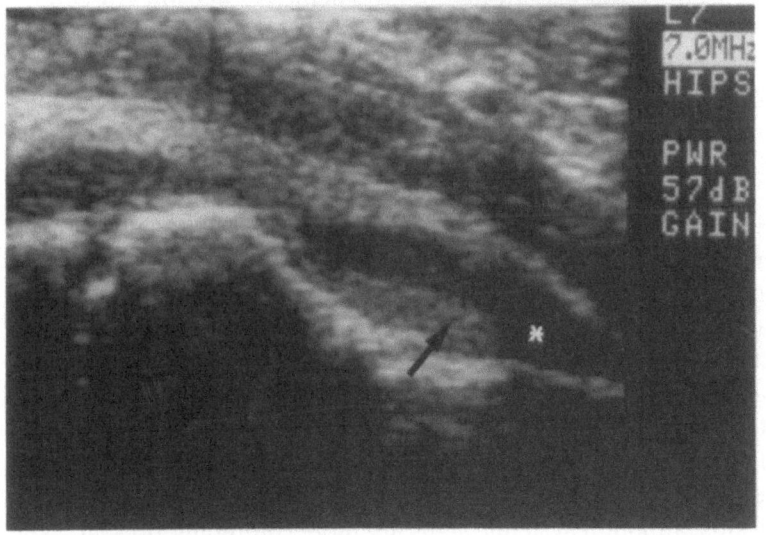

C

Vertebral Infection

Diskitis, vertebral osteomyelitis, and epidural abscess constitute a spectrum of inflammatory disorders of the pediatric spine.

Diskitis is an inflammation of the intervertebral disk space. Although the etiology is controversial, it is generally regarded as a low-grade bacterial or viral infection. Organisms reach the intervertebral disk through vessels that originate in the marrow space of a contiguous vertebra, traverse the vertebral end plate, and enter the nucleus pulposus and annulus fibrosus. This vascular network is present in children through the age of 8 years, but may persist through 30 years of age.[49,50,75]

Diskitis most commonly affects children between the ages of 6 months and 4 years and involves the lumbar spine, particularly L1–2, L2–3, and L3–4. A second, lower, epidemiologic peak in the incidence of diskitis occurs between 10 and 14 years of age. The thoracic spine is more commonly involved in these older children.

The clinical presentation of children with diskitis is notoriously nonspecific. Fever is usually absent or minimal. Younger children frequently present with reluctance or refusal to walk and bear weight. This often results in more common disorders, particularly septic arthritis or acute osteomyelitis of a lower extremity or the pelvis, being the initial clinical impression. Back or abdominal pain may be present, especially in older children. Hematologic evaluation often reveals only an elevated ESR and mild leukocytosis. Blood and biopsy cultures are positive, usually for *S. aureus*, in one third to one half of all patients with diskitis. A course of antibiotics is generally employed successfully, even when blood or biopsy cultures are negative for growth.[74]

Radiographs are often normal at the time of presentation. Disk space narrowing with or without erosion of the adjacent end plates is demonstrated after inflammation has been present for 2 to 7 weeks.

Often, a diagnosis of diskitis is first suggested by skeletal scintigraphy performed to assess suspected acute osteomyelitis of a lower extremity or the pelvis. The time interval between symptom onset and the first scintigraphic abnormality varies, but is shorter than that required for the development of radiographic manifestations. Bone scintigraphy should be abnormal in all patients with symptoms for more than 7 days.[23,74] The typical scintigraphic manifestation of diskitis is increased tracer localization involving the two vertebral end plates and bodies adjacent to the inflamed disk (Figs. 2.17 and 2.18). The increased localization may reflect microtrauma related to loss of the cushioning effect of the disk with extrusion of disk material into the vertebral body. It does not necessarily imply infection of the vertebrae themselves.

Vertebral osteomyelitis differs from diskitis in that there is involvement and eventual loss of height of a vertebral body. In children, it is predominantly seen prior to the age of 10 years. The clinical presentation is often identical to that described for diskitis, although systemic signs are more commonly present. Skeletal scintigraphy typically reveals increased tracer localization in a single vertebra (Fig. 2.19).[60] The scintigraphic appearance may resemble that of diskitis, however. Without frank loss of vertebral body height or direct bacterial culture from bone, it is often not possible to clearly differentiate vertebral osteomyelitis from diskitis.

SPECT increases the sensitivity of scintigraphy for the diagnosis of diskitis and vertebral osteomyelitis.[64] It is an essential part of the examination whenever spinal infection is considered likely and planar images are normal or equivocal.[60]

Paraspinal or epidural abscess may occur in association with diskitis or vertebral osteomyelitis. Less often, epidural abscess occurs in their absence.[60] Significant neurologic deficits may result from epidural abscess, necessitating a prompt diagnosis to prevent permanent damage. Since neurologic symptoms may be absent or minimal, early imaging with MRI is recommended whenever vertebral infection is suspected on clinical and/or scintigraphic grounds to exclude an associated soft tissue or epidural abscess, or, in cases of diskitis, to determine the effect of extruded disk material on the spinal canal (Fig. 2.17).[30] There are no scintigraphic findings that directly suggest an epidural abscess.

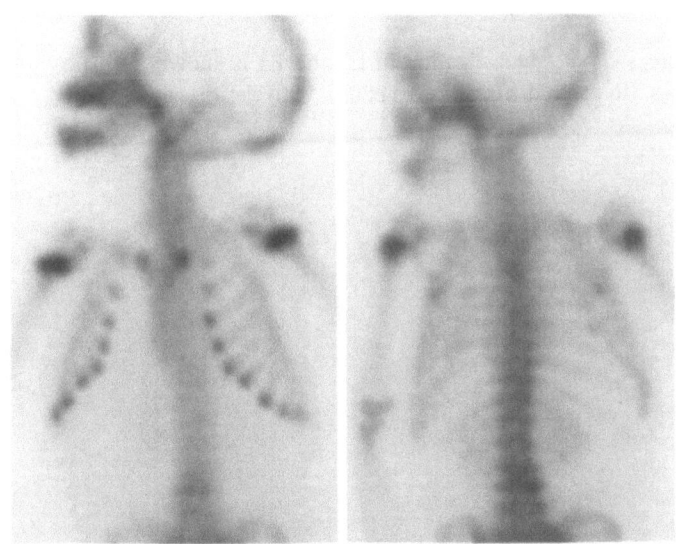

A

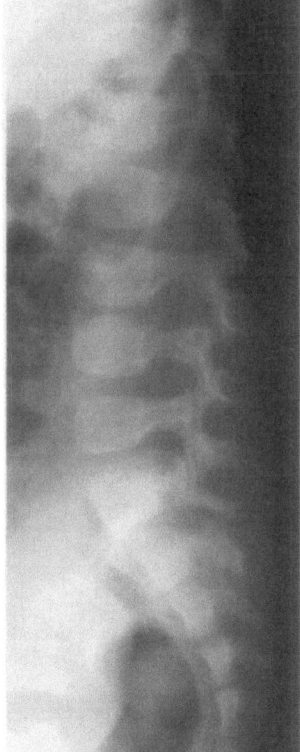

B

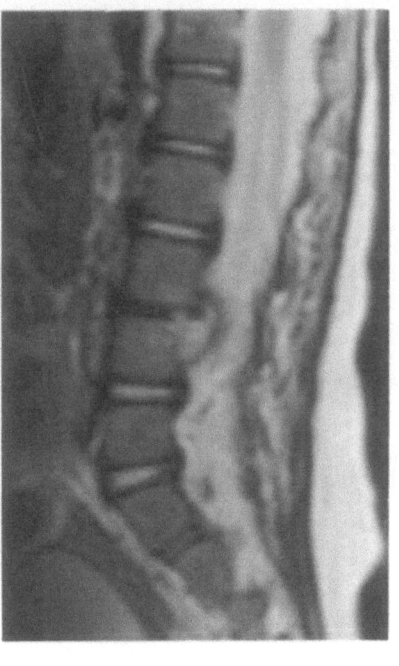

C

Figure 2.17. Diskitis. Anterior and posterior skeletal phase images of an 18-month-old girl with suspected lower extremity osteomyelitis reveal increased tracer localization in L3 and L4 (A). A radiograph obtained following scintigraphy shows decreased height to the L3–4 disk space (B). T2-weighted MRI demonstrates loss of normal signal in the L3–4 disk except at its right posterior aspect (C). An epidural tissue mass that produces mild impingement on the thecal sac extends from the mid-L3 to mid-L4 level. This may represent either extruded disk material or inflammatory tissue.

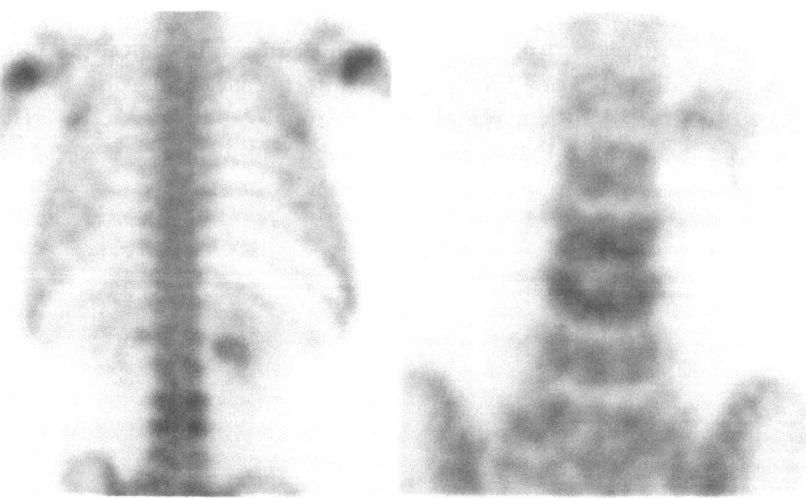

Figure 2.18. Diskitis. Increased tracer localization in L3 and L4 is shown with posterior planar and pinhole images. (Reprinted from Treves et al,[68] with permission.)

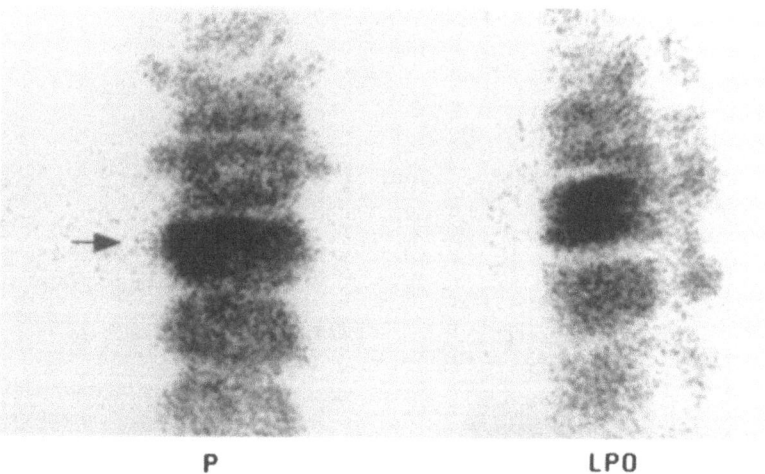

P   LPO

Figure 2.19. Vertebral osteomyelitis. Pinhole ^{99m}Tc-MDP images show intense tracer accumulation in the first lumbar vertebral body. (Reprinted from Treves, et al,[68] with permission.)

Acute Musculoskeletal Infection: Suggested Imaging Approach

With advances in cross-sectional imaging over the past decade, the relative merits of different imaging modalities for evaluating osteomyelitis have been debated. Whole-body skeletal scintigraphy is the most effective means of screening children with suspected osteomyelitis and normal radiographic evaluation. Although the sensitivity of MRI relative to that of scintigraphy has not been conclusively established,[27] MRI is useful when symptoms are sufficiently localized to direct the examination.[18,39] As noted previously, such symptom localization is frequently not present in young children. The need for sedation, as well as cost and availability, are also considered in choosing one modality over the other. At our institution, we rarely use sedation in performing skeletal scintigraphy but use sedation routinely in performing MRI of children under 6 years of age.

We have adopted the following strategy for the imaging evaluation of suspected osteomyelitis.[30,68] All infants and children with suspected osteomyelitis are initially evaluated with radiographs. When these are normal or equivocal, three-phase skeletal scintigraphy is performed. Antibiotic therapy, which may be initiated based on clinical suspicion prior to scintigraphy, is either continued or begun if scintigraphy is abnormal. In the few cases of acute osteomyelitis that do not respond to antibiotic therapy over a 48-hour interval, gadolinium-enhanced MRI is obtained to assess the possibility of intraosseous or soft tissue abscess. Due to the need to determine if an epidural or paraspinal abscess is present, MRI is performed immediately following scintigraphy when a vertebral abnormality is detected or rather than scintigraphy in the few cases with a clinical question limited to the spine. MRI or computed tomography (CT) is obtained in cases of pelvic osteomyelitis to establish the optimal anatomic approach when surgical drainage is planned. Ultrasonography is performed in cases of suspected septic arthritis of the hip.

Additional imaging may be beneficial in cases where skeletal scintigraphy is interpreted as normal or as equivocally positive but there is a persistent clinical suspicion of osteomyelitis. Theoretically, early in the course of osteomyelitis a balance between diminished radionuclide delivery due to microvascular occlusion and increased localization due to early osteoblastic repair may result in a normal skeletal scintigram. This occurs very rarely. False-normal interpretations may be rendered due to variations in the perception threshold of interpreting physicians for calling a study abnormal and in studies of inadequate technical quality. Whatever the cause, the rarely encountered normal scintigram in acute osteomyelitis indicates that a normal study is not an absolute guarantee that a patient does not have osteomyelitis. Repeat skeletal scintigraphy after 2 to 3 days, ^{67}Ga scintigraphy, labeled leukocyte imaging, and, if symptoms are sufficiently localized, MRI are appropriate imaging studies when clinical suspicion persists.

Subacute and Chronic Osteomyelitis

Subacute osteomyelitis may result from inadequate antibiotic treatment of acute osteomyelitis.[62] It also may occur in the absence of prior antibiotic therapy.[34] The long bones are predominantly affected.

The onset of pain or limping is insidious in children with primary subacute osteomyelitis. There may be localized swelling. Systemic signs are usually absent. Hematologic analysis is even less revealing than in acute osteomyelitis. The ESR is usually elevated, but to a lesser degree than with acute osteomyelitis. The white blood cell count is usually normal and blood cultures typically do not yield growth of organisms. *S. aureus* is often cultured from the involved bone.[43] Subacute osteomyelitis is revealed radiographically. There are two common radiographic appearances. Both differ considerably from the radiographic appearance of acute osteomyelitis. The most common manifestation is a well-defined radiolucency that corresponds to a localized bone abscess (Brodie abscess). The radiolucency is often surrounded by a sclerotic rim and associated with little or no periosteal reaction. These lesions are most commonly metaphyseal. They may extend through the physis into the epiphysis, extend into the diaphysis, or arise primarily in either the epiphysis or diaphysis. The other common radiographic manifestation is irregular cortical resorption. This also usually affects the metaphysis but may extend into, or arise in, the epiphysis or diaphysis. Periosteal reaction, which is typically thick rather than laminated, is frequently present, and sclerosis may be associated. A soft tissue mass is usually not identified. This radiographic appearance of subacute osteomyelitis may be difficult to distinguish from that of Ewing sarcoma.[11,37,52]

Skeletal scintigraphy typically shows increased tracer localization at sites of subacute osteomyelitis (Fig. 2.20), but is rarely required as part of the diagnostic evaluation.

Subacute osteomyelitis may persist for months or years and be considered chronic.[19] A significant problem in evaluating patients with suspected or treated chronic osteomyelitis is discrimination between active infection and sterile reparative bone. Skeletal scintigraphy is not useful for making this distinction. Sequential skeletal scintigraphy and ^{67}Ga studies have been used for this purpose. When ^{67}Ga localization exceeds that of a skeletal tracer, active infection is implied.[70] Labeled leukocytes can be used in a similar fashion and offer a theoretical advantage in that, unlike ^{67}Ga, they do not avidly localize to sites of bone remodeling. As leukocytes migrate to sites of chronic infection less markedly than to sites of acute infection, the significance of a normal labeled leukocyte study in the context of chronic osteomyelitis is uncertain.[53–55]

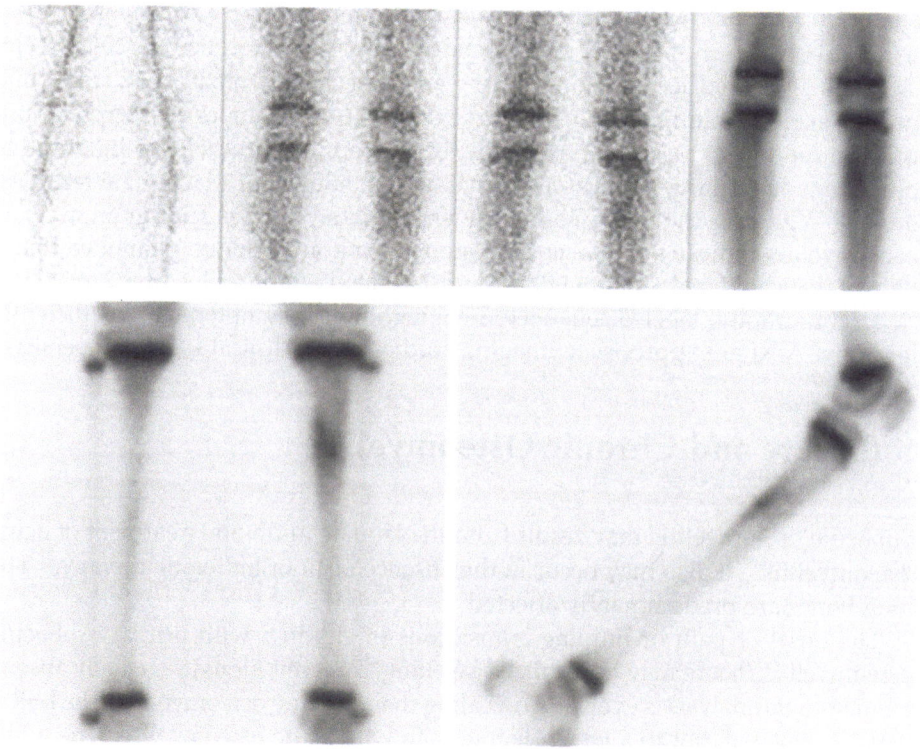

A

Figure 2.20. (A) Caption is on facing page.

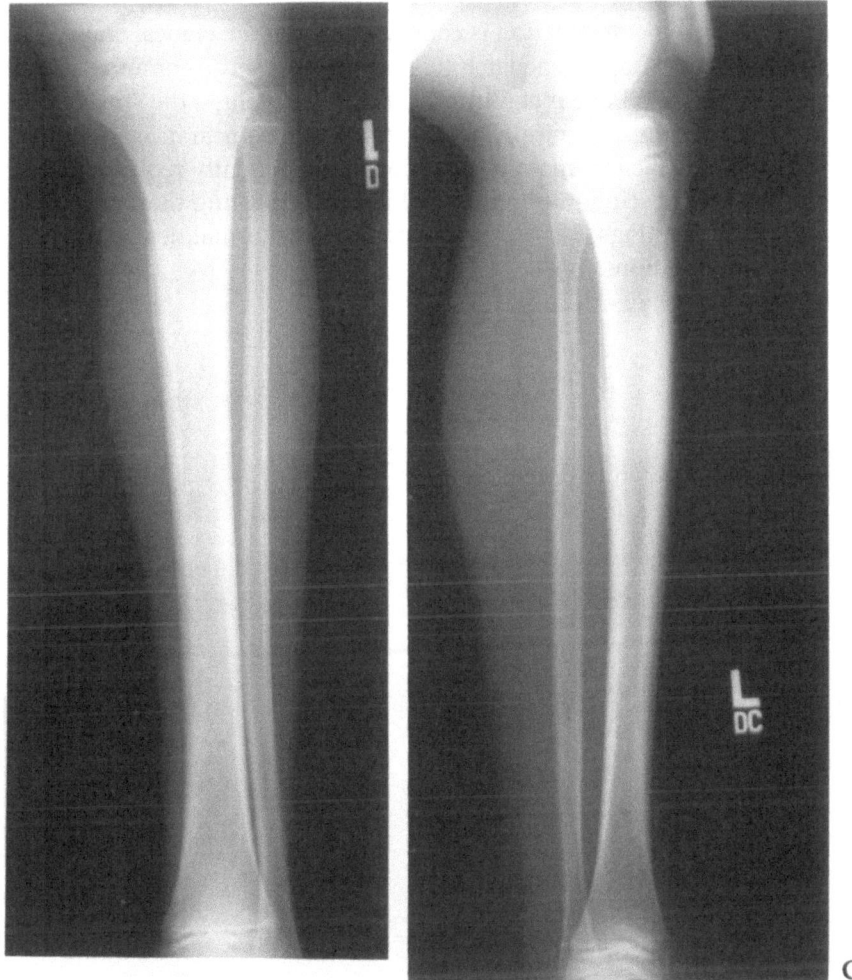

B

C

Figure 2.20. Subacute osteomyelitis. Radionuclide angiography shows that blood flow to the left calf is minimally increased (a, upper row). A tissue phase image (A, upper right panel) and skeletal phase images (A, lower panels) depict increased ^{99m}Tc-MDP accumulation in the posteromedial left proximal tibial diaphysis. Radiographically, there is smooth periosteal reaction corresponding to the scintigraphic abnormality. (B,C).

Chronic Recurrent Multifocal Osteomyelitis

Chronic recurrent multifocal osteomyelitis (CRMO) is a rare and poorly understood disease. It predominantly occurs in children between the ages of 7 and 14 years, but has been reported in children of other ages and in adults. Females are affected approximately twice as frequently as males. Symptom onset is insidious. Localized pain and soft tissue swelling are the most common complaints at presentation. Chronic recurrent multifocal osteomyelitis follows an unpredictable episodic but self-limited course over a period of months to years until spontaneous resolution occurs. Bone aspirates or biopsy specimens reveal nonspecific chronic inflammatory changes, but organisms do not grow from culture. Antibiotics do not alter the course of the disease.[14,25]

Radiographically, lytic destruction is common early in the clinical course (Fig. 2.21). Sclerosis becomes apparent later (Fig. 2.22). The most common sites of involvement are the long bone metaphyses. Other sites include the spine, pelvis, and clavicles. Distribution is typically asymmetric.[14] The appearance and presentation often suggest a skeletal malignancy. Biopsy is frequently required for this differentiation. Skeletal scintigraphy is useful in demonstrating the multifocality of skeletal involvement (Figs. 2.21–2.23). Scintigraphic abnormalities may precede radiographic manifestations.

Figure 2.21. Chronic recurrent multifocal osteomyelitis. Increased accumulation of ^{99m}Tc-MDP is present in the right clavicle, L4, the sacrum, and the distal right radius (A). A region of lower tracer localization adjacent to the focal concentration in the radius is better demonstrated with the pinhole image (A, lower right) than the high-resolution planar image. Pinhole imaging also shows abnormal tracer concentration in the distal right radial epiphysis. With SPECT, the L4 abnormality is shown to involve the posteromedial vertebral body (B).

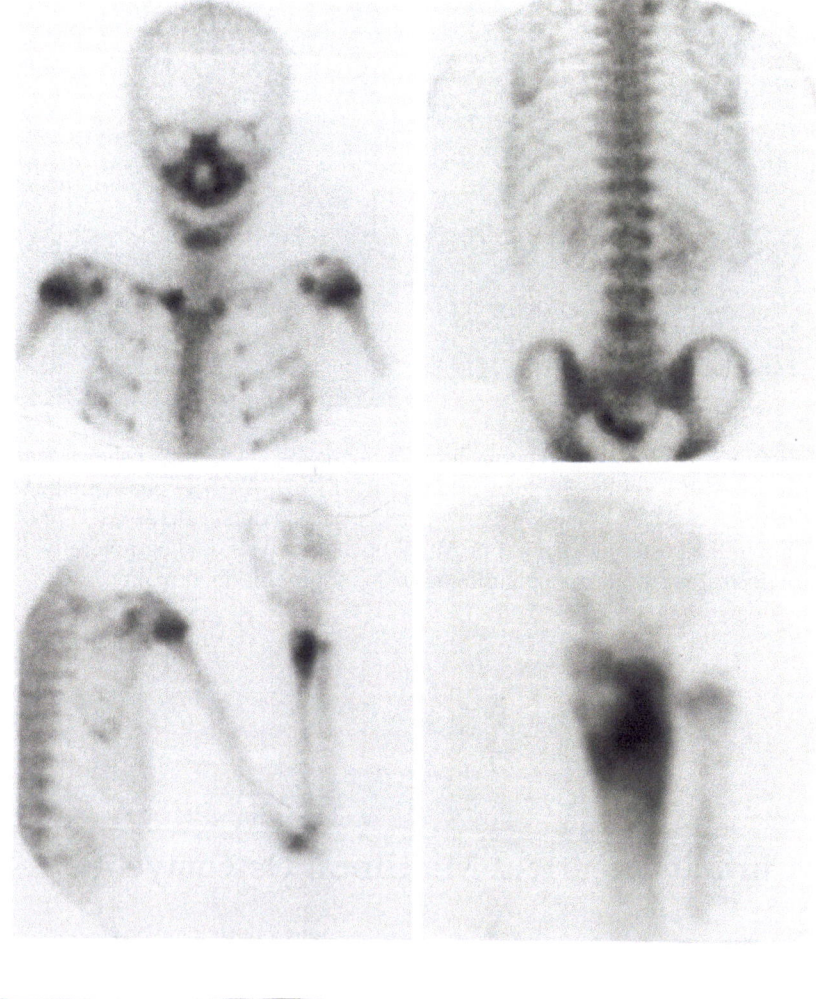

A

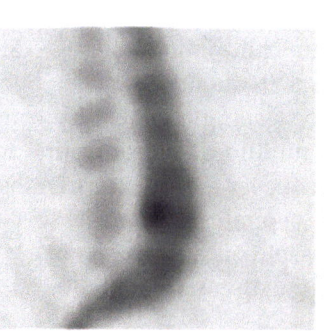
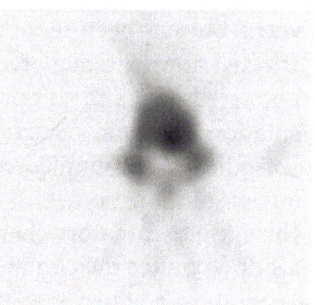

B

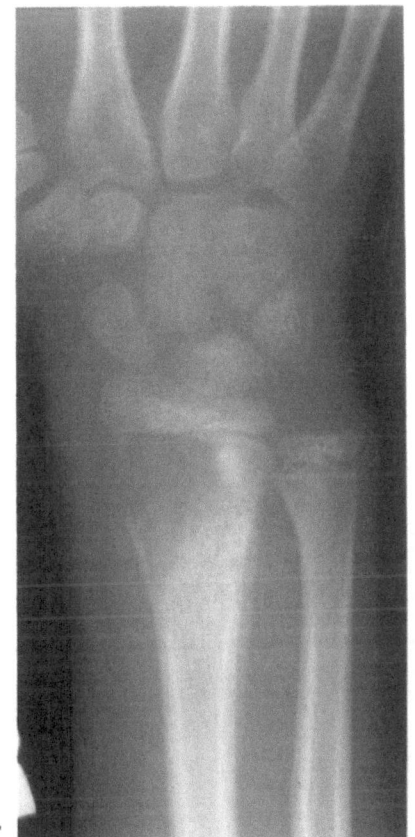

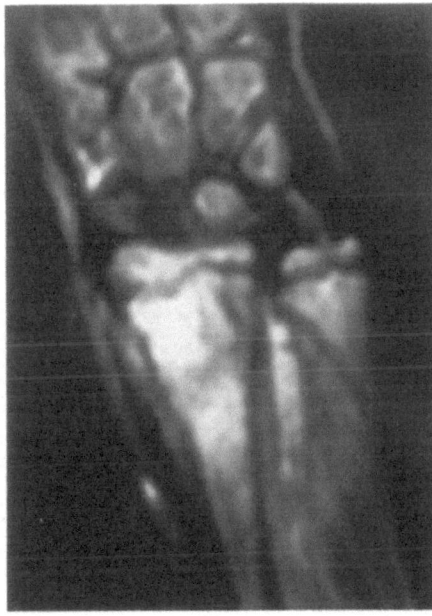
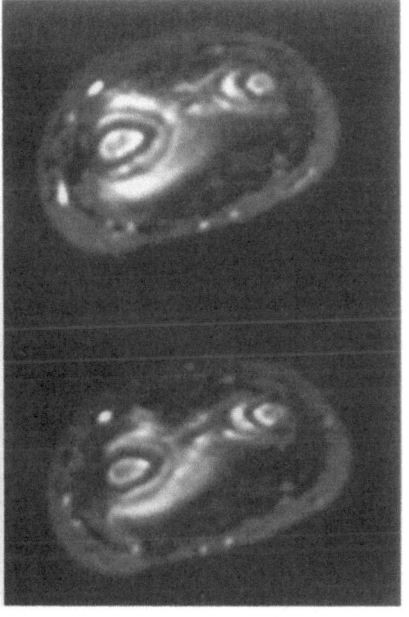

C

D

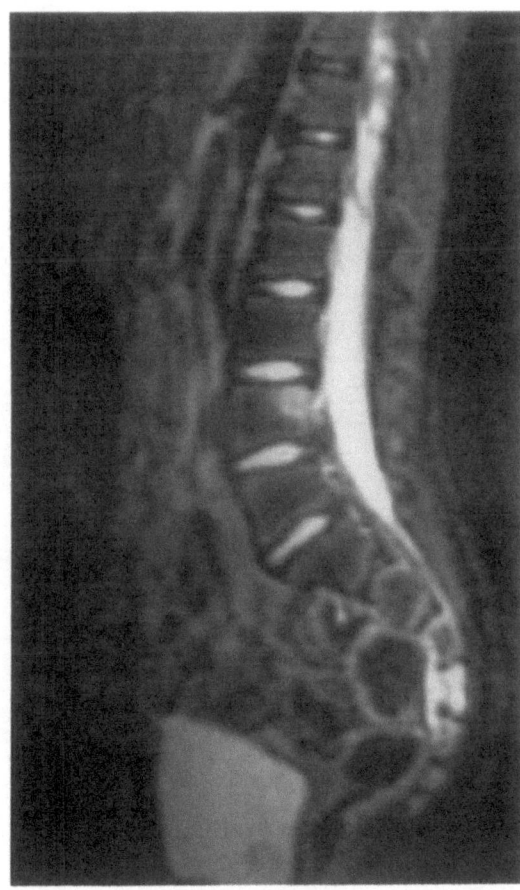

Figure 2.21 (*cont'd.*) A radiograph shows an osteolytic lesion of the distal right radial metaphysis (C). The lytic lesion in the distal right radius exhibits increased T2 signal intensity and appears to extend across the physis into the epiphysis, which is heterogeneously T2 bright (D). There is near circumferential periosteal reaction with evidence of cortical destruction along the radial aspect of the metaphysis as depicted on the transaxial images (D, right panel). There is abnormal high T2 signal involving L4 and the S4 segment (E).

E

Figure 2.22. Chronic recurrent multifocal osteomyelitis. Increased tracer localization is present in the left acromion process of the scapula and the left iliac bone (A).

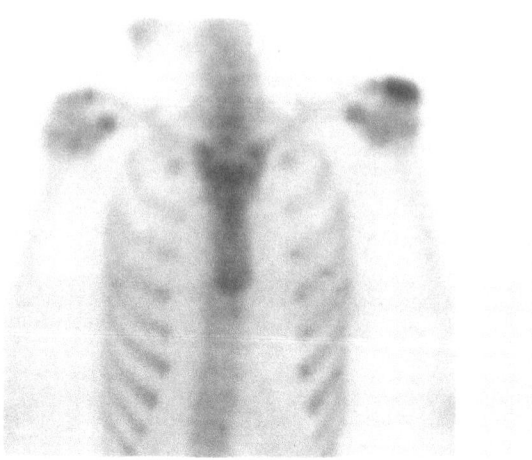
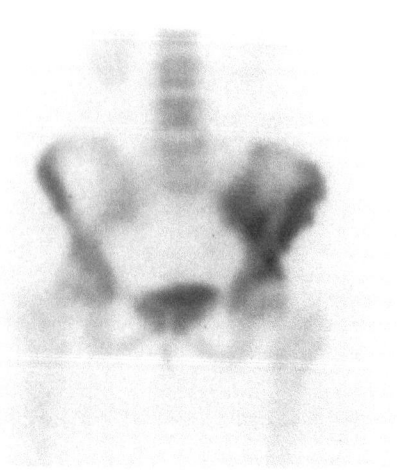

A

Figure 2.22 (*cont'd.*) Radiographically, there is sclerosis with interspersed foci of radiolucency involving the left acromion (B).

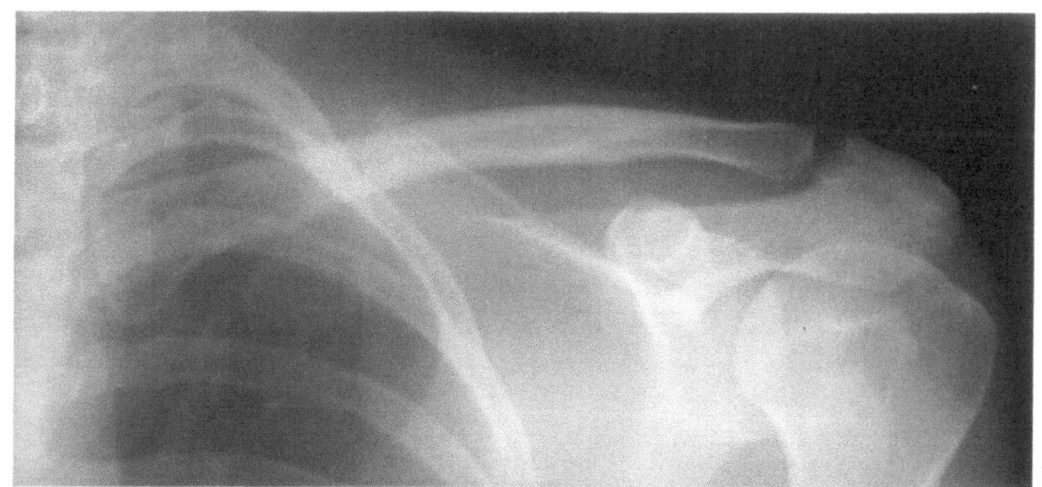

B

Figure 2.22 (*cont'd.*) Intense sclerosis and bone overgrowth affects the inferolateral left iliac wing (C).

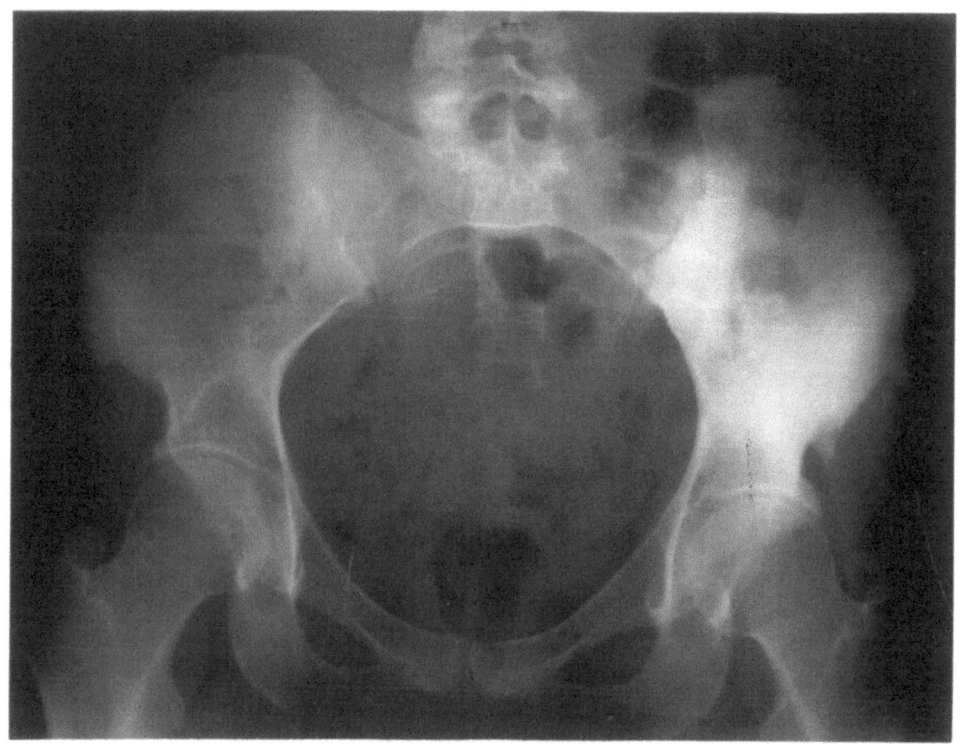

C

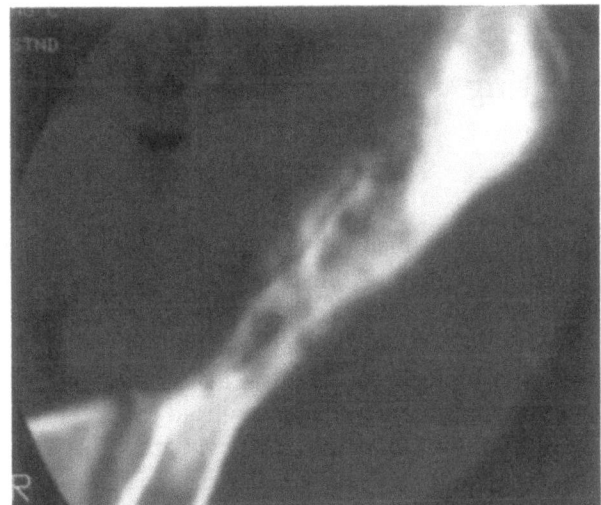

Figure 2.22 (*cont'd.*) Computed tomography shows sclerosis and permeative lysis of the left iliac wing (D).

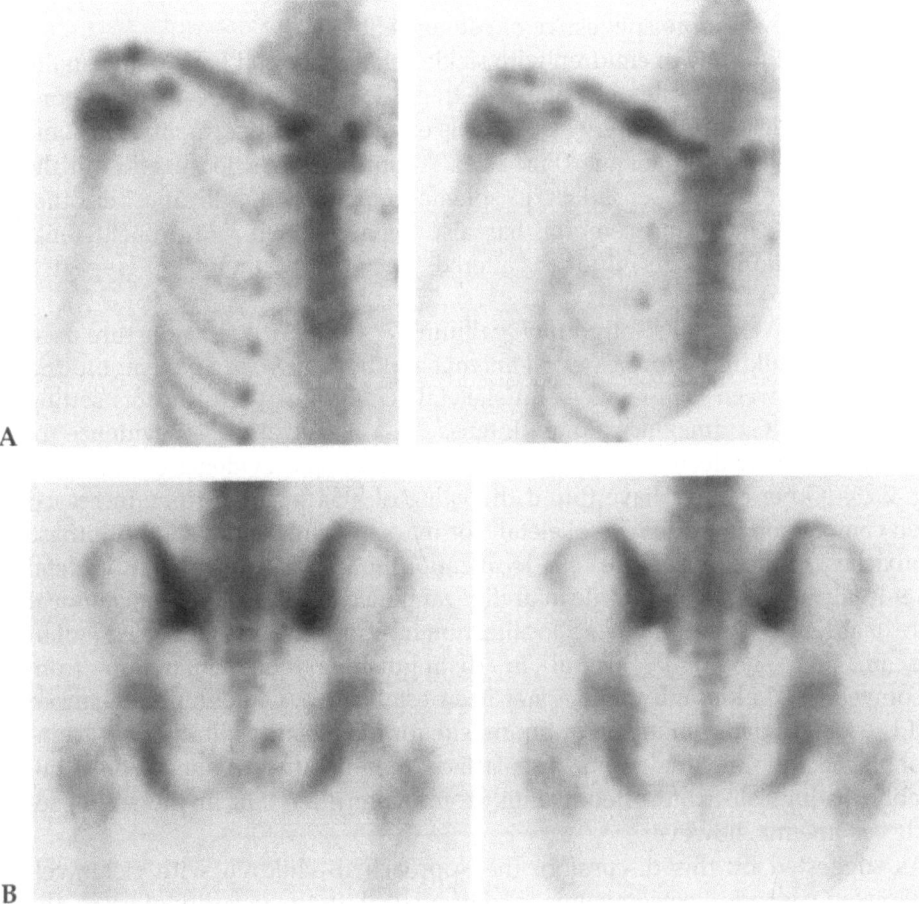

Figure 2.23. Chronic recurrent multifocal osteomyelitis. Increased ^{99m}Tc-MDP localization in the right clavicle (left panel) on a study performed at diagnosis is more intense 8 months later (right panel) during a period of local symptom exacerbation (A). Posterior images of the pelvis obtained synchronously with those of the clavicle show increased localization along the right sacroiliac joint that remains constant in intensity (B).

Osteomyelitis Complicating Other Diseases

Sickle Cell Anemia

Sickle cell anemia is a hemoglobinopathy in which valine replaces glutamic acid at the sixth position of the β-globulin chain (hemoglobin S). Changes in deoxygenated hemoglobin S result in erythrocyte rigidity and fragility. Children with sickle cell anemia are at increased risk for infections, including osteomyelitis and septic arthritis, as well as avascular necrosis of bone caused by vascular occlusion (Figs. 2.24–2.26). Skeletal pain in these children is more frequently related to a sickle cell crisis with bone infarction than it is to infection. Differentiation between osteomyelitis and bone infarction presents a clinical challenge in some cases. The degree of fever and leukocytosis may be similar. The ESR is a less reliable parameter in children with sickle cell disease. It may be falsely low but may be elevated with either bone infarction or osteomyelitis. Elevations over 20 mm/hour suggest infection.[26] Radiographs are usually either normal or reveal only soft tissue swelling acutely with both of these clinical entities. Bone destruction and periosteal reaction are the initial osseous manifestations of each.

Skeletal scintigraphy does not reliably distinguish osteomyelitis from bone infarction in sickle cell patients. Increased or decreased tracer delivery and localization are observed with either. This reflects the previously discussed mechanisms of ischemic osteomyelitis and the occurrence of bone remodeling within 3 to 7 days of infarction. Early in the course of symptoms, increased tracer delivery and uptake is, however, more suggestive of osteomyelitis.

Skeletal scintigraphy of children with sickle cell disease and bone pain usually demonstrates multiple sites of abnormal tracer localization due to prior bone infarctions. Skeletal scintigraphy also reveals extraosseous abnormalities in some children with sickle cell anemia (Fig. 2.24). Abnormal tracer localization in the spleen may be observed secondary to splenic infarction.[24] Localization in other infarcted tissue, including cerebral, has also been reported.[29] Prominent renal tracer localization occurs due to altered iron distribution and repeated transfusions.[59]

In addition to skeletal scintigraphy, gallium-67 and marrow imaging are used in evaluating children with sickle cell anemia and bone pain. We have not found comparison between ^{67}Ga images and skeletal scintigrams useful in this setting and rely on ^{67}Ga imaging alone. Intense ^{67}Ga localization is evidence of osteomyelitis while decreased or absent ^{67}Ga localization is evidence of infarction (Fig. 2.26). Other centers have found the value of ^{67}Ga imaging to be increased when comparison is made with skeletal[2,4] or marrow scintigraphy.[32,57] With these approaches, reduced or absent ^{67}Ga localization in an area of increased skeletal tracer localization indicates sterile infarction, and increased gallium localization at a site of absent ^{99m}Tc sulfur colloid localization indicates infection. Labeled leukocyte imaging should be useful in distinguishing bone infarction from osteomyelitis,[21,76] although this has not been established. Gadolinium-enhanced MRI is useful in determining an optimum site for diagnostic aspiration by distinguishing necrotic material from vascularized inflammatory tissue. It does not reliably distinguish acute osteomyelitis from acute infarction in the setting of sickle cell anemia, however.[12]

As suggested by this discussion, the approach to children with sickle cell disease and suspected osteomyelitis is controversial. In the majority of cases, the diagnosis must be made clinically. Blood cultures and bone aspiration have been suggested for cases where the temperature exceeds 39°C. Antibiotics are begun empirically when osteomyelitis is clinically likely. These must be chosen to include coverage of Salmonella species, the infective organisms in a significant number of cases.[26]

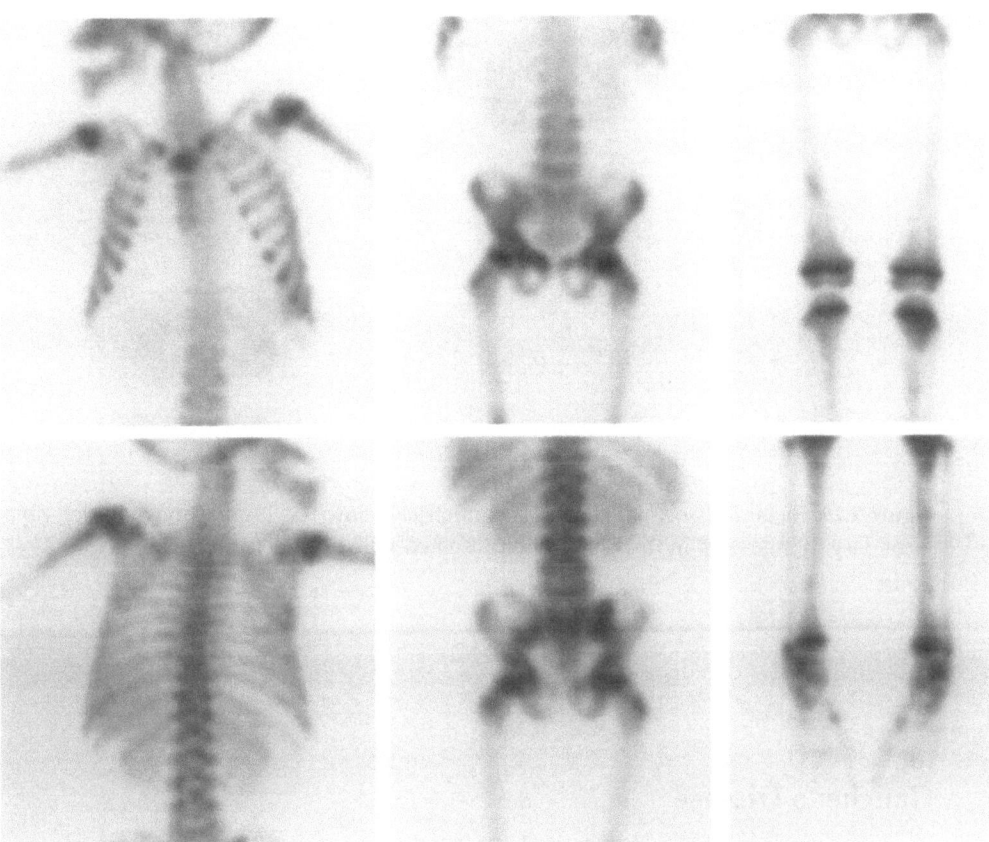

Figure 2.24. Sickle cell anemia. Multiple sites of abnormal ^{99m}Tc-MDP localization are demonstrated in the long bones and pelvis. The most intense focus of increased localization in the right pubis corresponds to a pathologic fracture through infarcted bone. There is tracer accumulation in the left upper quadrant within the spleen. This is best appreciated on the posterior images (lower row).

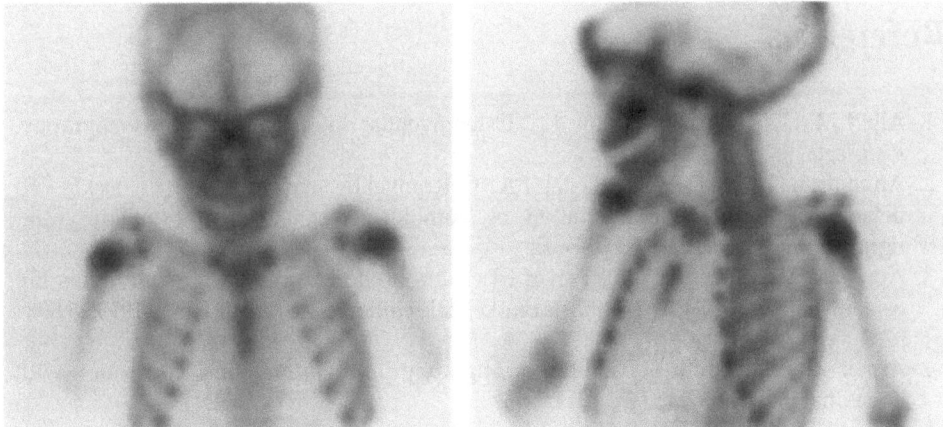

Figure 2.25. Sickle cell anemia. Absence of ^{99m}Tc-MDP localization in the upper sternum secondary to an acute infarction is depicted.

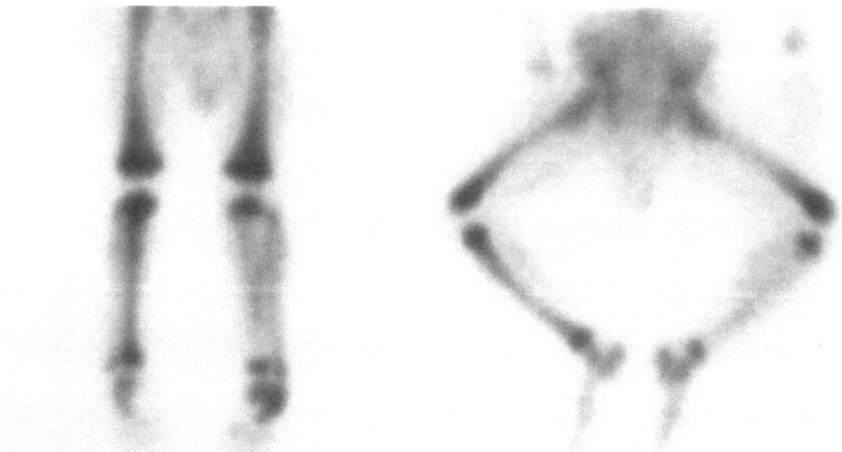

Figure 2.26. Sickle cell anemia. There is asymmetrically low ^{67}Ga localization in the left tibia secondary to infarction in this child who presented with actue left tibial pain.

Gaucher's Disease

Gaucher's disease is an autosomal recessive disease caused by glucocerebrosidase deficiency. It is characterized by the accumulation of lipid laden macrophages in the liver, spleen, and bone marrow and other sites. A significant percentage of patients are Ashkenazic Jews. A diagnosis of Gaucher's disease is most often reached in childhood and early adulthood. Skeletal manifestations include modeling deformities of the long bones, osteopenia, cortical thickening, and avascular necrosis. Differentiation between bone infarction and osteomyelitis is difficult in some children who present with acute localized pain, leukocytosis, and an elevated ESR due to bone infarction (Gaucher crisis or pseudoosteomyelitis). With a Gaucher crisis, skeletal scintigraphy typically reveals decreased tracer localization in cases studied within 3 days of symptom onset.[10,33] While this pattern is suggestive of infarction rather than osteomyelitis, further investigation with ^{67}Ga, marrow scintigraphy, or MRI may be useful in cases where the clinical diagnosis is uncertain.

References

1. Albiri MM, Kirpekar M, Ablow RC. Osteomyelitis: detection with ultrasonography. *Radiology* 1989;172:509–514.
2. Amundsen TR, Siegel MJ, Siegel BA. Osteomyelitis and infarction in sickle cell hemoglobinopathies; differentiation by combined technetium and gallium scintigraphy. *Radiology* 1984;153:807–812.
3. Applegate KA, Connolly LP, Treves ST. Neuroblastoma presenting clinically as hip osteomyelitis: a signature diagnosis on skeletal scintigraphy. *Pediatr Radiol* 1995;25:S93–97.
4. Armas RR, Goldsmith SJ. Gallium scintigraphy in bone infarction: correlation with bone imaging. *Clin Nucl Med* 1984;9:1–3.
5. Ash JM, Gilday DL. The futility of bone scanning in neonatal osteomyelitis: concise communication. *J Nucl Med* 1980;21:417–420.

6. Asmar BI. Osteomyelitis in the neonate. *Infect Dis Clin North Am* 1992;6:117–132.

7. Baldassare AR, Chang F, Zuckner J. Markedly raised synovial leucocyte counts not associated with infectious arthritis in children. *Ann Rheum Dis* 1978;37:404–409.

8. Barton LL, Dunkin LM, Habib FH. Septic arthritis in childhood: a 13 year review. *Am J Dis Child* 1987;141:898–900.

9. Bickerstaff DR, Neal LM, Booth AJ, et al. Ultrasound examination of the irritable hip. *J Bone Joint Surg [B]* 1990;72:549–553.

10. Bilchik TR, Heyman S. Skeletal scintigraphy of pseudo-osteomyelitis in Gaucher's disease. Two case reports and a review of the literature. *Clin Nucl Med* 1992;17:279–282.

11. Bogoch E, Thompson G, Salter RB. Foci of chronic circumscribed osteomyelitis (Brodie's abscess) that traverse the epiphyseal plate. *J Pediatr Orthop* 1984;4:162–169.

12. Bonnerot V, Sebag G, De Montalembert M, et al. Gadolinium-DOTA enhanced MRI of painful osseous crises in children with sickle cell anemia. *Pediatr Radiol* 1994;24:92–95.

13. Bressler L, Conway JJ, Weiss SC. Neonatal osteomyelitis examined by bone scintigraphy. *Radiology* 1984;152:685–688.

14. Brown T, Wilkinson RH. Chronic recurrent multifocal osteomyelitis. *Radiology* 1988;166:493–496.

15. Canale ST, Harkness RM, Thomas PA, et al. Does aspiration of bones and joints affect results of later bone scanning? *J Pediatr Orthop* 1985;5:23–26.

16. Capitanio M, Kirkpatrick JA. Early roentgen observations in acute osteomyelitis. *AJR* 1970;108:488–496.

17. Cohen MD. *Imaging of Children with Cancer.* St. Louis: Mosby Year Book; 1992.

18. Dangman BC, Hoffer FA, Rand FF, et al. Osteomyelitis in children: gadolinium enhanced MR imaging. *Radiology* 1992;182:743–747.

19. David R, Barron BJ, Madewell JE. Osteomyelitis, acute and chronic. *Radiol Clin North Am* 1987;25:1171–1201.

20. Faden H, Grossi M. Acute osteomyelitis in children. *Am J Dis Child* 1991;145:65–69.

21. Fernandez-Ulloa M, Vasavada PJ, Black RR. Detection of acute osteomyelitis with indium-111 labeled white blood cells in a patient with sickle cell disease. *Clin Nucl Med* 1989;14:97–100.

22. Fink CW, Nelson JD. Septic arthritis and osteomyelitis in children. *Clin Rheum Dis* 1986;12:423–435.

23. Fischer GW, Popich GA, Sullivan DE, et al. Diskitis: a prospective diagnostic analysis. *Pediatrics* 1978;62:543–548.

24. Fischer KC, Shapir S, Treves ST. Visualization of the spleen with a bone seeking radionuclide in a child with sickle cell anemia. *Radiology* 1977;122:398.

25. Giedion A, Holthusen W, Masel LF, et al. Subacute and chronic "symmetrical" osteomyelitis. *Ann Radiol* 1972;15:329–342.

26. Greene WB. Diseases related to the hematopoietic system. In: Morrisy R, Weinstein S, eds. *Lovell and Winter's Pediatric Orthopedics.* 4th ed. Philadelphia: Lippincott-Raven; 1996:345–391.

27. Harcke HT. Role of imaging in musculoskeletal infections in children [editorial]. *J Pediatr Orthop* 1995;15:141–143.

28. Hasegawa Y, Wingstrand H, Gustafson T. Scintimetry in transient synovitis of the hip. *Acta Orthop Scand* 1988;59:520–525.

29. Hung GL, Stewart CA, Yeo E, et al. Incidental demonstration of cerebral infarction on bone scintigraphy in sickle cell disease. *Clin Nucl Med* 1990;15:671–672.

30. Jaramillo D, Treves ST, Kasser JR, et al. Osteomyelitis and septic arthritis in childhood: appropriate use of imaging to guide treatment. *AJR* 1995;165:399–404.

31. Jones DC, Cady RB. "Cold" bone scans in acute osteomyelitis. *J Bone Joint Surg [B]* 1981;63:376–378.

32. Kahn CE Jr, Ryan JW, Hatfield MK, et al. Combined bone marrow and gallium imaging. Differentiation of osteomyelitis and infarction in sickle hemoglobinopathy. *Clin Nucl Med* 1988;13:443–449.

33. Katz K, Mechlis-Frish S, Cohen IJ, et al. Bone scans in the diagnosis of bone crisis in patients who have Gaucher disease. *J Bone Joint Surg [A]* 1991;73:513–517.

34. King DM, Mayo KM. Subacute hematogenous osteomyelitis. *J Bone Joint Surg [B]* 1969;51:458–463.

35. Kloiber R, Pavlosky W, Portner O, et al. Bone scintigraphy of hip joint effusions in children. *AJR* 1983;140:995–999.

36. Landin LA, Danielsson LG, Wattsgard C. Transient synovitis of the hip: its incidence, epidemiology and relation to Perthes' disease. *J Bone Joint Surg [B]* 1987;69B:238–241.

37. Laor T, Jaramillo D, Oestrich A. Skeletal system. In: Kirks DR, ed. *Practical Pediatric Imaging. Diagnostic Radiology of Infants and Children.* 3rd ed. Philadelphia: Lippincott-Raven; 1997:327–510.

38. Majd M, Frankel RS. Radionuclide imaging in skeletal inflammatory and ischemic disease in children. *AJR* 1976;126:832–841.

39. Mazur JM, Ross G, Cummings RJ, et al. Usefulness of magnetic resonance imaging for the diagnosis of acute musculoskeletal infections in children. *J Pediatr Orthop* 1995; 15:144–147.

40. McCoy JR, Morrisy RT, Seibert J. Clinical experience with the technetium-99m scan in children. *Clin Orthop Rel Res* 1981;154:175–180.

41. Minikel J, Sty J, Simons G. Sequential radionuclide imaging in avascular pediatric hip conditions. *Clin Orthop* 1983;175:202–208.

42. Mok PM, Reilly BJ, Ash JM. Osteomyelitis in the neonate. *Radiology* 1982;145:677–682.

43. Morrisy RT. Bone and joint sepsis. In: Morrisy R, Weinstein S, eds. *Lovell and Winter's Pediatric Orthopedics.* 4th ed. Philadelphia: Lippincott-Raven; 1996:579–624.

44. Nelson JD. Acute osteomyelitis in children. *Infect Dis Clin North Am* 1990;4:513–522.

45. Nelson JD, Bucholz RW, Kusmiesz H, et al. Benefits and risks of sequential parenteral-oral cephalosporin therapy for suppurative bone and joint infections. *J Pediatr Orthop* 1982;2:255–262.

46. Nixon G. Acute hematogenous osteomyelitis. *Pediatr Ann* 1976;5:64–81.

47. Ozonoff MB. Generalized orthopedic diseases of childhood. In: *Pediatric Orthopedic Radiology.* 2nd ed. Philadelphia: W.B. Saunders; 1992:461–568.

48. Peltola H, Vahvanen V. A comparative study of osteomyelitis and septic arthritis with special reference to aetiology and recovery. *Infection* 1984;25:75–79.

49. Ratcliffe JF. An evaluation of the intraosseous arterial anastomoses in the human vertebral body at different ages. Part 2. A microarteriographic study. *J Anat* 1982;34:373–382.

50. Ratcliffe JF. Anatomic basis for the pathologic and radiologic features of vertebral osteomyelitis and its differentiation from childhood discitis: a microarteriographic investigation. *Acta Radiol Diagn* 1985;26:137–143.

51. Riebel TW, Nasir R, Nazarenko O. The value of sonography in the detection of osteomyelitis. *Pediatr Radiol* 1996;26:291–297.

52. Roberts JM, Drummond DS, Breed AL, et al. Subacute hematogenous osteomyelitis in children: a retrospective study. *J Pediatr Orthop* 1982;2:249–254.

53. Schauwecker DS. Osteomyelitis: diagnosis with In-111 labeled leukocytes. *Radiology* 1989;171:141–146.

54. Schauwecker DS. The scintigraphic diagnosis of osteomyelitis. *AJR* 1992;158:9–18.

55. Schauwecker DS, Park HM, Mock BH, et al. Evaluation of complicating osteomyelitis with Tc-99m MDP, In-111 granulocytes, and Ga-67 citrate. *J Nucl Med* 1984;25:849–853.

56. Scott RJ, Christofersen MR, Robertson WW, et al. Acute osteomyelitis in children: a review of 116 cases. *J Pediatr Orthop* 1990;10:649–652.

57. Sebes JI. Diagnostic imaging of bone and joint abnormalities associated with sickle cell hemoglobinopathies. *AJR* 1989;152:1153–1159.

58. Spock A. Transient synovitis of the hip in children. *Pediatrics* 1959;24:1042–1049.

59. Sty JR, Babbitt DP, Sheth K. Abnormal ^{99m}Tc methylene diphosphonate accumulation in the kidneys of children with sickle cell disease. *Clin Nucl Med* 1980;5:445–447.

60. Sty JR, Wells RG, Conway JJ. Spine pain in children. *Semin Nucl Med* 1993;23:296–320.

61. Sty JR, Wells RG, Smith WD. The child with acute leg pain. *Semin Nucl Med* 1988;18:137–158.

62. Sty JR, Wells RG, Starshak RJ, Gregg D. The musculoskeletal system. In: Sty J, Wells R, Starshak R, Gregg D, eds. *Diagnostic Imaging of Infants and Children.* Vol. 3. Gaithesburg: Aspen; 1992:233–405.

63. Sullivan DC, Rosenfield NS, Ogden J, et al. Problems in the scintigraphic detection of osteomyelitis in children. *Radiology* 1980;135:731–736.

64. Swanson D, Blecker I, Gahbauer H, et al. Diagnosis of diskitis by SPECT technetium-99m MDP. A case report. *Clin Nucl Med* 1987;12:210–211.

65. Syrogiannopoulos GA, Nelson JD. Duration of antimicrobial therapy for acute suppurative osteoarticular infections. *Lancet* 1988;1(8575–6):37–40.

66. Teates CD, Williamson BRJ. "Hot and cold" bone lesion in acute osteomyelitis. *AJR* 1977;129:517–518.

67. Traughber PD, Manaster BJ, Murphy K, et al. Negative bone scans of joints after aspiration or arthrography: experimental studies. *AJR* 1986;146:87–91.

68. Treves ST, Connolly LP, Kirkpatrick JA, et al. Bone. In: Treves ST, ed. *Pediatric Nuclear Medicine*. 2nd ed. New York: Springer-Verlag; 1995:233–301.

69. Treves S, Khettry J, Broker FH, et al. Osteomyelitis: early scintigraphic detection in children. *Pediatrics* 1976;57:173–186.

70. Tumeh SS, Aliabadi P, Weissman BN, et al. Chronic osteomyelitis: bone and gallium scan patterns associated with active disease. *Radiology* 1986;158:685–688.

71. Vaughan PA, Newman NM, Rosman MA. Acute hematogenous osteomyelitis in children. *J Pediatr Orthop* 1987;7:652–655.

72. Volberg FM, Sumner TE, Abramson JS, et al. Unreliability of radiographic diagnosis of septic hip in children. *Pediatrics* 1984;73:118–120.

73. Welkon CJ, Long SS, Fisher MC, et al. Pyogenic arthritis in infants and children: a review of 95 cases. *Pediatr Infect Dis* 1986;5:669–676.

74. Wenger DR, Obechko WP, Gilday DL. The spectrum of intervertebral disk-space infection in children. *J Bone Joint Surg [A]* 1978;60:100–108.

75. Wiley AM, Trueta J. The vascular anatomy of the spine and its relationship to pyogenic vertebral osteomyelitis. *J Bone Joint Surg [B]* 1959;41:796–809.

76. Williamson SL, Williamson MR, Siebert JJ, et al. Indium-111 white blood cell scanning in the pediatric population. *Pediatr Radiol* 1986;16:493–497.

77. Wilson NI, Di Paola M. Acute septic arthritis in infancy and childhood. *J Bone Joint Surg [B]* 1986;68:584–587.

78. Zawin JA, Hoffer FA, Rand FF, et al. Joint effusion in children with an irritable hip: US diagnosis and aspiration. *Radiology* 1993;187:459–463.

79. Zieger MM, Dorr U, Schulz RD. Ultrasonography of hip joint effusions. *Skeletal Radiol* 1987;16:607–611.

3
Skeletal Trauma

Owing to its high sensitivity for detecting skeletal injury, skeletal scintigraphy is a valuable tool for evaluating traumatic conditions. This chapter addresses applications of skeletal scintigraphy for assessing skeletal injuries during childhood and adolescence: injuries associated with skeletal stress, injuries associated with learning to walk upright, and injuries associated with child abuse.

Stress Injuries

General Considerations

Repetitive submaximal musculoskeletal loading is required to build and sustain strength and endurance. Stress-induced forces on the skeleton trigger a coordinated response that involves bone resorption, mediated by osteoclasts, with bone repair and hypertrophy, mediated by osteoblasts.[45,46,53] Functional adaptive remodeling of bone results. A partial or complete disruption of bone, a stress fracture, may occur when there is a disproportion in favor of osteoclastic activity.

As few as 10% to 25% of stress fractures are detected radiographically at the initial clinical presentation.[56] Skeletal scintigraphy, by depicting changes in bone turnover at sites of stress, is abnormal as early as 2 weeks prior to the development of any radiographic abnormality. In some cases, radiographic abnormalities never develop. Increased skeletal tracer localization resulting from stress is, therefore, often present without a radiographically demonstrable fracture line or displacement in alignment. This localization is more accurately referred to as "stress reaction" than "stress fracture" in the context of stress injuries.

Increased tracer localization is frequently seen at asymptomatic sites of skeletal remodeling[55,73] (Figs. 3.1 and 3.2). In one series, skeletal scintigraphy demonstrated areas of increased localization that did not correlate with symptoms in just over one third of athletes studied.[55] Asymptomatic scintigraphic abnormalities reflect a spectrum of adaptive changes, including hypertrophy and microfracture, that occur in bone subjected to stress.[9,45,46,53] They generally do not warrant a modification in athletic activity.

Stress injuries related to sports are often the same in children as those that occur in adults. Injuries that are either more commonly or exclusively encountered in children are emphasized in this section.

Pars Interarticularis Stress

Spondylolysis, a defect in the pars interarticularis of a vertebra, is generally considered a stress fracture. Ethnic and familial variations in its incidence suggest that heredity plays a predisposing role in some cases.[1,19,99] This is due to either the angulation of the spinal lamina and facets or a congenital weakness in the pars interarticularis.[67,97]

Spondylolysis occurs in association with athletic activities ranging from ballet and gymnastics to football line play and weight lifting.[34,77,84] Hyperextension is the principal mechanism of injury. The L5-S1 and L4-L5 levels are most frequently

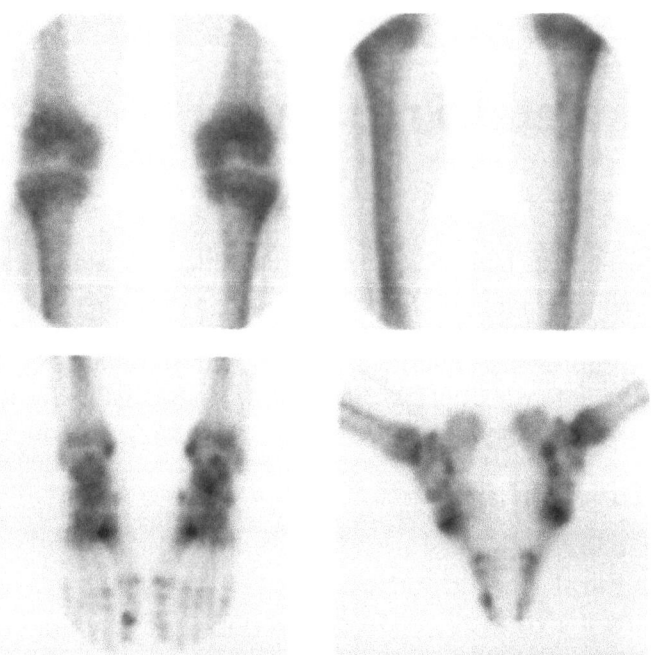

Figure 3.1. Asymptomatic skeletal stress. Skeletal scintigraphy reveals increased tracer localization involving the tibial diaphyses and multiple sites in the feet and ankles of a 19-year-old professional ballet dancer, whose only clinical complaint was low back pain.

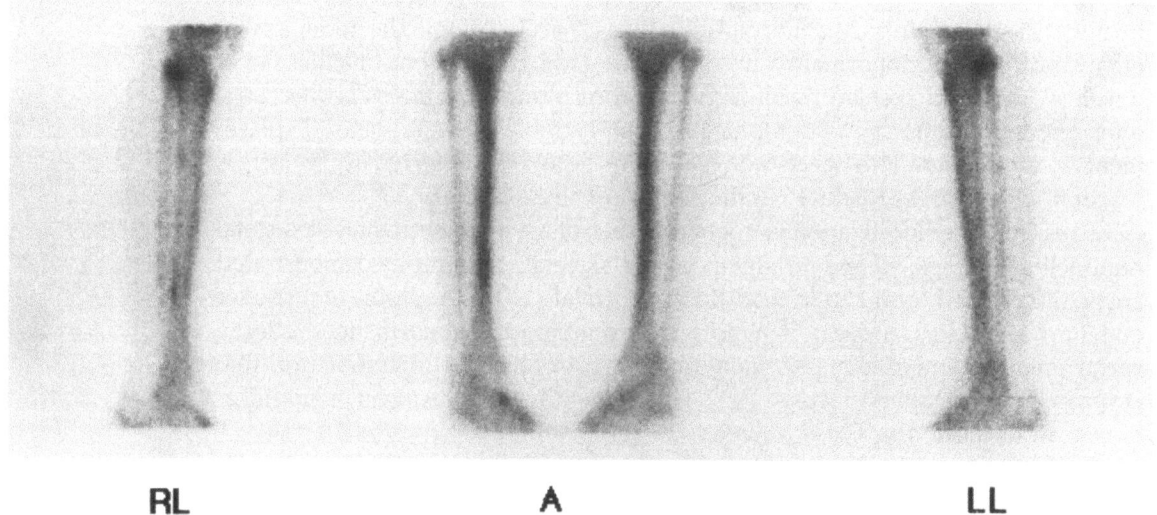

RL A LL

Figure 3.2. Asymptomatic tibial stress. Increased bilateral tibial tracer localization, particularly anteriorly, is seen in a runner with no associated lower extremity symptoms. RL, right lateral; A, anterior; LL, left lateral.

affected. Bilateral spondylolytic defects may be complicated by spondylolisthesis, anterior subluxation of the involved vertebra.[59]

The most common presenting complaint is pain, either chronic or acute. Pain is aggravated by hyperextension of the spine. Clinical presentation is usually during the adolescent growth spurt. Occasionally, spondylolysis is detected on a pelvic or abdominal radiograph obtained for unrelated reasons. Symptomatic cases are treated with activity modification and a back brace. Only rarely are further interventions, such as body casting or surgery, required. Spondylolisthesis is also treated nonoperatively providing that slippage has not exceeded 30% to 50% of the width of S1 or L5.[50]

Spondylolysis and spondylolisthesis are radiographic diagnoses. The typical radiographic appearance of spondylolysis is a radiolucency extending across the pars interarticularis (Fig. 3.3). This is best visualized with collimated lateral and 45° oblique views of the lumbosacral spine.[2] In cases of unilateral spondylolysis, contralateral stress remodeling may be apparent radiographically as sclerosis and enlargement of the contralateral pedicle.[96] Spondylolisthesis is demonstrated with a lateral radiograph. Various methods for quantitating the degree of slippage relative to the anterior-posterior dimension of S1 and L5 have been described. Radiographs in flexion and extension are useful to demonstrate any mobility of the affected vertebra.[67]

Spondylolysis can be demonstrated with computed tomography (CT) and magnetic resonance imaging (MRI). Differentiation of a pars interarticularis defect from the adjacent facet joints may be difficult with CT.[25] A zero degree gantry angle allows better delineation of a defect than does the angulation routinely used to evaluate potential disk herniation. Sagittal CT reconstruction and correlation with the lateral scout projection are useful.[67] In many cases, CT reveals sclerosis rather than a defect in the pars interarticularis (Fig. 3.4). Spondylolysis is suggested with MRI by interruption in the normal marrow signal between the superior and inferior facets.[36] Both CT and MRI provide information regarding associated neural foraminal narrowing and disk degeneration, bulge, or herniation.[4,25]

Skeletal scintigraphy is useful for demonstrating occult stress changes when radiographs are normal and for assessing metabolic activity in cases where spondylolysis is shown radiographically. This physiologic information is not available with radiographs, CT, or MRI. Low back pain can be ascribed to bone stress when scintigraphy shows increased tracer localization in the pars interarticularis of a symptomatic individual. This localization indicates ongoing stress-induced bone remodeling.[15,51,93]

Planar skeletal scintigraphy is more sensitive than radiography[68] and single photon emission computed tomography (SPECT) is more sensitive than planar scintigraphy[3,70] for demonstrating stress changes in the pars interarticularis (Figs. 3.4 and 3.5). SPECT increases the diagnostic yield of scintigraphy by approximately 50%. Its use is an essential part of the scintigraphic evaluation of children with low back pain.[3] Even in cases where planar scintigraphy reveals an abnormality, SPECT frequently shows associated stress changes contralaterally (Figs 3.3 and 3.6) or at additional spinal levels. Since spondylolisthesis is not identified scintigraphically, radiographic correlation should be considered in cases that first come to diagnosis with skeletal scintigraphy.

A spondylolytic defect may heal completely, persist in a quiescent state (usually filled with fibrocartilage), or fail to heal and exhibit continued osseous repair.[67] Tracer localization reverts toward normal except in cases where stress remodeling persists.[52] Scintigraphy, therefore, is valuable in the follow-up of children with pars interarticularis stress. A reduction in tracer localization demonstrated with serial studies during back brace therapy implies healing and assists in planning a return to athletic activity.[84]

Pelvic Apophyseal Injuries

Apophyses are growth centers that do not contribute directly to longitudinal growth. Apophyses appear in the iliac crest, anterior superior iliac spine, anterior inferior iliac spine, the ischium, the lesser trochanter, and the greater trochanter during the teenage years. Muscles that attach on these apophyses are the abdominal wall musculature (iliac crest), the sartorius (anterosuperior iliac spine), the rectus femoris (anteroinferior iliac spine), the hamstrings and adductors (ischium), the iliopsoas (lesser trochanter), and the external rotators (greater trochanter). Until ossified, the apophyseal growth cartilage constitutes the weakest point in the musculotendinous unit. Apophyses are therefore prone to being avulsed in response to sudden forceful or repetitive muscular traction.[18,39,88,94]

Pelvic and proximal femoral apophyseal avulsions occur most commonly in sprinters, football players, ballet dancers, and jumpers. The young athlete with a pelvic avulsion typically reports acute onset of pain during an episode of strenuous activity. Healing usually requires at least 6 weeks of reduced activity. Crutches and a partial weight-bearing gait are useful during the early part of this period.[8]

An apophyseal avulsion appears radiographically as displacement of an apophyseal center from its normal position. In some cases, considerable callus and bony reaction is present. Evaluation with CT or MRI may be useful to further define the separation or, in an occasional difficult case, to differentiate an avulsion injury from a neoplasm.[47]

Avulsions of the anterior inferior iliac spine and the iliac crest apophyses may show relatively little displacement and escape radiographic detection. Skeletal scintigraphy may be the first study to suggest the diagnosis in such cases and in cases where there is displacement but the evaluation has not included films of the pelvis. An avulsion fracture should be suspected in adolescents with hip, pelvic, or low back pain and asymmetrically increased skeletal tracer localization corresponding to a pelvic or hip apophysis (Figs. 3.7 and 3.8).

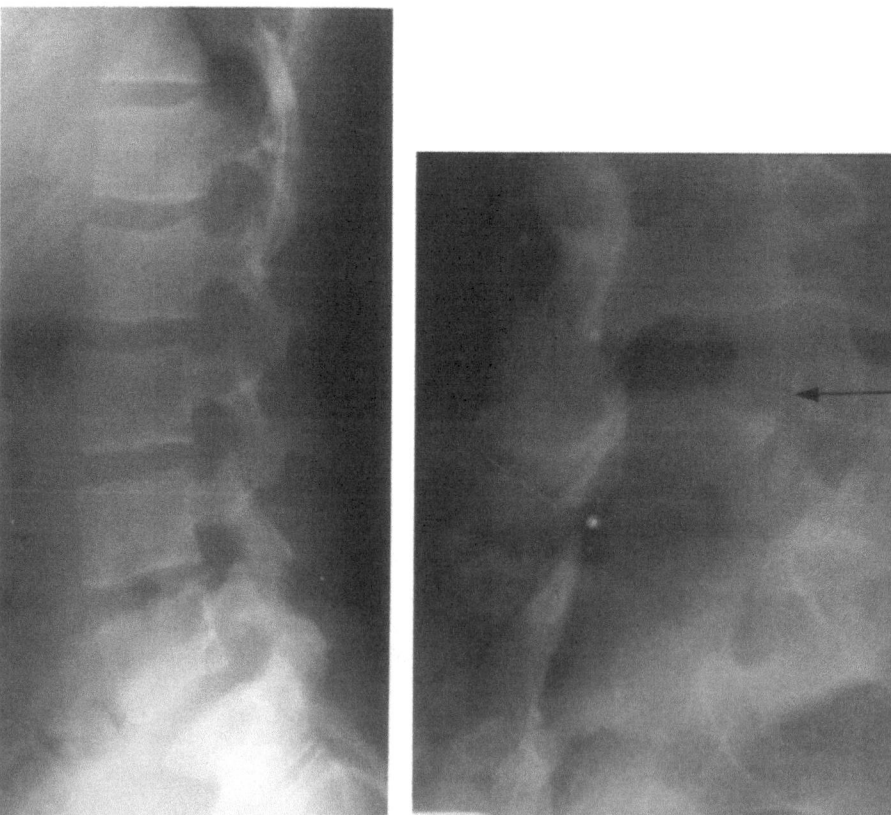

A   B

Figure 3.3. Spondylolysis and pars interarticularis stress. A lateral radiograph (A) demonstrates sclerosis and a linear lucency at the level of the L5 pars interarticularis. A left posterior oblique projection demonstrates a spondylolytic defect in the left L5 pars interarticularis (B).

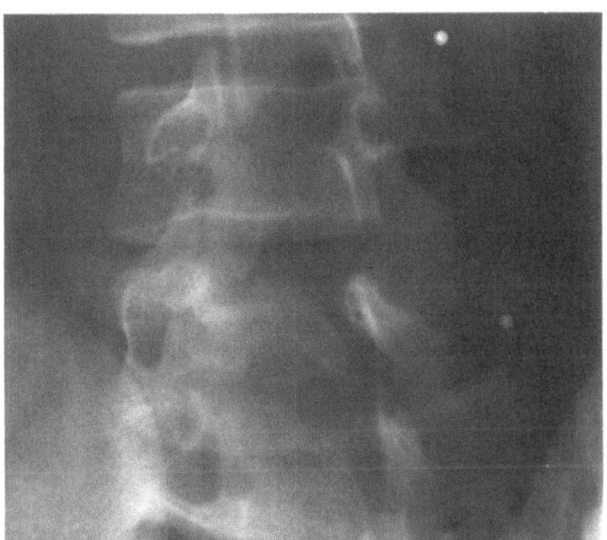

C

Figure 3.3 (*cont'd.*) Sclerosis involving the right L5 pedicle is noted on the right posterior oblique projection (C).

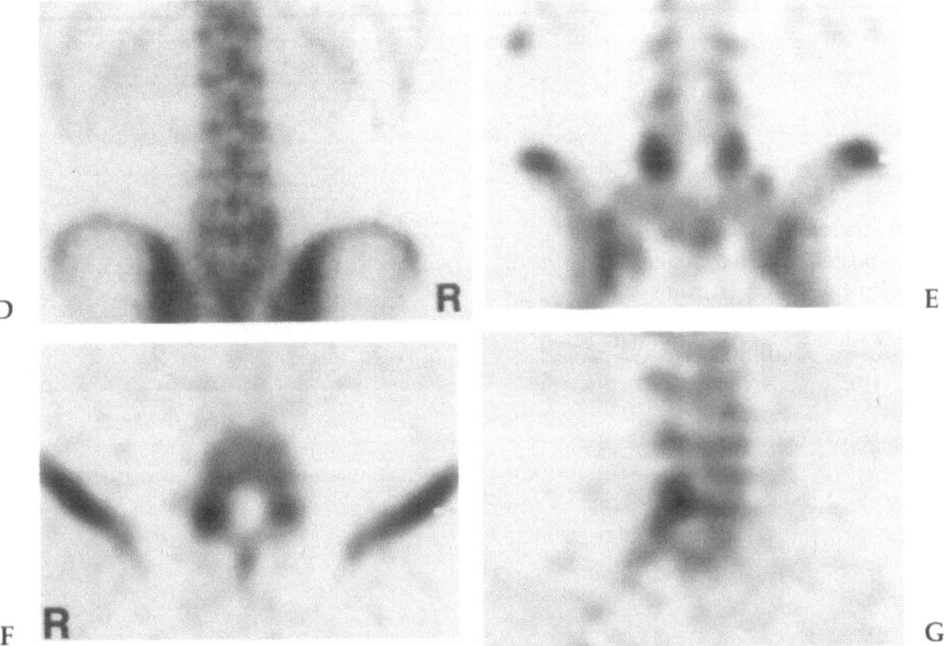

D R E

F R G

Figure 3.3 (*cont'd.*) Planar scintigraphy (D) and SPECT—coronal (E), transverse (F), sagittal (G)—reveal that there is active bone remodeling occurring at the radiographically abnormal sites. This determination can be useful in guiding therapy. Note that in this individual a greater degree of tracer localization is associated with the sclerotic changes than the radiographically observed defect.

Other sites of pelvic injury apart from apophyseal avulsions are the ilium adjacent to the sacroiliac joint and the pubic ramus (Figs. 3.9 and 3.10). Injuries to the pubis can occur at the origin of the adductor longus and brevis muscles, at the origin of the gracilis muscle, and at insertions of the rectus abdominal muscle.[11,28,65,69]

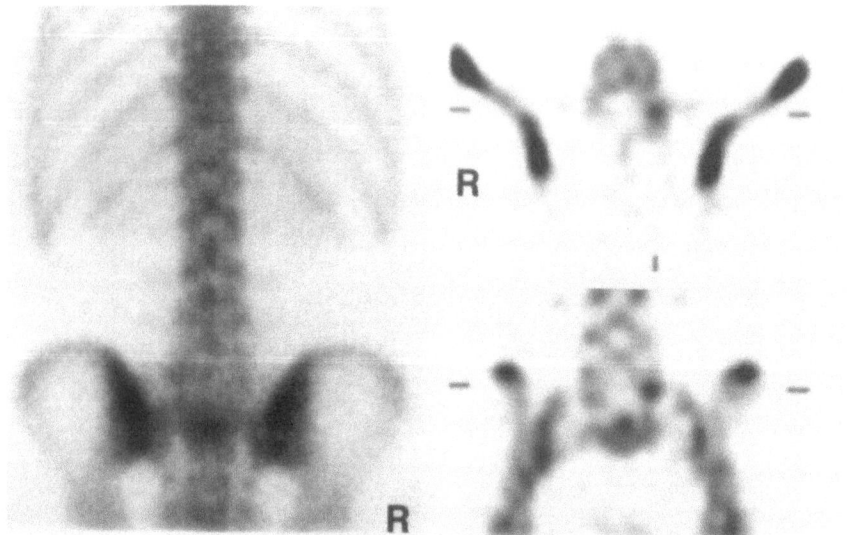

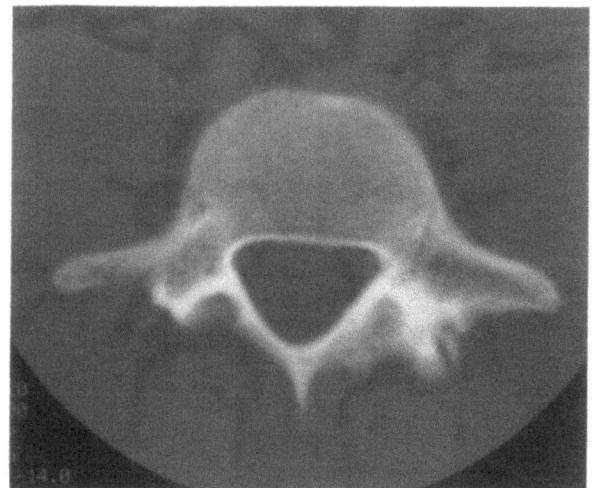

Figure 3.4. Pars interarticularis stress. Increased tracer localization at L5, which is suggested on a posterior planar image (A, left panel), is convincingly depicted by SPECT (A, transverse and coronal images) in the left L5 pars interarticularis. Computed tomography demonstrates corresponding sclerosis involving the left pars interarticularis (B).

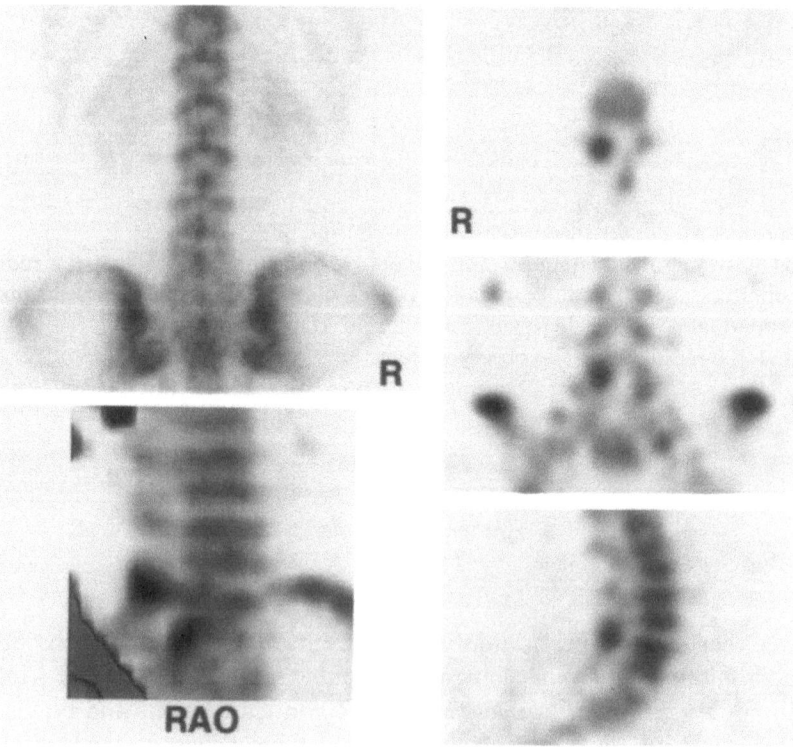

Figure 3.5. Pars interarticularis stress. A posterior planar image is normal. Increased tracer localization involving the right pars interarticularis of L4 is seen with transverse, coronal, sagittal, and volume rendered (displayed in the right anterior oblique [RAO] projection) SPECT.

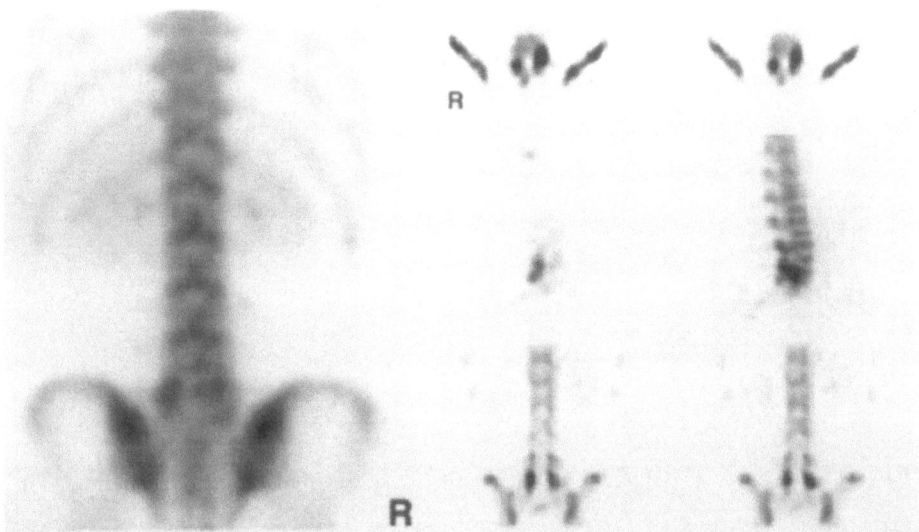

Figure 3.6. Pars interarticularis stress. A posterior planar image reveals increased tracer localization on the right and less prominently on the left at L5. Transverse, sagittal, and coronal SPECT show bilateral pars interarticularis stress.

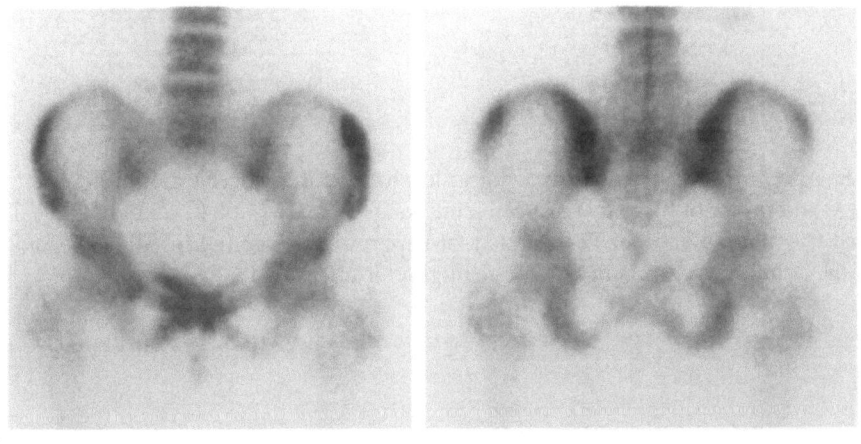

Figure 3.7. Apophyseal injury. Increased tracer localization is present in the left iliac crest at the origin of the abdominal wall musculature in a 16-year-old runner (A: anterior projection; B: posterior projection).

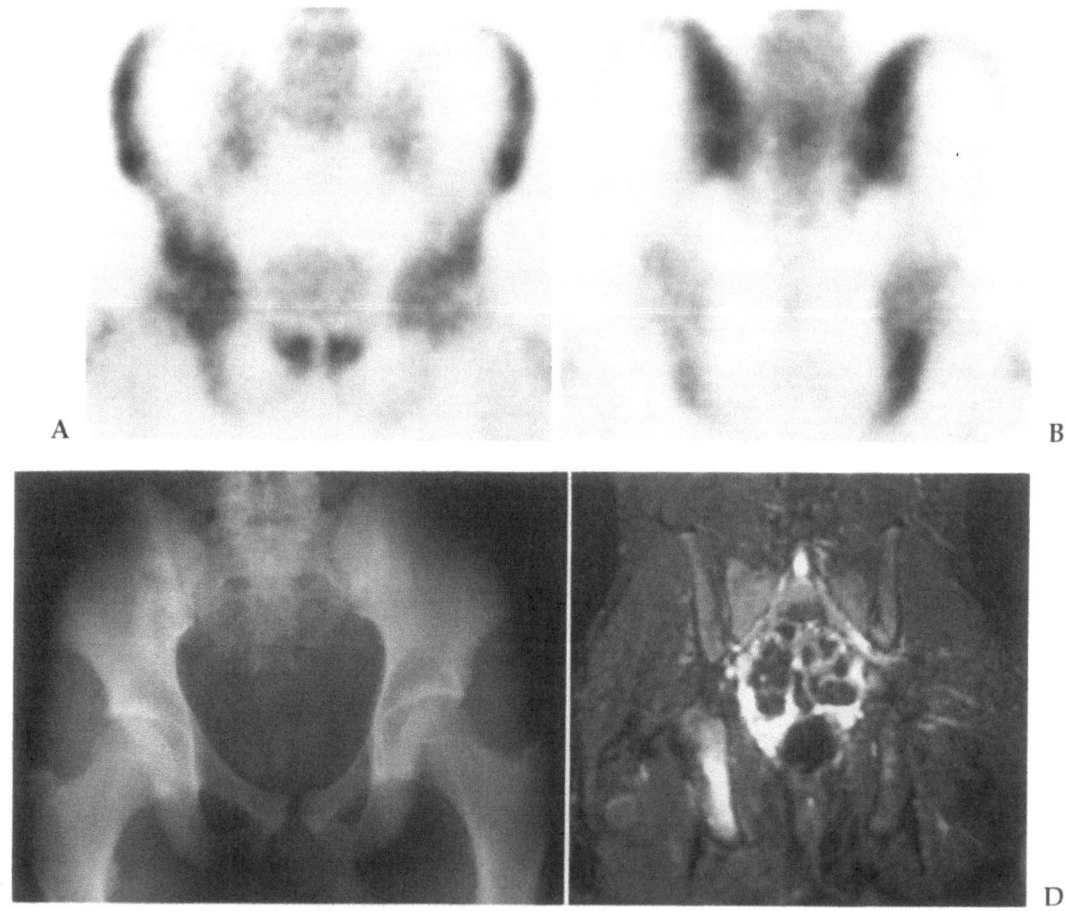

Figure 3.8. Apophyseal injury. Increased tracer localization in the ischium is seen on the anterior (A) and posterior (B) planar skeletal scintigrams. A radiograph (C) does not reveal an avulsed fragment. A coronal T2-weighted fat-suppressed image (D) reveals increased signal in the ischium corresponding to the scintigraphic abnormality.

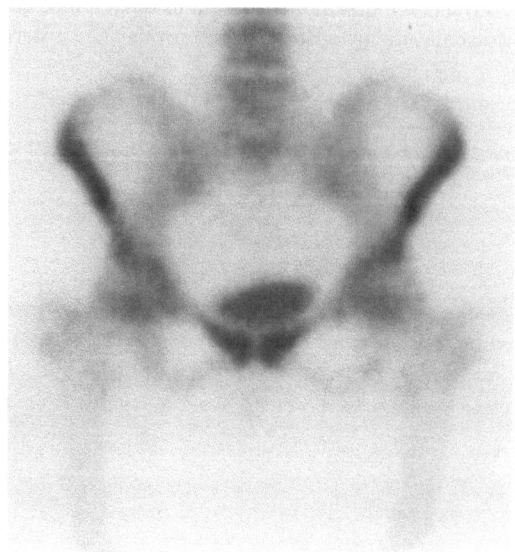

Figure 3.9. Pubic stress injury. Increased tracer localization is seen in the superior pubic rami, right greater than left.

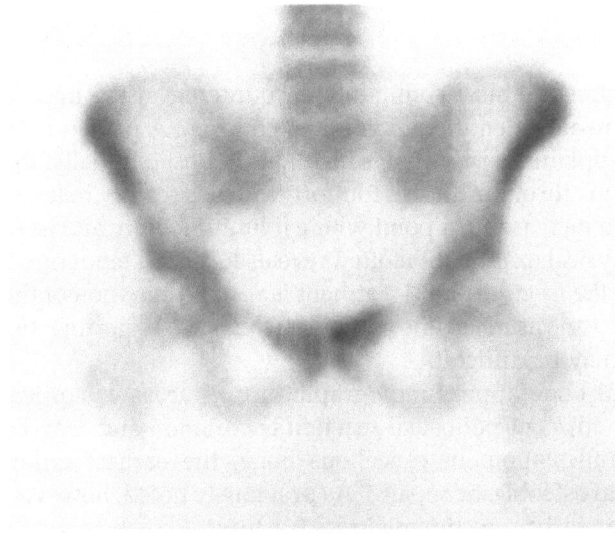

A

Figure 3.10. Pubic stress injury. Asymmetric tracer localization in the left superior pubic ramus is suggested by an anterior planar image (A).

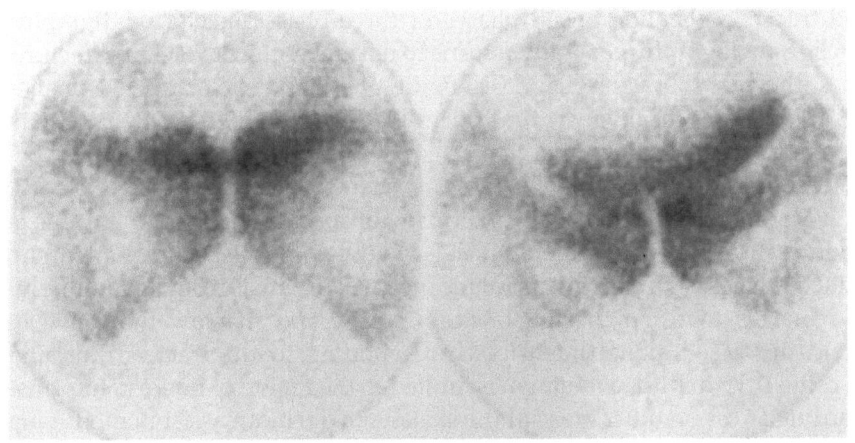

B   C

Figure 3.10 (*cont'd.*) Evaluation is difficult secondary to tracer within the urinary bladder on this and an anterior pinhole magnification image (B). A pinhole image with slight craniad camera angulation (C) depicts a linear area of increased tracer localization in the left superior pubic ramus.

Lower Extremity Stress Fractures

Stress fractures are fatigue fractures, that is, they result from the application of abnormal stress to normal bone. Although it is difficult to precisely define abnormal stress, it entails strenuous activity that is repetitive and/or new for a given individual. Stress fractures are distinguished from insufficiency fractures, which occur with the application of normal stress to bone with deficient elastic resistance, and from pathologic fractures, which occur in bone weakened by a preexisting disease or lesion.

In pediatrics, stress fractures are most commonly encountered in the middle and late teenage years but are also identified in younger children. A patient with a stress fracture typically complains of pain that is insidious in onset. Initially, the athlete may be able to perform "through" the discomfort, which is readily relieved with rest. Gradually, the pain increases to a point where it limits activity and is no longer relieved with rest. Physical examination often reveals localized tenderness. There may be swelling over the fracture site. Treatment is rest. Elimination of the inciting activity is required for variable time periods. Decisions regarding the timing of return to activity may be difficult.[8]

Stress fractures in cortical bone appear radiographically as areas of cortical resorption or infraction. An adjacent periosteal reaction is common and may be the initial radiographic manifestation. In cancellous bone, the earliest radiographic sign is sclerosis due to osteoblastic repair.[47] As previously noted, however, radiography is insensitive for early detection of stress fractures.[56]

Early in their course, stress fractures are typically depicted as focal areas of increased tracer localization on all phases of three-phase skeletal scintigraphy. Radionuclide angiography generally returns to normal within 4 weeks of fracture. For at least the year following diagnosis, tissue phase and skeletal phase images may reveal persistent focally increased tracer localization of lesser intensity than that noted at the time of diagnosis.[54]

An alternative to scintigraphy in cases of suspected stress fracture is MRI. Initially, MRI of stress fractures shows diffuse nonspecific changes. With time, a linear abnormality that is hypointense on T1-weighted images becomes apparent. T2-weighted images, short tau inversion recovery (STIR) images, and gadolinium-enhanced images reveal high signal within cortex and marrow indicative of edema and decreased signal intensity corresponding to the fracture line and adjacent callus.[47] With MRI, evaluation is limited to the region of interest. Information regarding stress on other areas of the skeleton, which can assist in modifying an individual's activity, is not provided.

While scintigraphy does not differentiate stress reaction from stress fracture, focal increased tracer localization at characteristic sites can confidently be regarded and treated as a stress fracture. This is particularly true when a focal abnormality appears to involve more than just the superficial cortex. Overall, the most common location of stress fractures is the tibia, where the vast majority involve the posterior cortex (Figs. 3.11–3.13).[56,66,74] The less frequently encountered stress fractures of the anterior tibia are noteworthy, however, in that they are prone to complications such as nonunion and avascular necrosis (AVN). Anterior tibial stress fractures usually result in increased tracer localization, but are occasionally manifested scintigraphically as focally decreased localization. This is presumably due to ischemia.[5,71] Other relatively common sites of stress fracture in children and adolescents include the fibula (Fig. 3.14), the tarsal bones, and the metatarsals.[56,66,74]

Stress fractures of the femoral neck are rare in the immature skeleton and are more frequently seen after physeal closure.[21,26,37,98] Femoral neck stress fractures result from forces exerted through the femoral calcar that can approach 20 times body weight during running.[91] Although uncommon in children, these fractures are particularly important to recognize as they have potential for displacement, malunion, and AVN.[21,30,37] Focally increased tracer localization in the medial femoral neck is typically quite apparent, especially with pinhole magnification (Fig. 3.15). A less common scintigraphic appearance is that of a transverse zone of increased tracer localization extending across the femoral neck (Fig. 3.16). Since stress fractures of the femoral neck may present insidiously, significant concern should be raised in an asymptomatic individual, when increased tracer localization involving the femoral neck is detected (Fig. 3.17).

Stress injuries of the accessory ossicles about the ankle and midfoot and the sesamoids of the great toe are often overlooked as potential sources for localized pain. Of the accessory ossicles, the os trigonum, an accessory ossicle that results from failure of fusion of the posterior process of the talus to the talus, and the accessory navicular are the most frequently injured (Figs. 3.18–3.20). Stress fracture of the os trigonum can occur due to its impaction between the calcaneus and posterior tibial rim with repeated plantar flexion. This occurs with activities such as downhill running, gymnastics, and ballet.[7,27] The accessory navicular, a common anatomic variant, is separated from the tarsal navicular by a synchondrosis. Pressure from shoes or the action of the tibialis posterior muscle may injure this fibrous union or the accessory navicular itself. Microscopic changes similar to those noted with physeal fractures result.[76] Increased tracer localization in an accessory ossicle of a symptomatic child indicates a stress injury.[49,76] Injuries of the great toe sesamoids occur with activities associated with toe pointing, such as ballet, or prolonged standing. Scintigraphy reveals focally increased tracer localization (Figs. 3.21 and 3.22).[89]

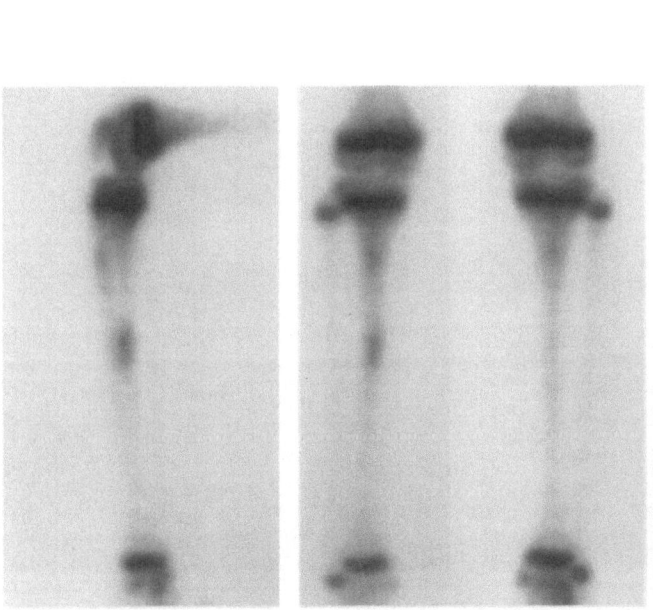
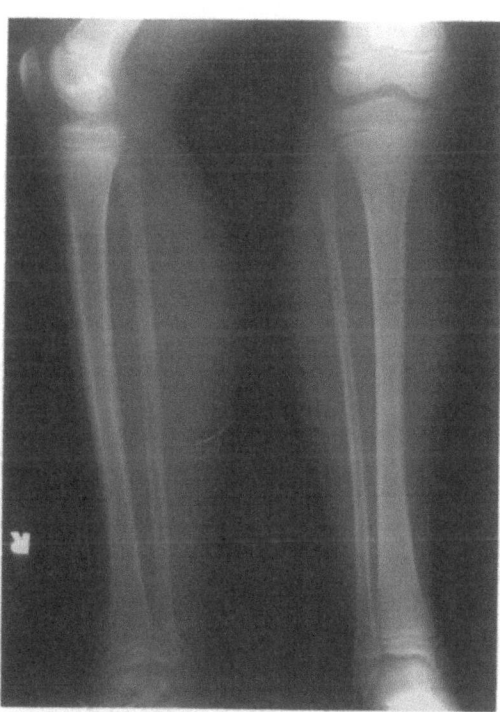

A   B

Figure 3.11. Tibial stress injury. Skeletal scintigraphy (medial and anterior projections) demonstrates focally increased ^{99m}Tc-MDP localization in the posterior right tibial diaphysis (A). It extends across nearly the entire width of the tibia. Prominent tracer localization in the anterior proximal tibiae corresponds to the tibial tuberosities. Radiographs (B) of this 14-year-old runner with right calf pain are normal. This was treated as a stress fracture.

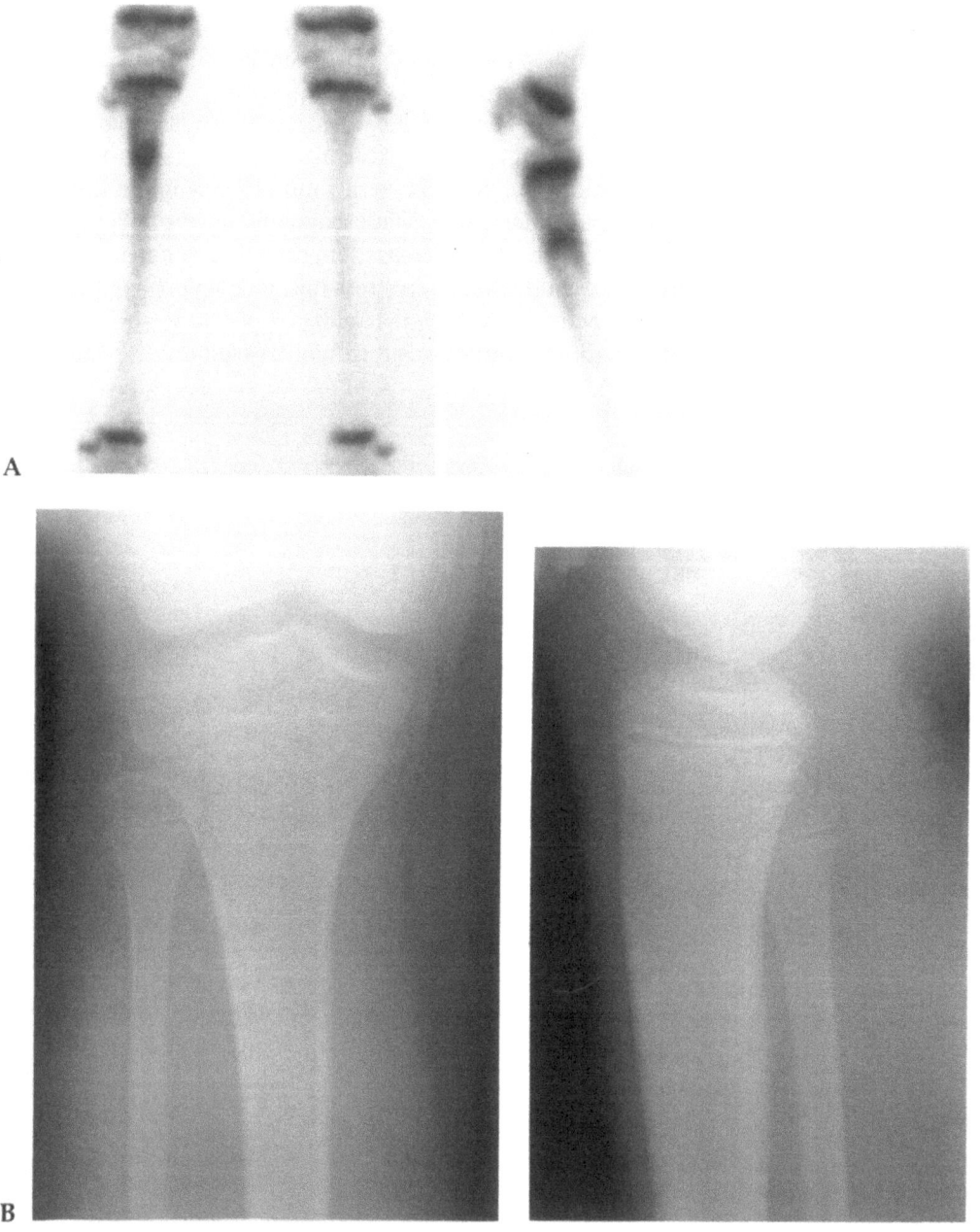

Figure 3.12. Tibial stress fracture. Increased ^{99m}Tc-MDP localization involves and extends across the proximal right tibial diaphysis (A, anterior and medial projections). Anteroposterior (B) and lateral (C) radiographs reveal a fracture of the posteromedial tibial diaphysis.

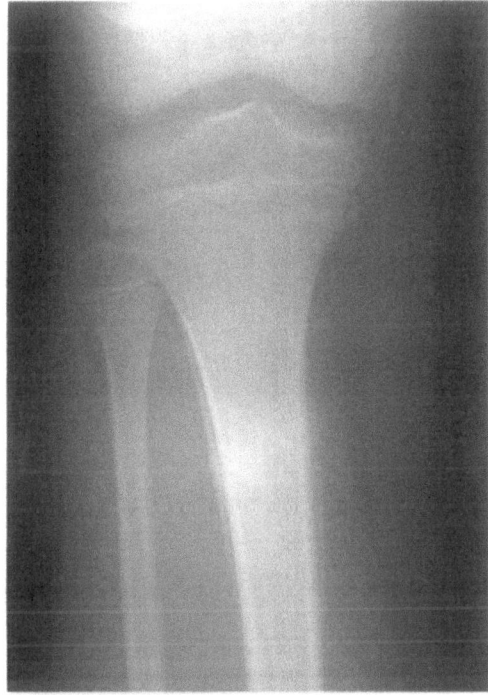

D

Figure 3.12 (cont'd). One month later, an anteroposterior radiograph shows extensive periosteal reaction and sclerosis associated with the fracture (D).

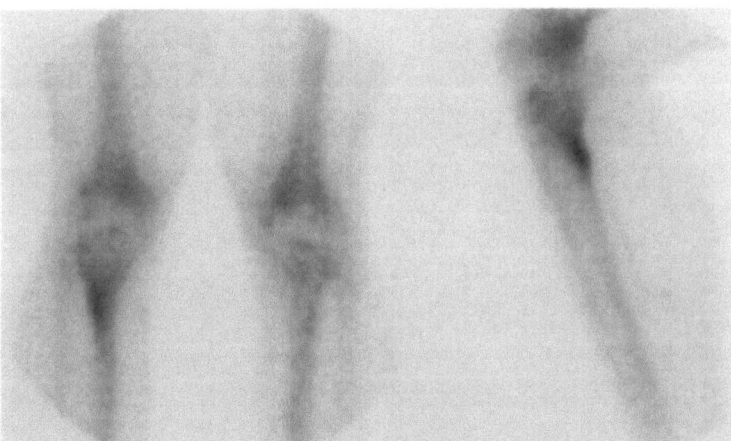

Figure 3.13. Tibial stress injury. Focally increased tracer localization involving the posterior proximal right tibial metaphysis is depicted on anterior and medial scintigraphic images. This symptomatic 19-year-old runner was treated for a stress fracture.

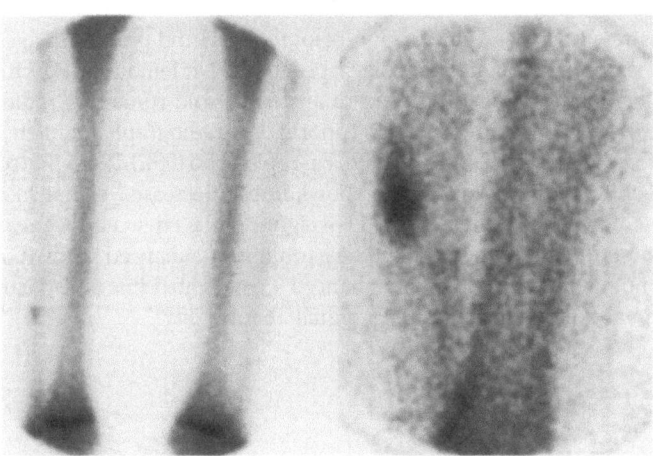

Figure 3.14. Fibular stress injury. Planar and pinhole images reveal a distal right fibular focus of increased tracer localization in a teenage runner.

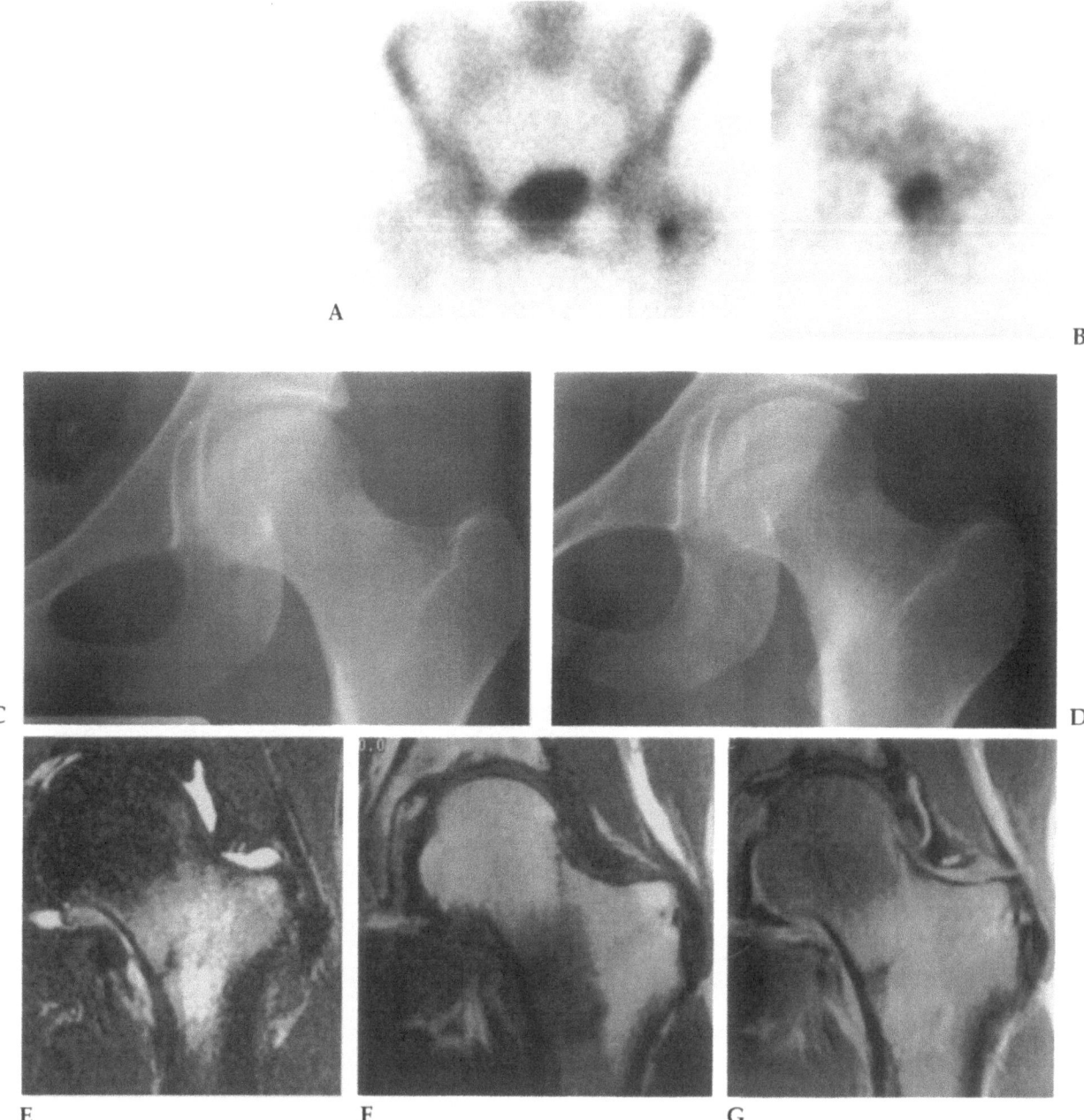

Figure 3.15. Femoral neck stress fracture. Anterior high-resolution (A) and pinhole images (B) show focally intense tracer localization in the medial aspect of the left femoral neck with preservation of tracer localization in the femoral head of an 18-year-old runner. A radiograph, obtained at the time of skeletal scintigraphy (C) is normal. A radiograph obtained 4 weeks later (D) demonstrates sclerosis at the fracture site. Fast spin echo (FSE) T2-weighted image (E) performed 1 week following scintigraphy shows linear decreased signal in a fracture line surrounded by high signal edema. With T1-weighting, the edema appears as low signal on the nonenhanced (F) and high signal on the gadolinium-enhanced study (G). The fracture line, which is not identified on the nonenhanced T1-weighted image, is visualized following gadolinium as a nonenhancing linear signal abnormality.

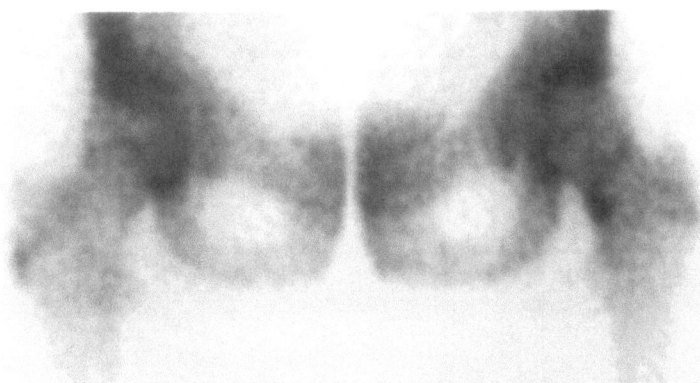

Figure 3.16. Femoral neck stress injury. Pinhole magnification images of a 17-year-old cross-country runner shows focally intense tracer localization in the medial aspect of the left femoral neck with a linear zone of less prominently increased tracer localization extending across the femoral neck. The physes are nearly completely closed. Tracer localization in the epiphysis is preserved.

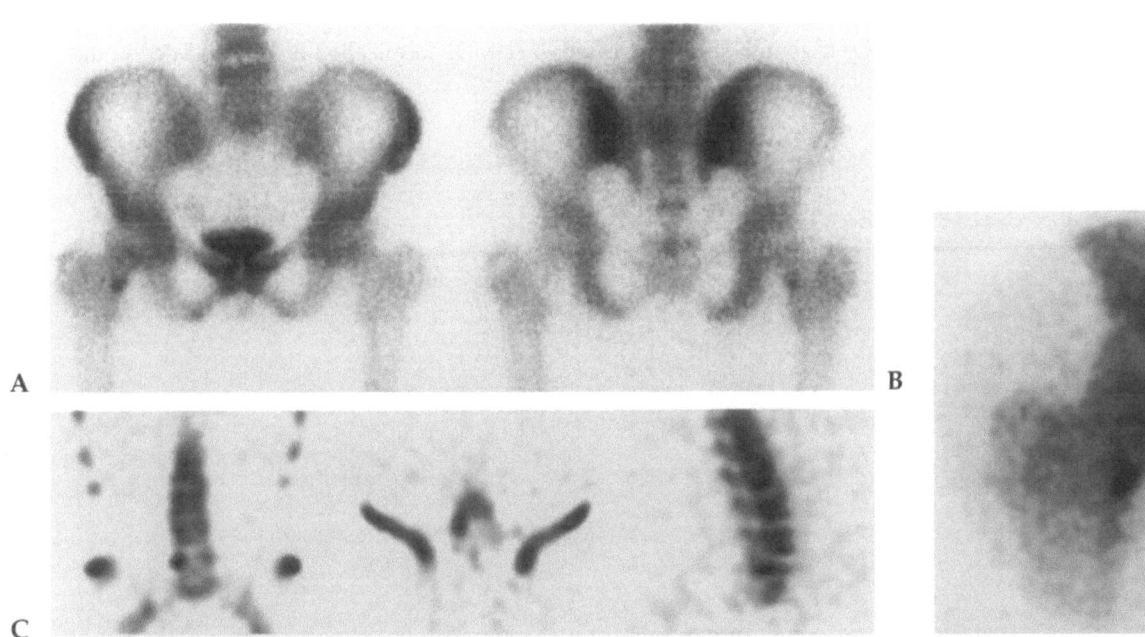

Figure 3.17. Pars interarticularis and femoral neck stress injuries. This 16-year-old gymnast, who was referred for low back pain, reported intermittent right hip discomfort when questioned following skeletal scintigraphy. Anterior (A) and posterior (B) planar images reveal increased tracer localization at L5 and in the proximal right femur. Stress reaction in the right L5 pars interarticularis was confirmed with SPECT (C). Pinhole magnification imaging shows focally intense tracer localization along the medial aspect of the right femoral neck (D).

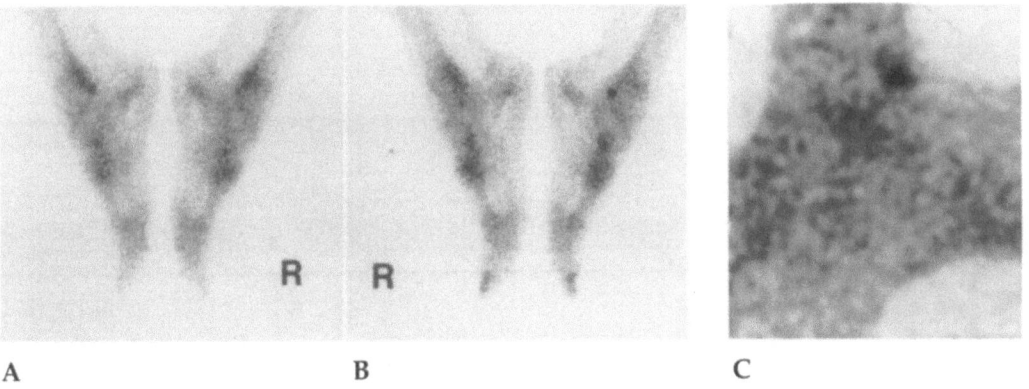

Figure 3.18. Os trigonum stress. Increased tracer localization in the os trigonum of a ballet dancer's left ankle is shown by lateral (A) and medial (B) planar imaging. Pinhole imaging (C) confirms the finding.

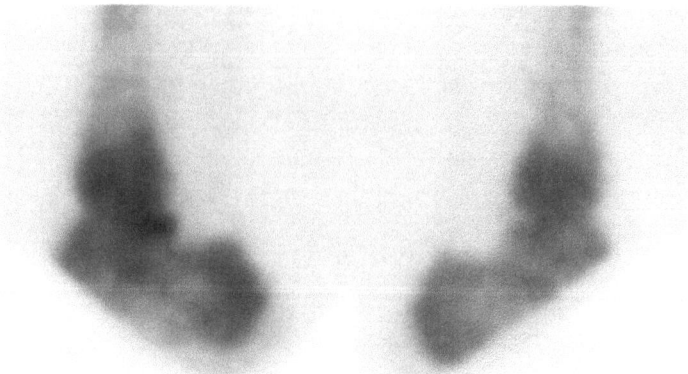

Figure 3.19. Os trigonum stress. Increased ^{99m}Tc-MDP localization is demonstrated in the os trigonum of a runner's right ankle.

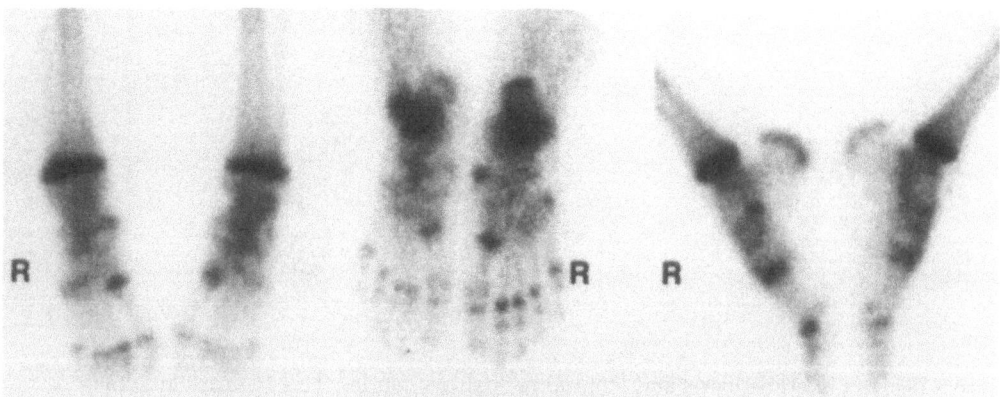

Figure 3.20. Accessory navicular stress injury. Increased tracer localization medial to the right navicular indicates a stress injury to an accessory navicular (anterior, plantar, and medial projections).

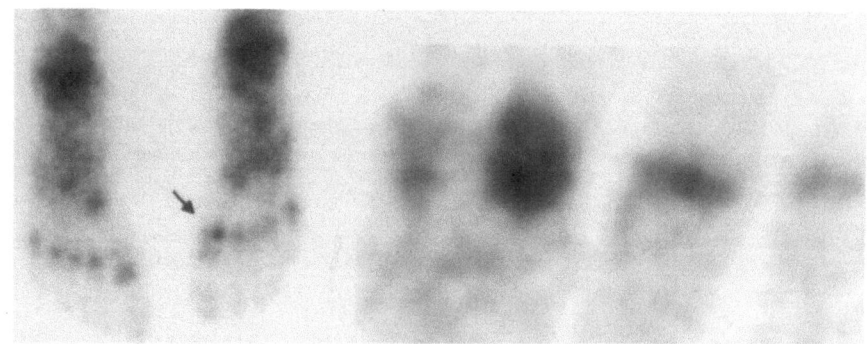

Figure 3.21. Sesamoid stress injury. Increased tracer localization in the right lateral sesamoid is shown on plantar planar (A) and pinhole (B) magnification images of a ballet dancer.

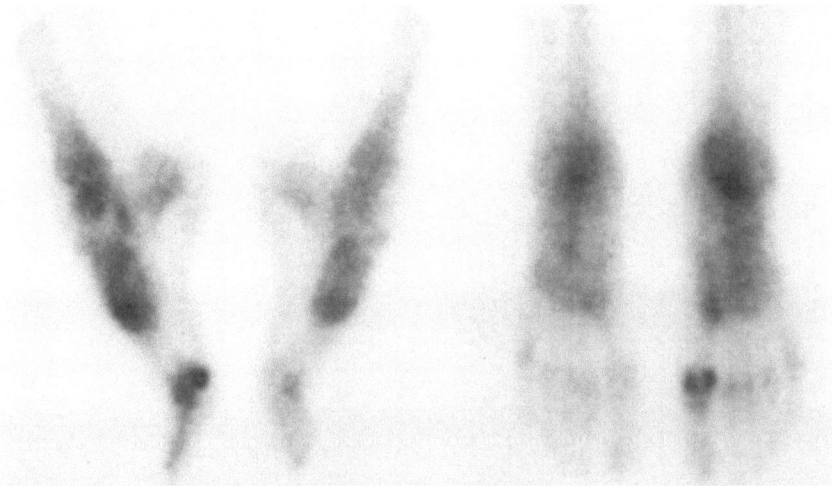

Figure 3.22. Sesamoid stress injury. Medial and anterior images reveal intense tracer localization in the medial and lateral sesamoids of a ballet dancer's left great toe.

Tibial Periostitis

While the primary role of scintigraphy in assessing young athletes with shin pain is to demonstrate or exclude the presence of a stress fracture, scintigraphy is also useful in showing findings associated with what has been labeled the medial tibial stress syndrome or soleus syndrome.[32,61,64] This frequent cause of shin pain in athletes is due to periostitis incited by the soleus and/or tibialis posterior muscles.[32,61,64] These two muscles plantar flex the foot. The tibialis posterior also supports the arch.

The typical presenting complaint is lower leg pain, often anterior in location, that is brought on by exercise. The pain is frequently bilateral. The medial tibial stress syndrome is most commonly seen in runners, particularly those with excessive pronation. Rest or exercise modification, orthotics, and nonsteroidal antiinflammatory medications are useful in treatment.[8]

Skeletal scintigraphy demonstrates increased tracer localization along the posterior tibial cortex. This extends vertically along the diaphysis. Radionuclide angiography typically is normal, although slightly increased tracer delivery is occasionally demonstrated (Fig. 3.23).[32,61]

Less commonly, increased tracer localization is noted vertically along the anterior tibial cortex. This is also most likely related to a periostitis, probably related to the transmission of forces from a hard running surface. Commonly, both anterior and posterior tibial stress changes are present in the same individual (Figs. 3.24 and 3.25).

Differentiation between tibial periostitis and stress fracture, which may coexist, is difficult in some cases. Elongated increased tracer localization affecting the posteromedial or anterolateral tibia suggests periostitis, while focal fusiform increased localization suggests fracture. Increased tracer delivery, intense localization on skeletal phase images, and involvement of more than the superficial cortex are also more worrisome for early fracture (Figs. 3.26–3.28).[58,74,100]

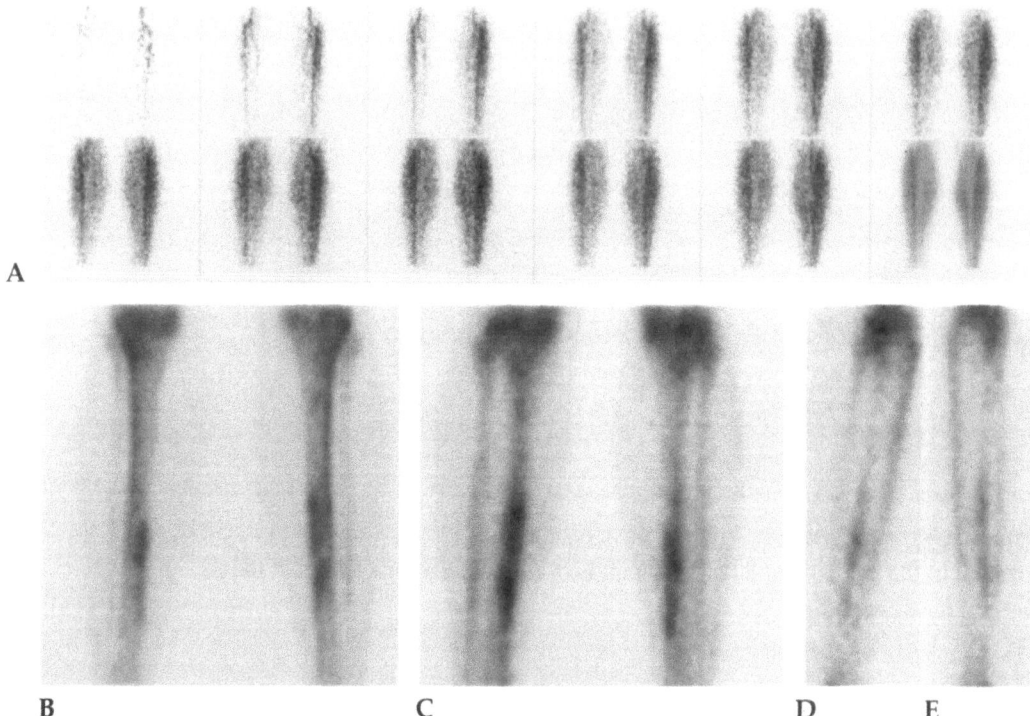

Figure 3.23. Posterior tibial stress reaction (soleus syndrome). Anterior radionuclide angiography (A) and tissue phase imaging (A, lower right panel) show mild diffusely increased tracer delivery to the tibias. Anterior (B), posterior (C), right lateral (D), and left lateral (E) skeletal phase images depict increased ^{99m}Tc-MDP localization in long segments of the posterior tibial diaphyses bilaterally.

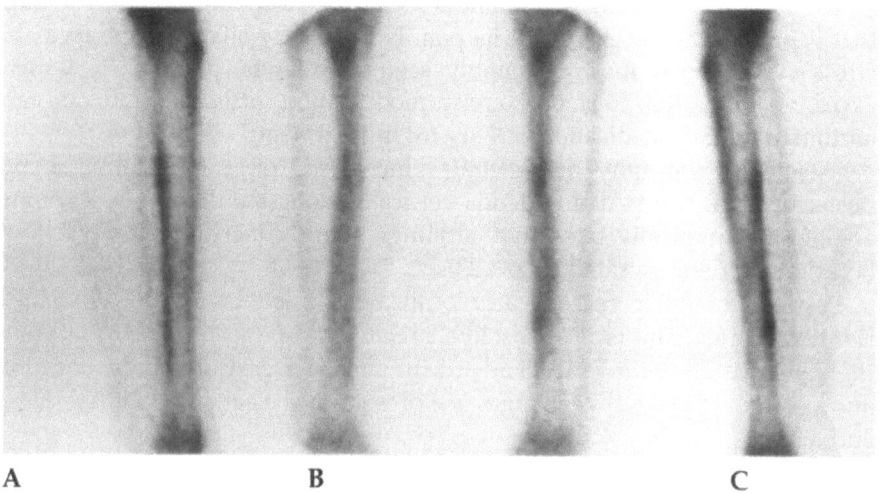

Figure 3.24. Tibial stress reactions. Increased ^{99m}Tc-MDP localization involving long segments of the anterior and posterior tibial cortex bilaterally are depicted in a runner with bilateral foreleg pain (A: right lateral projection; B: anterior projection; c: left lateral projection).

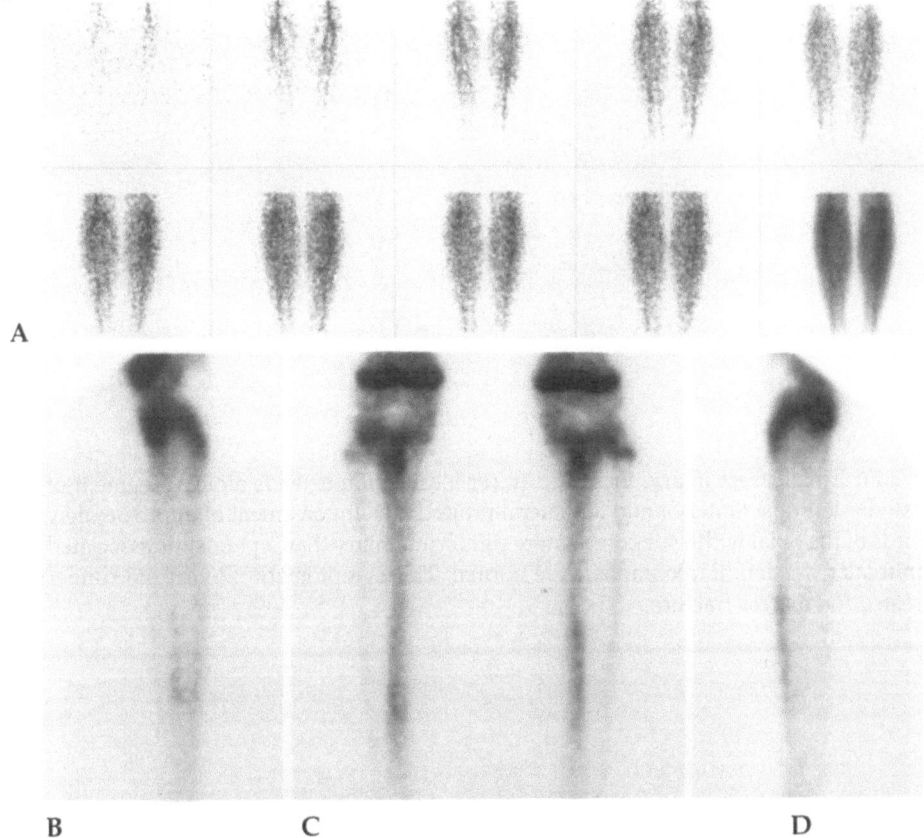

Figure 3.25. Tibial stress reactions. Anterior radionuclide angiography (A) and a tissue phase image (A, lower right panel) reveal slight increase in tracer delivery to the soft tissues and muscles of the left calf. Increased tracer localization involving the anterior and posterior right and the anterior left tibial diaphysis is depicted on a lateral image of the right tibia (B), an anterior image of both tibiae (C), and a lateral image of the left tibia (D).

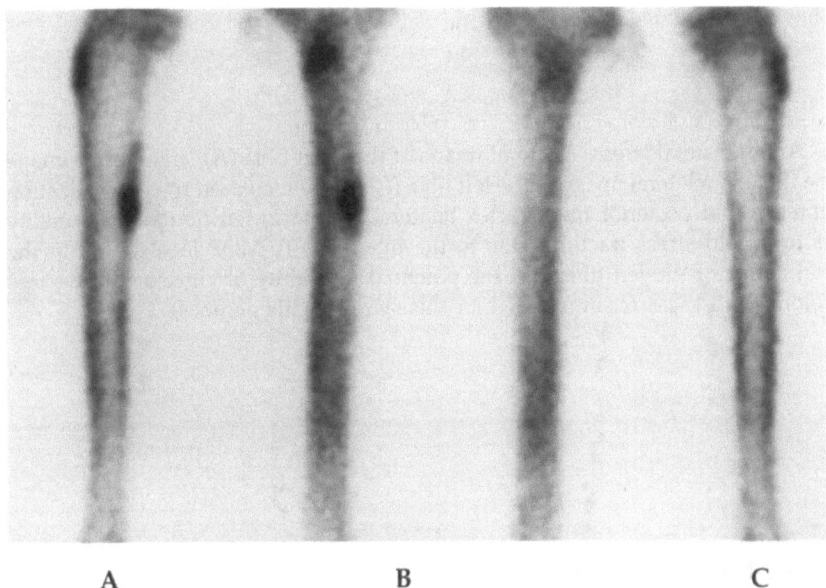

Figure 3.26. Focal and diffuse tibial stress reactions. Focally increased tracer localization involving the right posteromedial tibial cortex is depicted with right medial (A) and anterior (B) skeletal phase images. Diffusely increased tracer localization involving the anterior and posterior tibial cortices bilaterally is also shown with these and a left medial (C) image. Prominent ^{99m}Tc-MDP localization in the proximal anterior tibias corresponds to the tibial tubercles. The intense focal abnormality in the right tibia suggests early stress fracture in this 14-year-old runner, whose radiographs were normal.

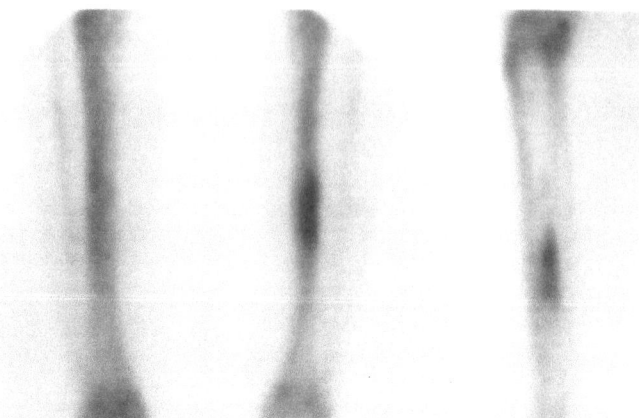

Figure 3.27. Tibial stress injury. Increased tracer localization extends along a segment of the posterior left tibia (anterior and left lateral projections). Involvement of approximately two thirds of the tibial width suggests a more significant injury than a periostitis associated with muscular traction. Radiographs were normal. This symptomatic 17-year-old runner was treated for a stress fracture.

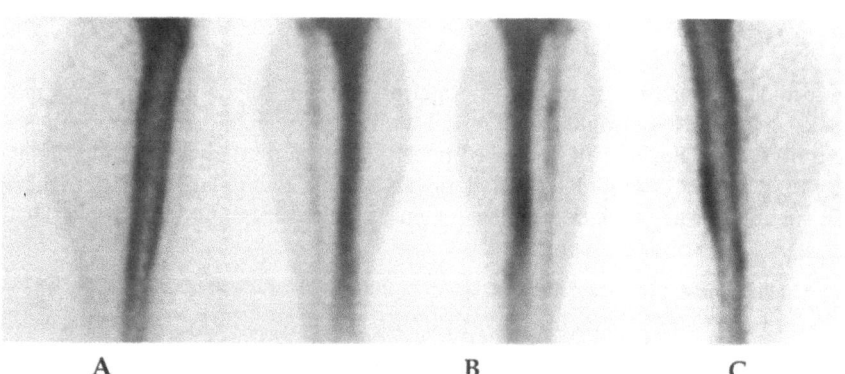

A	B	C

Figure 3.28. Anterior tibial stress. A lateral image of the right tibia (A), an anterior image of both tibiae (B), and a lateral image of the left tibia (C) reveal increased tracer localization along the anterior and posterior tibial cortex bilaterally. A focal left fibular abnormality corresponds to an old stress fracture. Due to the intense ^{99m}Tc-MDP localization in the anterior tibial cortex of the left tibia and the potential morbidity of anterior tibial stress fracture, prolonged rest was recommended for this symptomatic gymnast.

Slipped Capital Femoral Epiphysis

Slipped capital femoral epiphysis (SCFE) is an epiphyseal separation that results from stress injury to the proximal femoral physis. Muscular traction displaces the femoral neck anterolaterally relative to the separated epiphysis. The epiphysis, which is held in the acetabulum, rotates medially and posteriorly. Males are affected more frequently than females. The incidence is highest in individuals of African ancestry. Children with SCFE usually are overweight, slightly tall for their age, and tend to have delayed skeletal maturation. The incidence of SCFE is highest during the pubertal growth spurt. A combination of mechanical shearing forces (accentuated by obesity) and a predisposing hormonal influence have been implicated in the pathogenesis of SCFE. Other settings in which SCFE occurs include renal osteodystrophy, hypothyroidism, hypopituitarism with growth hormone therapy, and following pelvic and femoral irradiation. These associations are particularly common in SCFE developing prior to 10 years of age. Bilateral slippage occurs in as many as 30% of cases.[47,85]

Children with SCFE typically present with hip or groin pain. A change in gait or range of motion at the involved hip may be present. Treatment of SCFE is aimed primarily at preventing further slippage. Operative pin fixation generally provides the best long-term functional outcome. Techniques to reduce the degree of slippage that are employed in cases where the slip is severe carry a significant risk of complications including AVN, chondrolysis, and late degenerative changes.[38]

The diagnosis of SCFE is made radiographically with classification based on the posterior and medial position of the epiphysis relative to the femoral neck. Radiographic signs of slippage may be subtle on the anteroposterior projection. This reflects the fact that major posterior displacement of the epiphysis is present in 99% of SCFE cases, whereas major medial displacement is present in 75% of cases.[47] This mandates the use of a lateral radiograph (true lateral or frog-leg) in assessing suspected SCFE. With medial slippage of the femoral head, less than one sixth of its width lies lateral to a line drawn tangential to the lateral border of the femoral neck on an anteroposterior radiograph. The femoral head and neck may appear osteopenic and reduced in height. The physis may appear widened. The metaphysis is frequently displaced relative to the acetabulum and its proximal margin often appears indistinct or blurred. Normally, a frog-leg lateral radiograph shows the anterior and posterior margins of the epiphysis and metaphysis to closely align with each other. Their junction appears smooth. With posterior slippage, the lateral radiograph reveals a metaphyseal-epiphyseal step-off due to posterior epiphyseal displacement.

Slippage is classified as minimal when epiphyseal displacement is less than one third the width of the femoral neck, moderate when it is one third to one half this width, and severe when it exceeds one half this width.[38] If the epiphyseal slip is chronic, reactive bone is present at the medial and posterior femoral neck. This reflects an effort to buttress the displaced epiphysis. Only about 50% of patients with eventual bilateral SCFE have radiographic changes involving both hips at presentation. When present, these findings are typically asymmetric.[47]

Although SCFE is a radiographic and not a scintigraphic diagnosis, skeletal scintigraphy may provide valuable information at diagnosis and during follow-up. An uncomplicated acute slip typically appears as increased tracer localization in the physis and adjacent metaphysis with preserved localization in the epiphysis (Figs. 3.29 and 3.30).[23] Since a small percentage of cases with minimal slippage elude radiographic detection, this diagnosis should be considered in the appropriate clinical setting, when this scintigraphic pattern is seen. Femoral head ischemia complicating untreated SCFE or after internal pin fixation results in decreased or absent tracer localization in the femoral head (Fig. 3.31). This pattern identifies children at increased risk for AVN.[22,23] Chondrolysis is suggested scintigraphically when there is prominent periarticular tracer localization involving the acetabular roof or early closure of the physis at the greater trochanter. In patients with continued pain following treatment, scintigraphic assessment of the physiologic status of the proximal femoral physis helps determine if slippage has recurred. When scintigraphy demonstrates closure of the proximal femoral physis during conservative treatment or following surgery, a recurrent SCFE is unlikely (Fig. 3.32).[78]

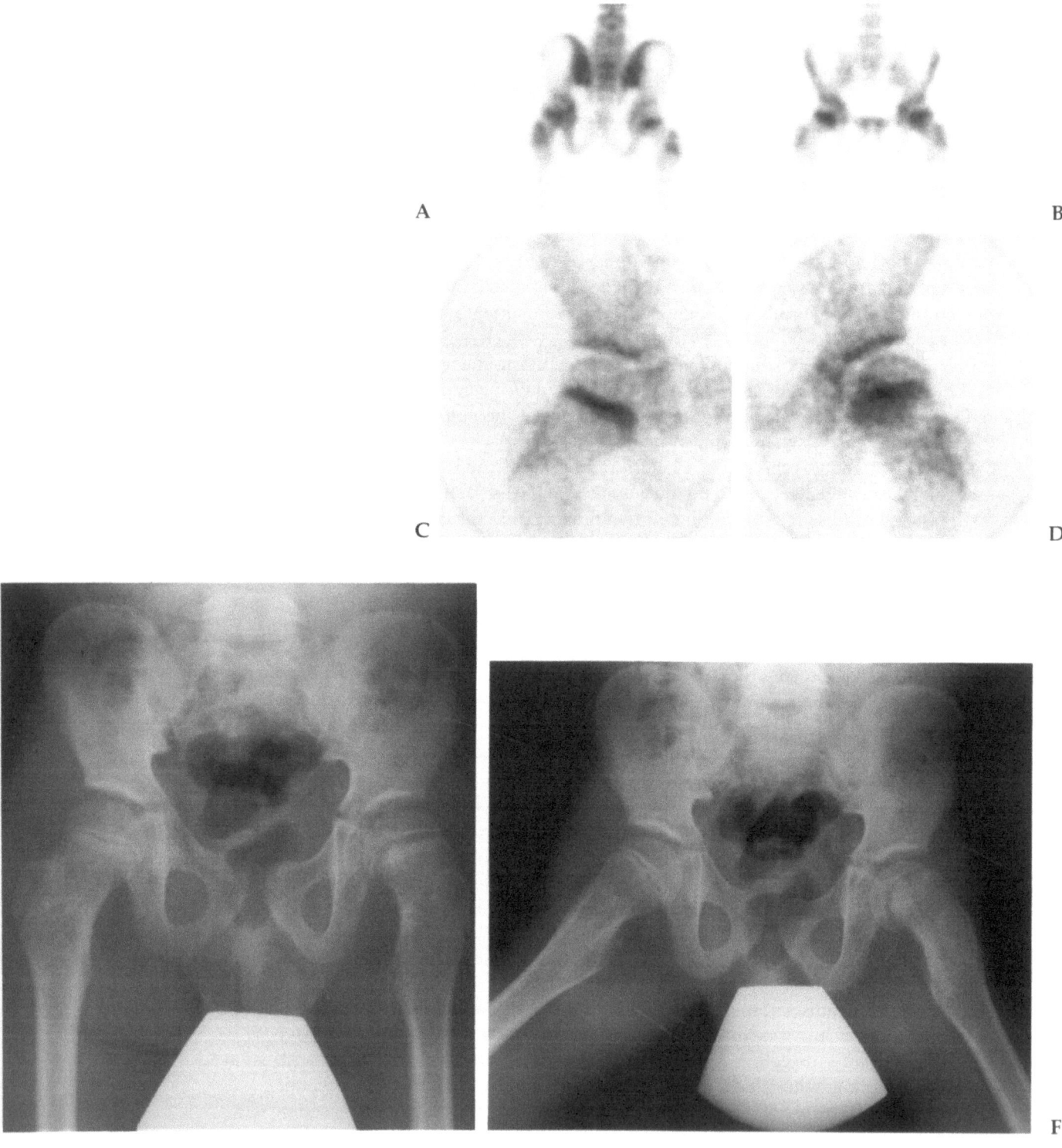

Figure 3.29. Slipped capital femoral epiphysis. Posterior (A) and anterior (B) skeletal phase planar images reveal increased tracer localization in the left femoral metaphysis. This finding, which was detected incidentally on a study performed for long-term neuroblastoma follow-up, is better demonstrated with pinhole magnification (C: right hip, D: left hip). An anteroposterior radiograph (E) reveals widening of the left proximal femoral physis and joint space. Medial displacement of the femoral capital epiphysis relative to the metaphysis is confirmed by a frog leg lateral radiograph (F).

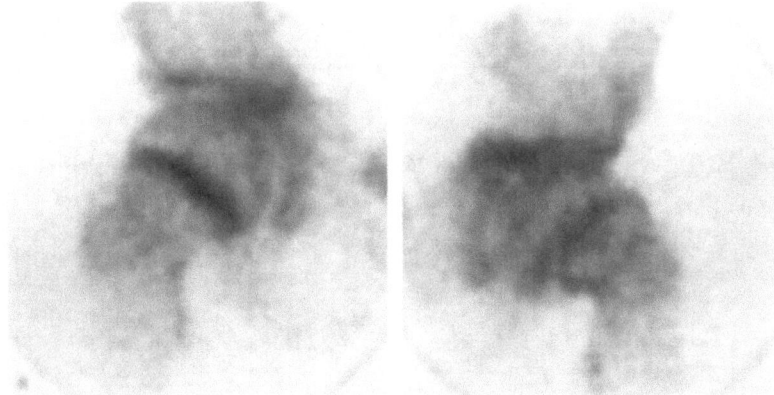

Figure 3.30. Slipped capital femoral epiphysis. Medial displacement of the left femoral capital epiphysis relative to the metaphysis is shown with pinhole magnification. (Reprinted from Treves et al,[91a] with permission.)

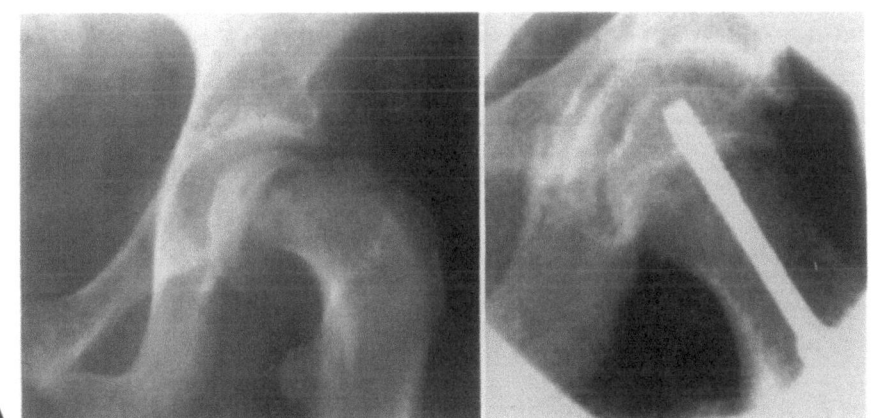

A   B

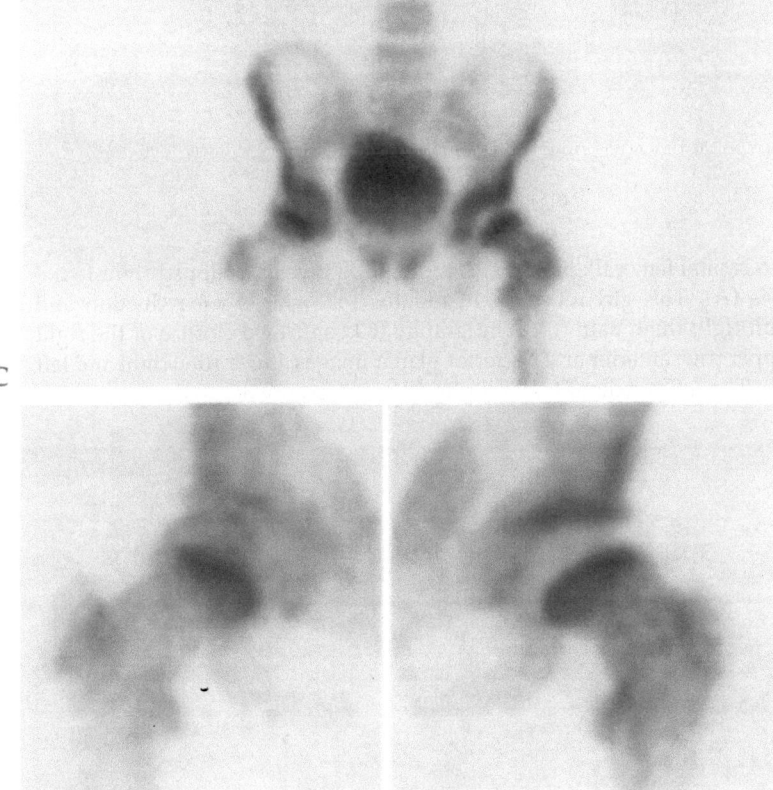

C

D   E

Figure 3.31. Slipped capital femoral epiphysis. An anteroposterior radiograph (A) reveals marked displacement of the left femoral capital epiphysis relative to the metaphysis. Following open reduction and internal fixation (B), anterior planar (C) and pinhole magnification images (D: normal right hip; E: left hip) show absence of tracer localization in the left femoral capital epiphysis.

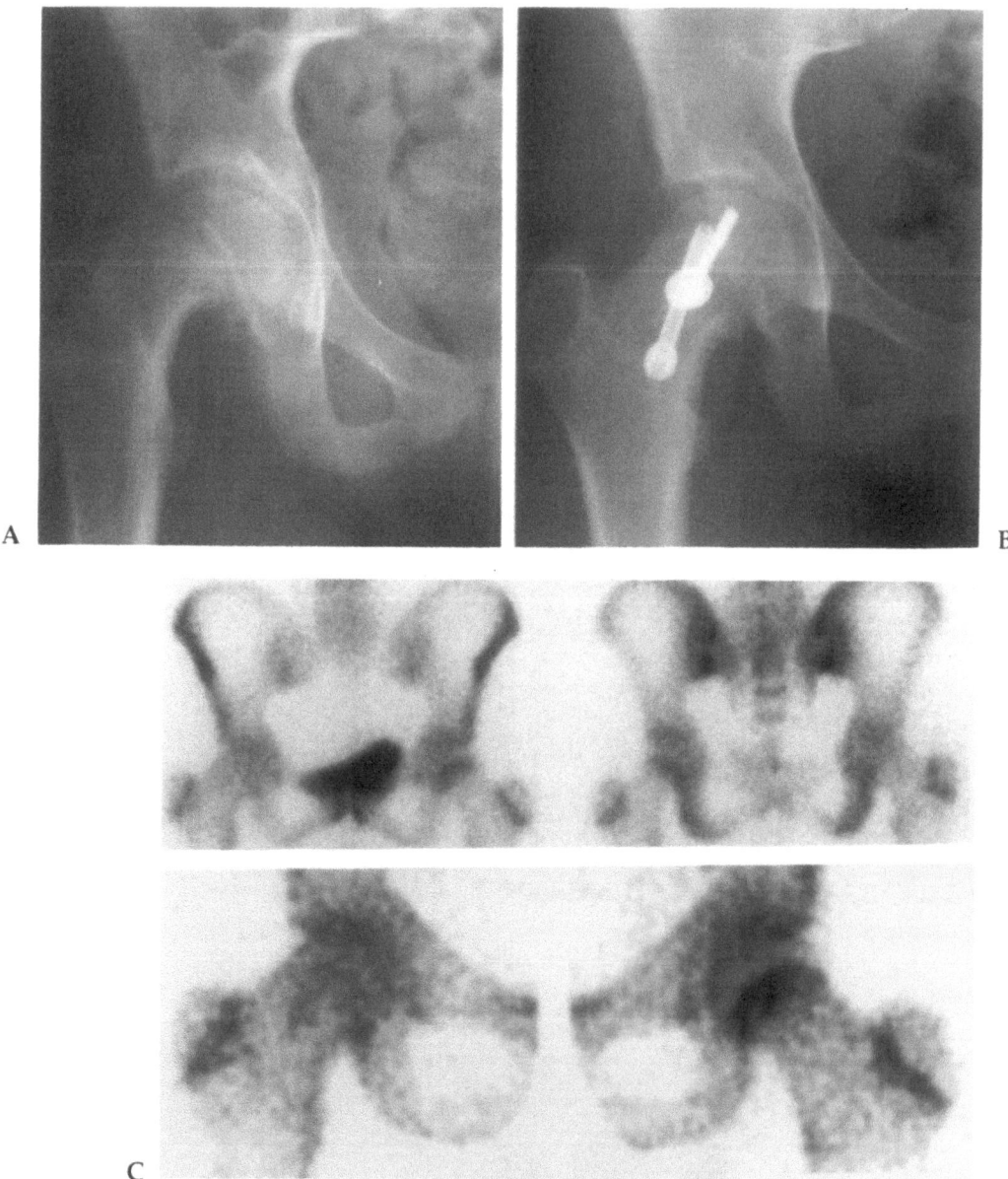

Figure 3.32. Slipped capital femoral epiphysis. A radiograph reveals a slipped right femoral capital epiphysis (A). This girl returned 14 months following open reduction and internal fixation with right thigh pain (B). Scintigraphy (C) confirmed closure of the right proximal physis (upper row: anterior and posterior planar images; lower row: right and left hip pinhole images). The left proximal femoral physis remained open.

Tarsal Coalition

Tarsal coalition is an important cause of foot or ankle pain in children and adolescents. This condition is due to failure of segmentation or abnormal fusion between tarsal bones, most commonly the calcaneus with the navicular (calcaneonavicular coalition) or the talus (talocalcaneal coalition). Other types (talonavicular, calcaneocuboid, cuboidonavicular, navicular-cuneiform) are rare. The union is fibrous, cartilaginous, or osseous. The fusion typically becomes rigid during adolescence, presumably due to ossification of a fibrous union.[47] The typical presentation is peroneal spastic flatfoot. Pain results from fracture of the coalition or ankle injuries secondary to diminished mobility caused by the coalition. Most cases of tarsal coalition respond to nonoperative management, including rest, orthotics, and casting. Surgical resection of the bar forming the coalition is performed in cases where symptoms persist.[87]

Talocalcaneal coalition (Fig. 3.33) is manifested radiographically by secondary signs of dorsal talar beaking, broadening and rounding of the lateral process of the talus, narrowing of the posterior talocalcaneal joint, a concave appearance to the undersurface of the talar neck, rounding of the tibial articulation of the ankle joint,[20] and the "C sign," which is an abnormal outline formed by the medial talar dome and inferior sustentaculum tali.[48] These findings, which are also associated with other causes of limited subtalar motion, are demonstrated with conventional anteroposterior and lateral views. When secondary changes are present, a 45° posterior axial oblique projection (of Harris) may show an osseous talocalcaneal coalition. Calcaneonavicular coalition typically does not produce secondary signs on standard radiographic projections. A 30° to 45° oblique projection of the foot is diagnostic in most cases.[47]

Coronal CT is useful in cases of high clinical suspicion when radiographs are normal and for anatomic definition when surgery is planned. Osseous bars, irregular and sclerotic joint surfaces, and abnormal subtalar joint alignment can be demonstrated with CT.[81] Magnetic resonance imaging is useful for demonstrating nonosseous coalitions, which are difficult to detect with CT.[95] Since as many as 60% of tarsal coalitions are bilateral,[63] cross-sectional imaging should include both feet.

In some cases, the diagnosis is first suggested when skeletal scintigraphy demonstrates increased tracer localization corresponding to the coalition.[24] The incidence of bilaterality requires that images of the contralateral foot and ankle be carefully scrutinized.

Figure 3.33. Tarsal coalition. A Harris projection reveals an osseous talocalcaneal coalition (A, arrow). Skeletal phase images show poor tracer localization in the bones of the feet of a 13 year-old girl who had been unable to exercise secondary to discomfort. Intense tracer localization at the right ankle medially (B) corresponds to a fracture (arrowhead) through a talocalcaneal coalition (T, talus; C, calcaneus) seen with MRI (C,D). A contralateral coalition is suggested by the increased localization seen medially with scintigraphy.

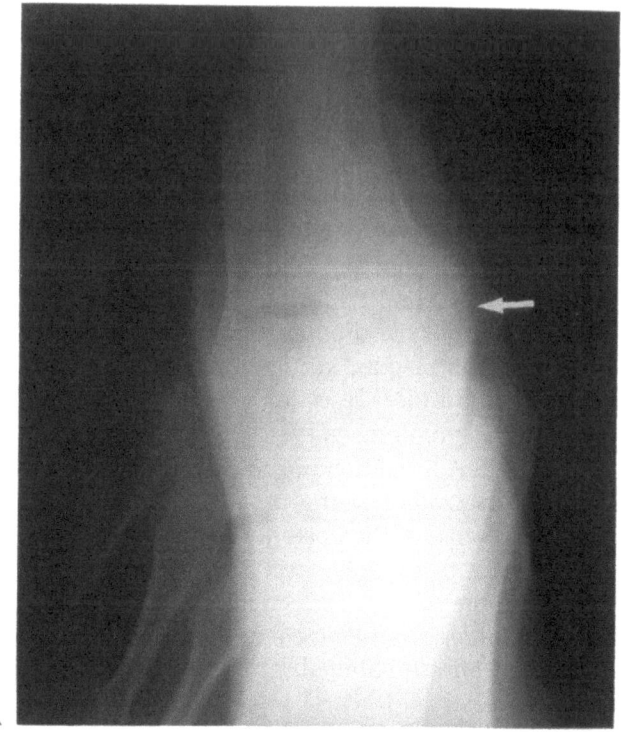

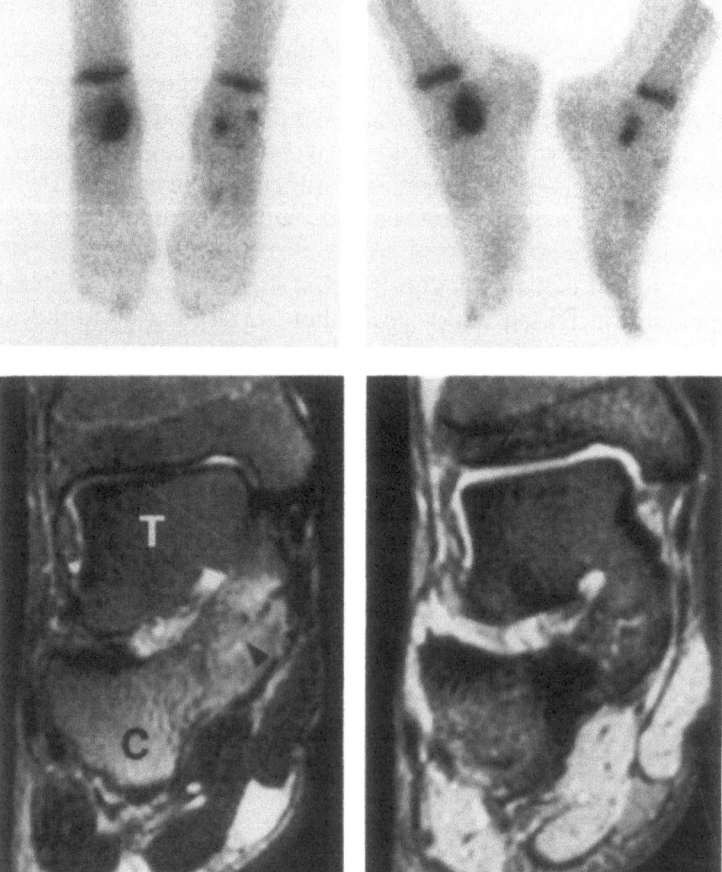

Upper Extremity Stress Injuries

While the preponderance of stress injuries affect the low back, pelvis, and lower extremities, stress injuries to the upper extremities and thorax occur in sports that involve repetitive or strenuous upper body activity. Examples include stress fractures of the ribs in rowing, of the humerus and ulna in baseball, and of finger phalanges in bowling.[16,29,54,92] Increased tracer localization due to periostitis also occurs along muscular insertions in the upper extremity.[72]

The medial epicondyle of the humerus is a relatively common site of upper extremity apophyseal avulsion in children. Traction by flexor and pronator muscles, such as occurs with baseball pitching, renders this structure vulnerable to avulsion until it fuses with the humerus between the ages of 18 and 20 years.[67] Radiographs are usually diagnostic of this injury ("Little Leaguers elbow"). In cases where displacement is minimal, skeletal scintigraphy is useful to demonstrate increased radionuclide localization in the medial epicondyle. Suspected cases of medial epicondylar avulsion are also assessed with MRI, which can reveal osteochondral fragmentation.[86] Other upper body apophyses that are occasionally injured are the olecranon, the coracoid, and the acromion.[85]

Differential Diagnosis of Stress Injuries

A variety of skeletal conditions may present with a history that suggests a stress injury. These include malignancies, such as osteosarcoma and Ewing sarcoma, benign tumors, such as osteoid osteoma, and acute or chronic osteomyelitis. Imaging specialists must bear this in mind when interpreting studies of young athletes, although each of these diseases typically has a distinct scintigraphic appearance from that of sports injuries. Correlation between skeletal scintigraphy and any other imaging study that has been obtained is always valuable. In cases where the scintigraphic pattern or the clinical examination is atypical for an athletic injury, additional correlative studies must be obtained.

Injuries of Toddlers

Fractures of the lower extremity are associated with children beginning to walk upright and bear weight on their lower extremities between the ages of 9 months to 3 years. These fractures may either be directly attributable to a fall or stress injuries. The most characteristic injury is a spiral fracture of the tibia (toddler's fracture).[14]

The child with a toddler's fracture usually refuses or is reluctant to bear weight on the affected extremity. Physical examination may reveal point tenderness and minimal soft tissue swelling but is frequently nonlocalizing. Treatment is with a below-knee walking cast.

Radiographically, a toddler's fracture is spiral or oblique in orientation and involves the lower one third of the tibia. Due to its orientation, the fracture may be difficult to identify. Internal oblique radiographs are helpful but are not routinely obtained unless the diagnosis is specifically questioned. In some cases, a fracture line or periosteal reaction only becomes apparent days or weeks after clinical presentation.[47]

Due to its greater sensitivity for early fracture diagnosis,[57,58] skeletal scintigraphy is useful when radiographs do not confirm the presence of a suspected toddler's fracture. Poor localization of signs and symptoms may result in a child with a toddler's fracture being referred for scintigraphy with a clinical question concerning a site remote from the tibia. In such cases, the initial radiographs may not have included the injured area. Skeletal scintigraphy demonstrates either focal, linear, or diffuse radionuclide localization in the fractured tibia (Figs. 3.34–3.37).[62]

Scintigraphy is also valuable in the diagnosis of other related fractures seen in this age group. These include fractures of the fibula, cuboid (Figs. 3.37 and 3.38), calcaneus (Figs. 3.39 and 3.40), and metatarsal bases.[6,80] Occult fractures should be considered and searched for when interpreting skeletal scintigraphy of a "limping" toddler. Although complications from a delay in diagnosis of these fractures are not likely, a correct diagnosis allays parental concern, obviates the need for further evaluation, and allows the prompt institution of appropriate therapy.

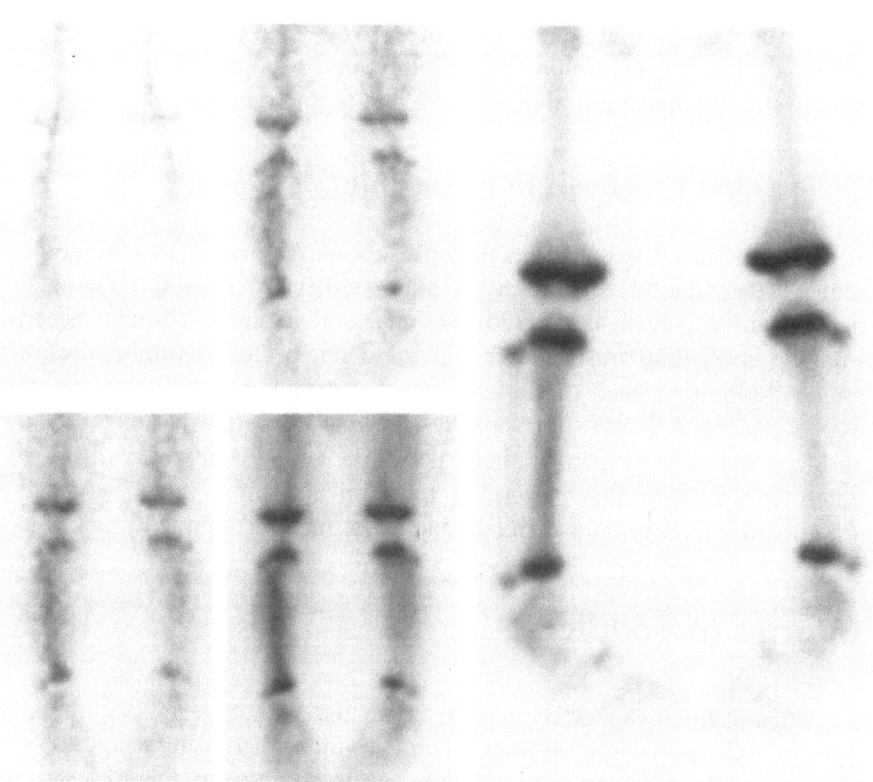

Figure 3.34. Toddler's fracture. Selected images from radionuclide angiography and a tissue phase image demonstrate increased tracer delivery to the right calf of a 22-month-old girl. The skeletal phase image shows diffusely increased ^{99m}Tc-MDP localization in the right tibial diaphysis.

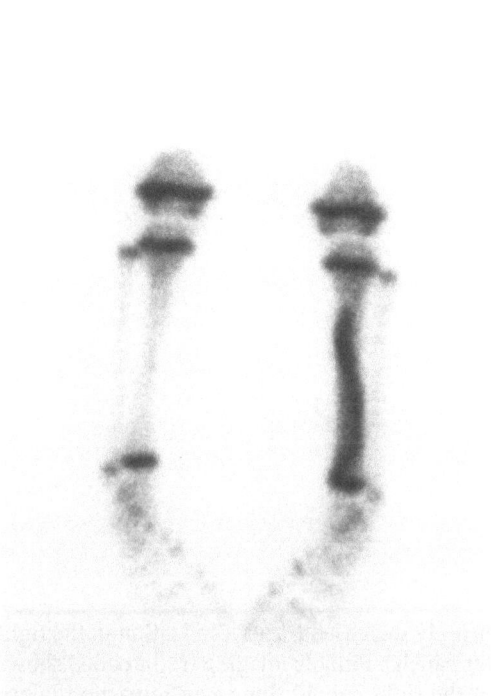

Figure 3.35. Toddler's fracture. A well-defined region of markedly increased ^{99m}Tc-MDP localization delineates a spiral fracture in a 2-year-old boy. (Reprinted from Treves,[91a] with permission.)

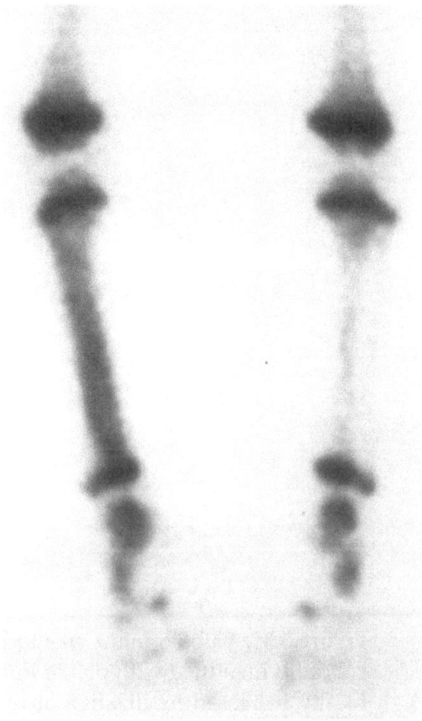

Figure 3.36. Toddler's fracture. Diffusely increased tracer localization is noted in the right tibia of a 20-month-old boy, who was evaluated for reluctance to bear weight.

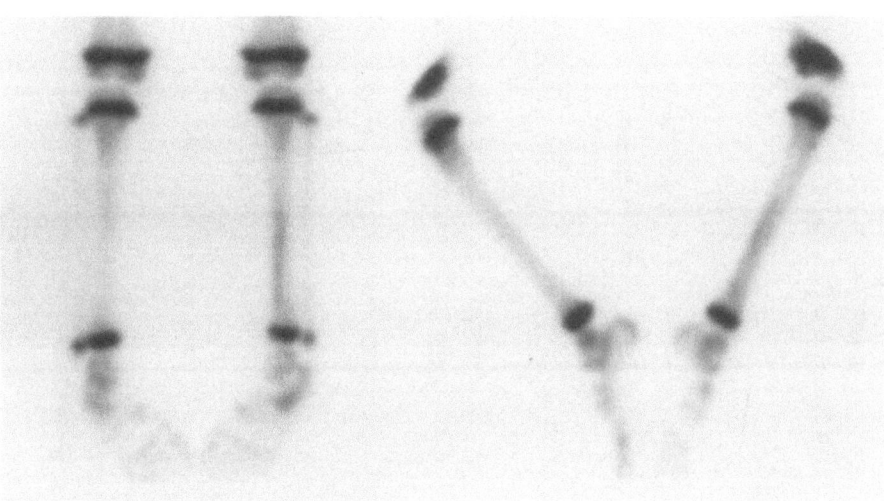

Figure 3.37. Toddler's injuries of the tibia and cuboid. Increased tracer localization is demonstrated in the left tibial diaphysis and left cuboid of a 2-year-old boy.

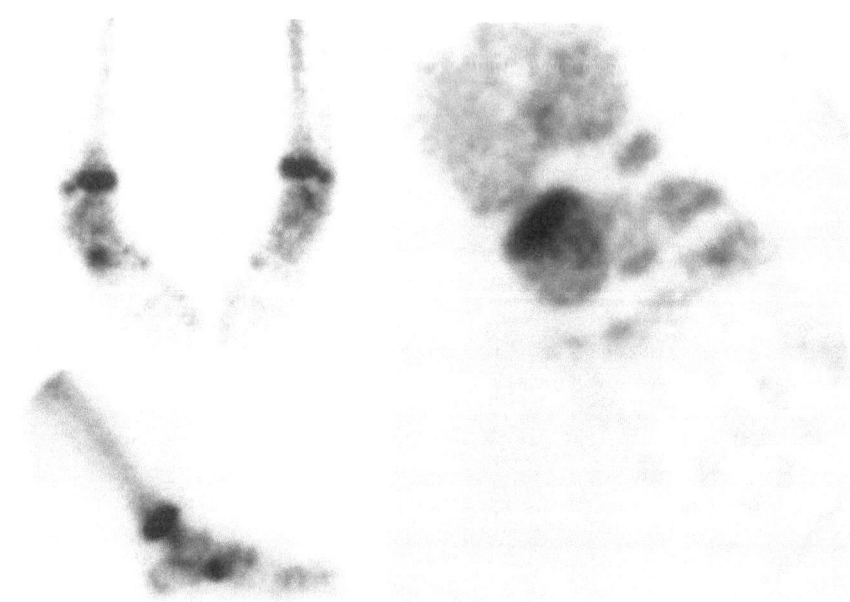

Figure 3.38. Cuboid injury in a toddler. Diffusely increased tracer localization in the right cuboid is identified with planar imaging (left panels). Pinhole imaging (right panel) shows focally increased localization at the base of the right cuboid due to an impaction injury related to a fall.

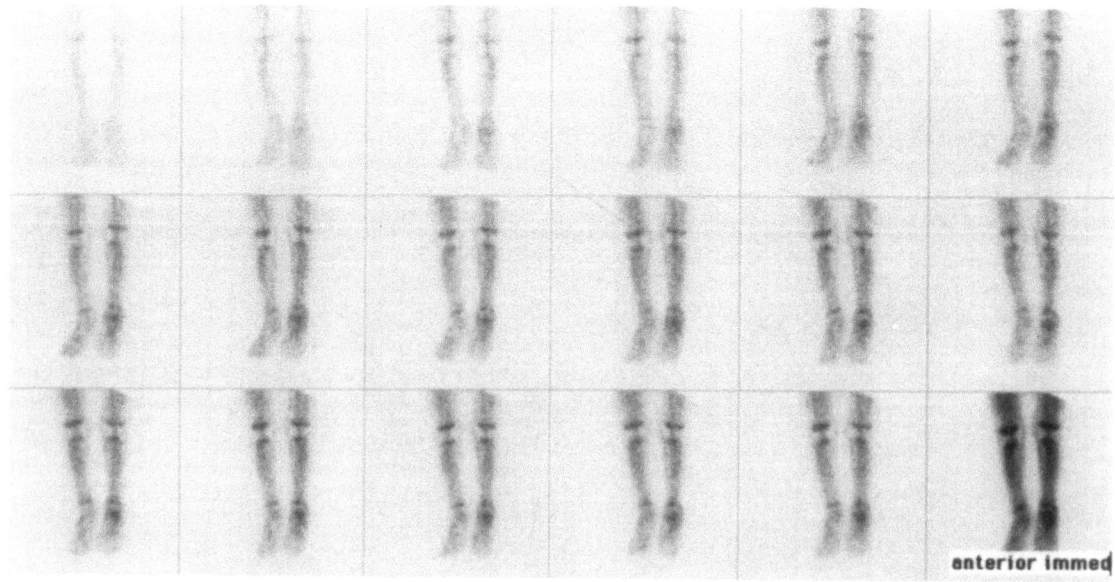

A

Figure 3.39. Calcaneal injury in a toddler. Increased tracer delivery and early localization to the left calcaneal region are depicted with radionuclide angiography and tissue phase imaging (A).

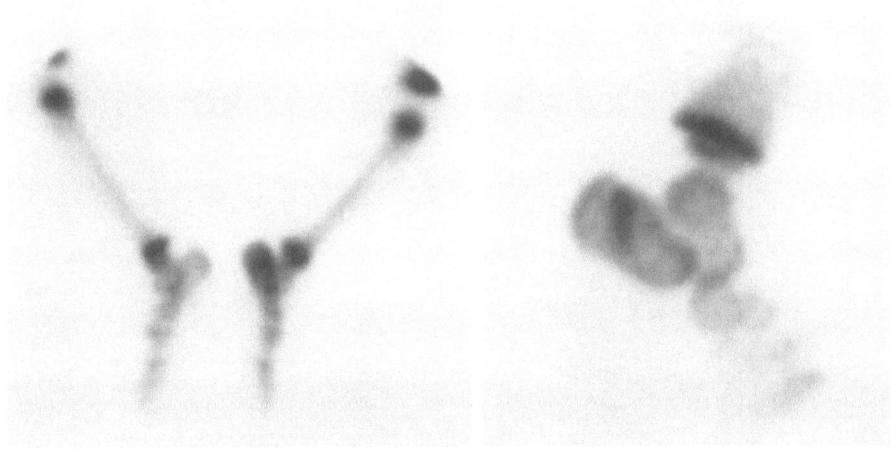

B

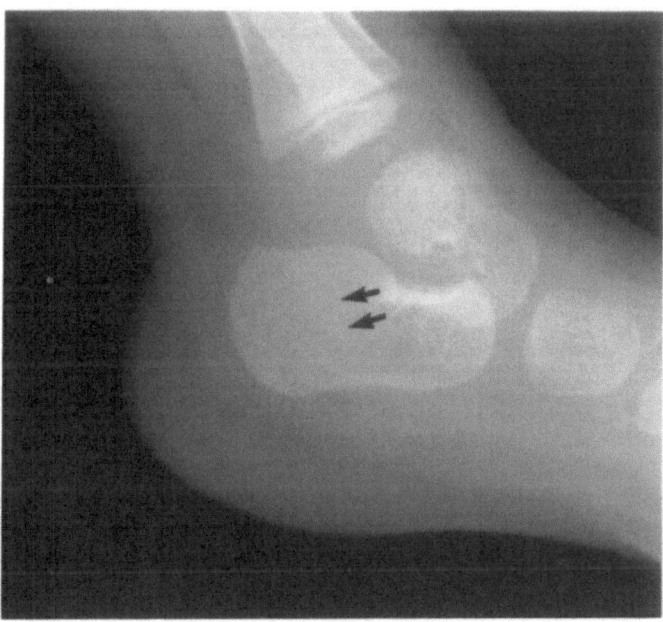

C

Figure 3.39. (*cont'd.*) Increased ^{99m}Tc-MDP localization is demonstrated diffusely in the left calcaneus (B, planar and pinhole images). A focal component is better depicted with pinhole imaging. A faint band of sclerosis is identified in the calcaneus radiographically (C).

Figure 3.40. Calcaneal injury in a toddler. Tissue phase (upper panels) and skeletal phase (lower panels) images demonstrate diffusely increased ^{99m}Tc-MDP localization in the left calcaneus of a 25-month-old girl who was favoring her left lower extremity.

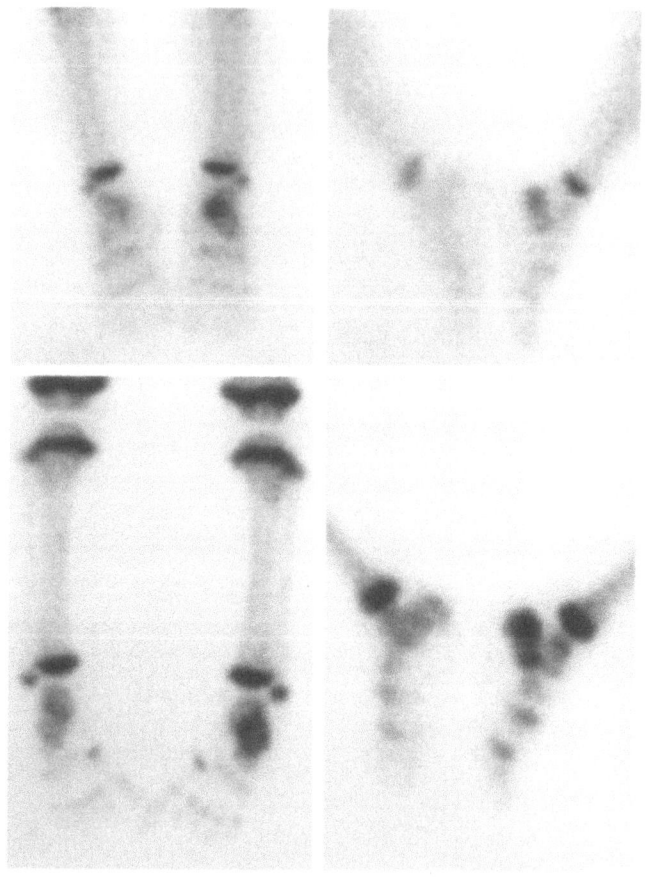

Child Abuse

General Considerations

Physical, sexual, and emotional abuse or neglect of children is a significant societal problem, the gravity of which is grasped by reviewing data from the National Incidence Study (NIS) of Child Abuse and Neglect in the United States. The National Center of Child Abuse and Neglect (NCCAN) has issued three reports in fulfilling this congressionally mandated periodic surveillance effort. The first (NIS-1) dealt with data collected during 1979 and 1980, the second (NIS-2) with data obtained in 1986 and 1987, and the most recent (NIS-3) with data from 1993 and 1994.

The NCCAN reports a conservative estimate of 1,553,800 abused or neglected children in NIS-3. This represents a 149% increase from NIS-1 and a 67% increase from NIS-2. The estimated number of children who suffered serious harm or injury increased from 141,700 in NIS-2 to 565,000 in NIS-3. Of the abused or neglected children in NIS-3, 381,700 were victims of physical abuse (a 42% increase from NIS-2). The increase in the incidence of child abuse and neglect, reflected in the preceding numbers, is believed to reflect a true increase and not just heightened societal sensitivity concerning the problem.[75]

Abuse may occur at the hands of any authority figure. Birth parents are perpetrators in over 70% of cases. A child who is physically abused by a birth parent is more likely to be a victim of the mother than the father reflecting a higher number of homes where the mother as opposed to the father serves as a single parent. Conversely, males account for over 80% of nonparental perpetrators. Child abuse knows no ethnic, racial, or class boundaries.[75]

Greater than 50% of all cases of physical abuse occur during the first year of life and virtually all cases occur before the age of 6 years.[10,47] Abused children are often subjected to repeated trauma. Early identification of abused children is essential if they are to be removed from a situation in which further, perhaps fatal, injury is all too likely. Imaging, particularly by demonstrating occult skeletal trauma, plays an important part in this process.

The typical victims of abuse, infants and young children, are often not of an age where they are able to verbally localize the sites of trauma or pain. Subsequently, evaluation of the entire skeleton is an essential component of the evaluation of suspected child abuse. Radiographic skeletal surveys performed for this purpose include anteroposterior and lateral views of the skull and thorax, lateral views of the spine, an anteroposterior view of the abdomen and pelvis, and anteroposterior views of the three segments of each extremity.[41] Following review of these radiographs, additional films are obtained of any site deemed suspicious for injury. Skeletal scintigraphy is performed with multiple-spot imaging of the entire skeleton. This is supplemented with pinhole magnification and SPECT as necessary. With both radiography and scintigraphy, careful patient positioning, use of high-quality imaging systems, and strict attention to detail are essential.

Mechanisms of Injury and Their Manifestations

Interpretation of imaging studies is facilitated by awareness of the types and patterns of skeletal injury associated with child abuse. These can be understood by considering the two primary mechanisms of injury: shaking and blunt trauma.

The assault of an infant younger than 1 year of age frequently entails the victim being grasped about the thorax, facing the assailant, and violently shaken to and fro. Metaphyseal and rib fractures are characteristic of this form of abuse. Scapular fractures, particularly involving the acromion, also occur.

Metaphyseal fractures result from shearing forces that are generated by rapid acceleration and deceleration. Metaphyseal fractures account for almost 90% of the long bone fractures in infants who die as a result of child abuse.[44] The metaphyseal predilection reflects weakness of newly formed bone adjacent to the physis during a period of rapid growth. These fractures most frequently involve the tibia, distal femur, and proximal humerus. They are often bilateral. The fracture plane is close to the physis centrally. Peripherally, it undercuts a larger fragment incorporating the subperiosteal collar of Laval-Jeantet. Histologically, a planar series of microfractures through the immature primary spongiosa is present.[43] The radiographic appearance of these fractures depends on the orientation of the x-ray beam to the metaphyseal fragment. A metaphyseal fracture appears as a crescent ("bucket-handle" fracture) when imaged obliquely, and as two peripheral triangles ("corner" fracture) when imaged tangentially.[41,43,47] Metaphyseal injuries, which appear scintigraphically as alterations in the normal shape of the physis (Figs. 3.41 and 3.42) or as increased intensity of physeal tracer localization that may extend to affect the metaphysis (Figs. 3.42–3.45),[82] may be difficult to detect with skeletal scintigraphy. Modern equipment, meticulous care in patient positioning, a high level of suspicion for any irregularity in the shape of the physis, and experience in interpreting pediatric skeletal scintigraphy enhance the sensitivity of skeletal scintigraphy in detecting metaphyseal injuries. Experienced interpreters of pediatric skeletal scintigraphy have found scintigraphy to be more sensitive than radiographs for detecting metaphyseal injuries.[13,82] It is our opinion, however, that scintigraphy should not be used as the sole means of detecting metaphyseal injuries. When scintigraphy is interpreted as normal, particularly by less experienced practitioners, a metaphyseal injury is not excluded. When metaphyseal injuries are detected scintigraphically, radiographic correlation is valuable in depicting this characteristic type of injury for medicolegal purposes and in excluding underlying pathology.

Rib fractures should always raise the suspicion of inflicted injury. Rib fractures occur at sites of compression, posteriorly near the costovertebral junction (where the rib is compressed against the transverse process), laterally, and anteriorly.[40] In considering the violent force required to fracture a rib, it is important to note that the compliance of the rib cage prevents rib fractures from occurring during cardiopulmonary resuscitation (CPR) in infants despite the variable training of CPR providers.[17] Rib fractures are difficult to detect radiographically and are often only apparent when callus develops. Acutely fractured ribs at the costovertebral junction may appear normal or show only minor widening of the rib neck. Laterally located acute fractures are more likely to be detected but are also often radiographically occult. Acute costochondral fractures are usually not associated with radiographic abnormalities. Skeletal scintigraphy has proven to be especially useful for detecting rib fractures in their acute stage.[40,79,82] These fractures are typically multiple and appear as focal areas of increased tracer localization (Figs. 3.42, 3.44, and 3.46–3.48). The superimposition of prominent tracer localization in the costochondral junctions over the posterior ribs on a posterior projection requires that oblique projections be obtained regularly to confirm or exclude posterior rib fractures. Costochondral injuries are difficult to detect scintigraphically due to intense tracer localization in the adjacent growth centers.

Abused children who are older and heavier than infants of 6 months of age are often grasped by an extremity and shaken. With this type of abuse, torsional forces may cause a metaphyseal fracture while direct pressure may result in a diaphyseal fracture or a periosteal injury.[13] Diaphyseal injuries are the most common injuries demonstrated in victims of child abuse.[60] They are suggestive of abuse in infants younger than 1 year of age. Once a child begins to walk, diaphyseal injuries are more often due to accidental trauma.[90] Since there is no demarcating age above which all diaphyseal injuries are accidental and below which all diaphyseal injuries are nonaccidental, close clinical correlation is always required. Radiographically, a fracture line, often spiral in configuration, may be demonstrated. Periosteal reaction due to subperiosteal hemorrhage may be the only radiographic manifestation. Scintigraphy is highly reliable in detecting diaphyseal injuries, and frequently demonstrates radiographically occult injuries.[13,35,82] Although a focal abnormality is occasionally identified, it is more common to see diffusely increased diaphyseal tracer localization (Figs. 3.41, 3.42, 3.44–3.46, and 3.49).

Abused infants and children are also subject to blunt trauma, either in the form of a direct blow or by being thrown against an object. Any bone can be injured in this fashion. Skull fractures are common. These fractures are typically linear and nondepressed. They incite minimal osteoblastic response and are therefore difficult to demonstrate with skeletal scintigraphy (Figs. 3.45 and 3.50). Other common sites of fractures associated with blunt trauma include the long bone diaphyses, body of the scapula (Fig. 3.43), sternum, clavicle (Fig. 3.42), and the tubular bones of the hands and feet.

Often, more than one mechanism of injury is present. For example, after shaking an infant, the assailant may hurl the victim against an object.[40] Additionally, the episode for which the child is brought to medical attention is frequently not an isolated event. Hyperflexion-extension injuries of the spine, particularly spinous process and vertebral body fractures, occur with each mechanism.

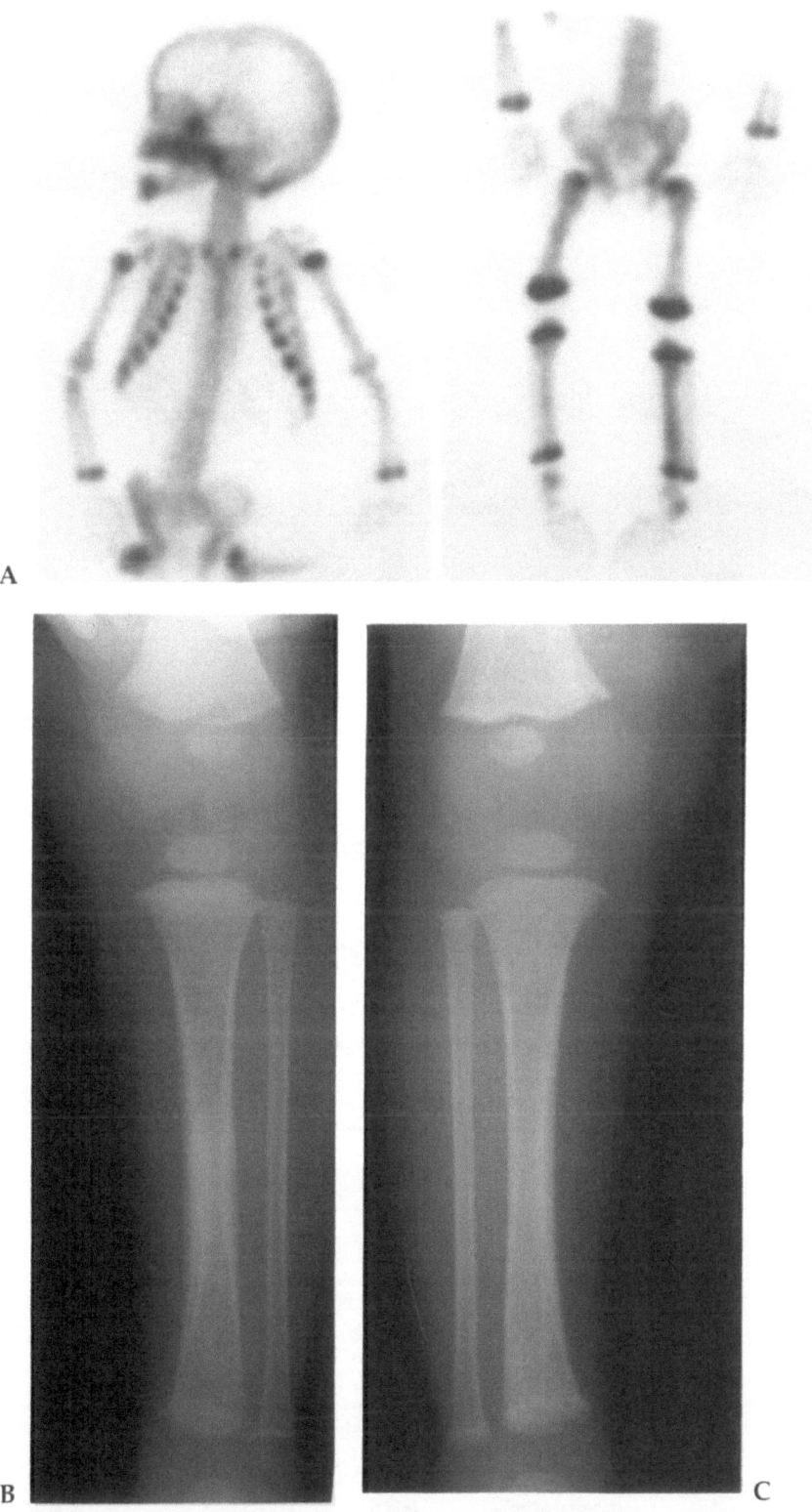

Figure 3.41. Child abuse. Skeletal scintigraphy depicts diffusely increased tracer localization in the humeral, femoral, and tibial diaphyses bilaterally (A). Poor physeal definition, particularly of the distal femoral physes, suggests the presence of metaphyseal fractures. Right (B) and left (C) lower extremity radiographs definitively depict fractures of the distal femoral as well as the proximal and distal tibial and fibular metaphyses bilaterally. Smooth periosteal reaction is noted along the left tibial diaphysis. The right tibial diaphyseal injury is not apparent.

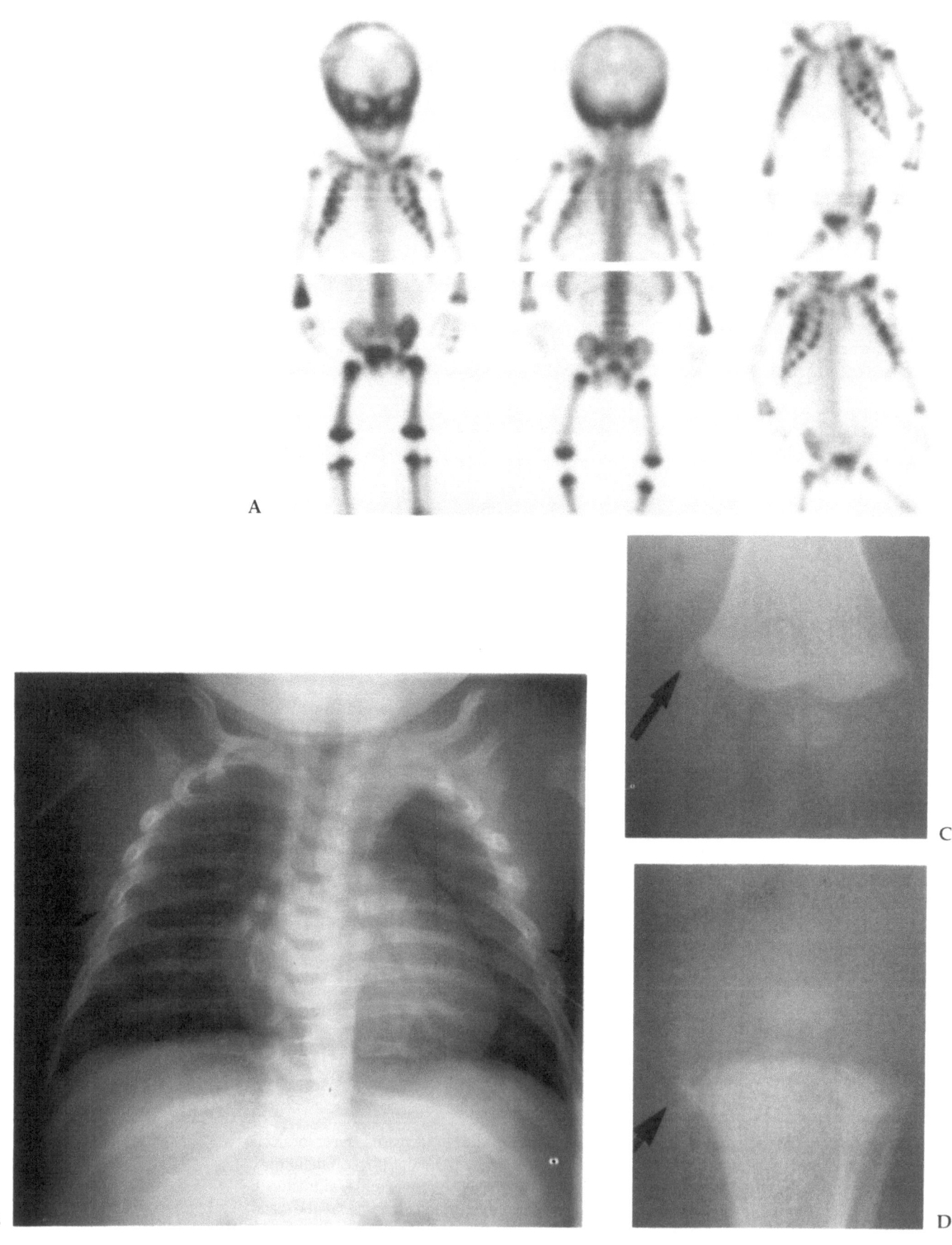

A

B

C

D

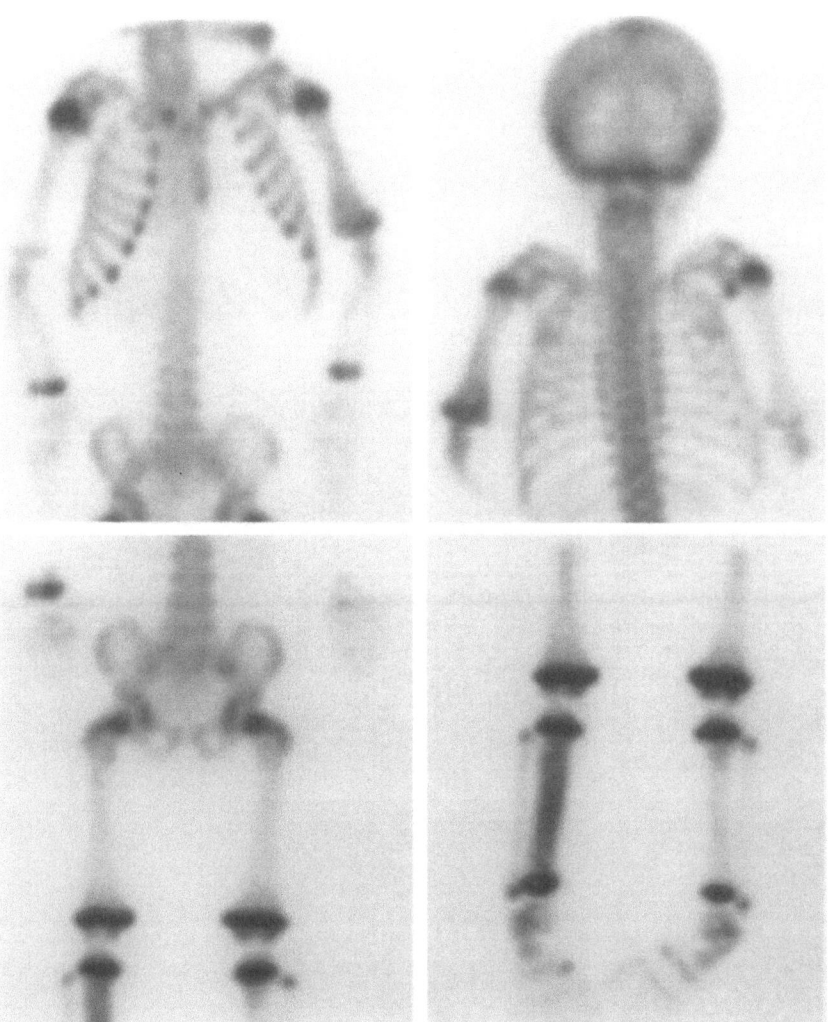

Figure 3.43. Child abuse. Skeletal scintigraphy reveals mildly increased tracer localization in the fourth through ninth ribs at the costovertebral junctions, the right glenoid, the left distal humerus, and the right tibia (A).

Figure 3.42. Child abuse. Skeletal scintigraphy (A, anterior, posterior, and anterior oblique projections) reveals increased tracer localization in the left clavicle, multiple right and left ribs laterally, multiple left ribs at the costovertebral junctions, the left ilium and the femoral, tibial and humeral diaphyses bilaterally. The appearance of the physes and adjacent metaphyses indicates definite injuries to the distal right radius, both proximal femorae and the left proximal tibia and possible injuries of the distal femoral and right proximal tibial metaphyses. A chest radiograph shows fractures of the right fifth and sixth and left fifth ribs. The other rib injuries and the left clavicular injury are not identified (B). Fractures of the left distal femoral (C) and proximal tibial metaphyses are depicted radiographically (D).

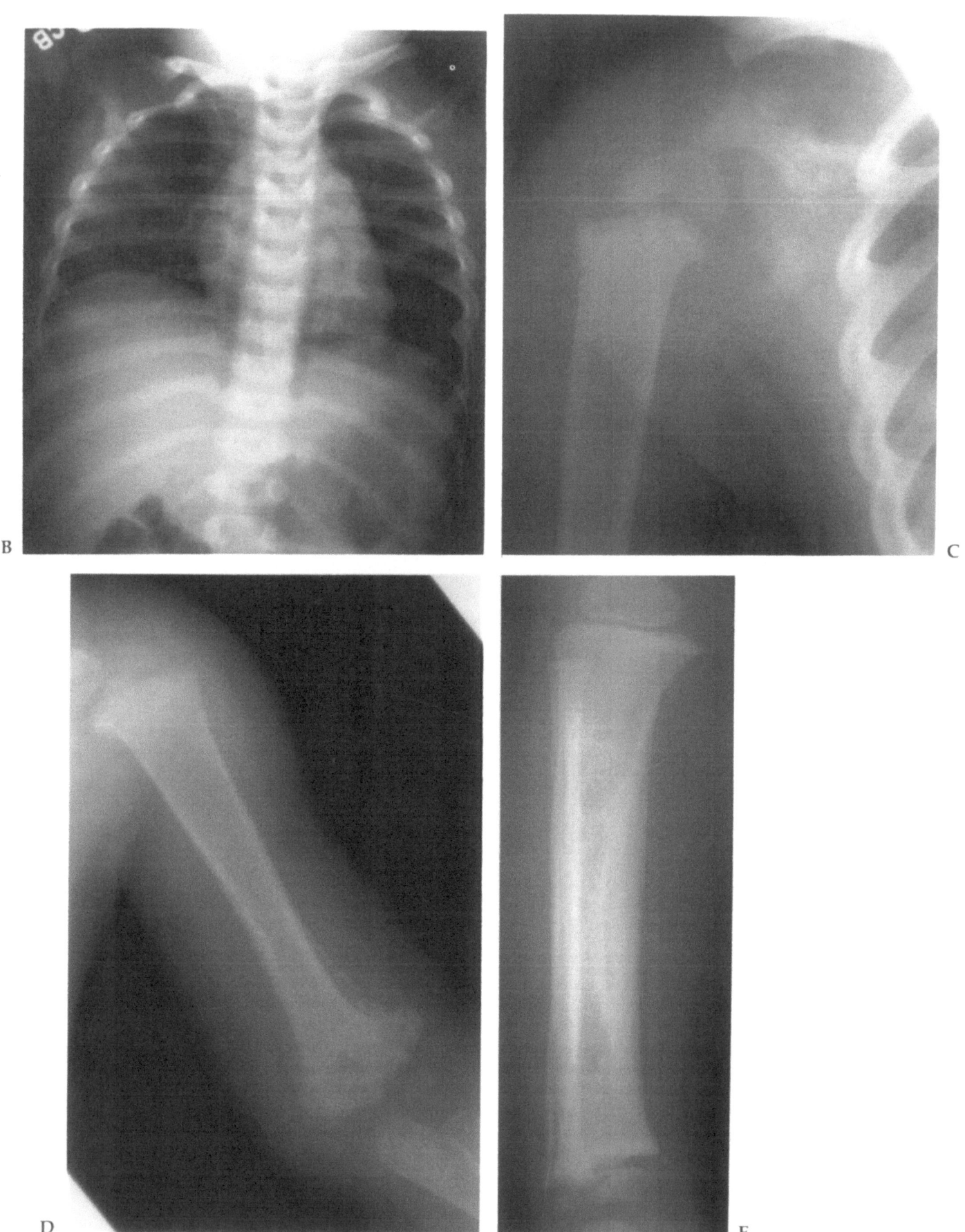

B

C

D

E

120

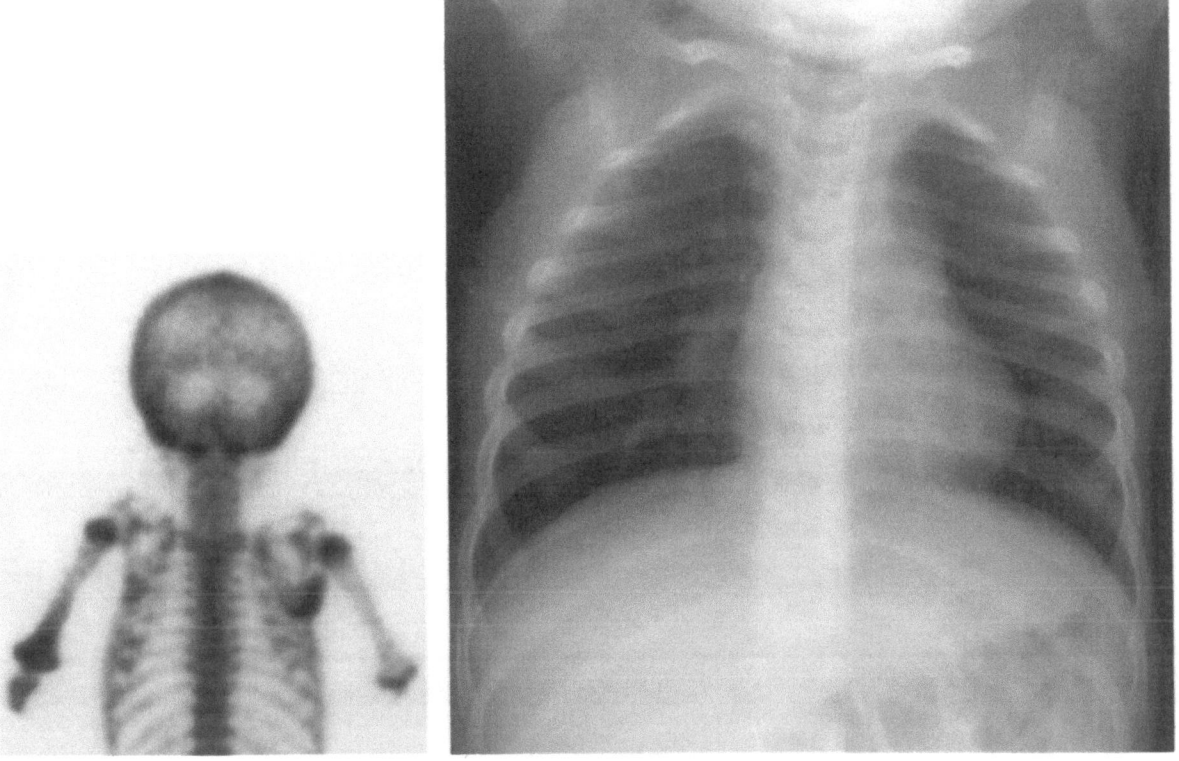

A
B

Figure 3.44. Child abuse. Skeletal scintigraphy (A, posterior image) of a 13-month-old boy shows increased tracer localization in the right scapula, left distal humerus and the left third, seventh, and eighth ribs. These fractures are not clearly identified on a chest radiograph (B).

◄──────

Figure 3.43. (*cont'd.*) The posterior rib fractures are not identified on a chest radiograph (B). Healing fractures are demonstrated radiographically in the right glenoid (C), left distal humerus (D), and right tibia (E). Note that there is a metaphyseal fracture involving the distal tibia as well as diaphyseal new bone formation that correlates with the scintigraphic abnormality.

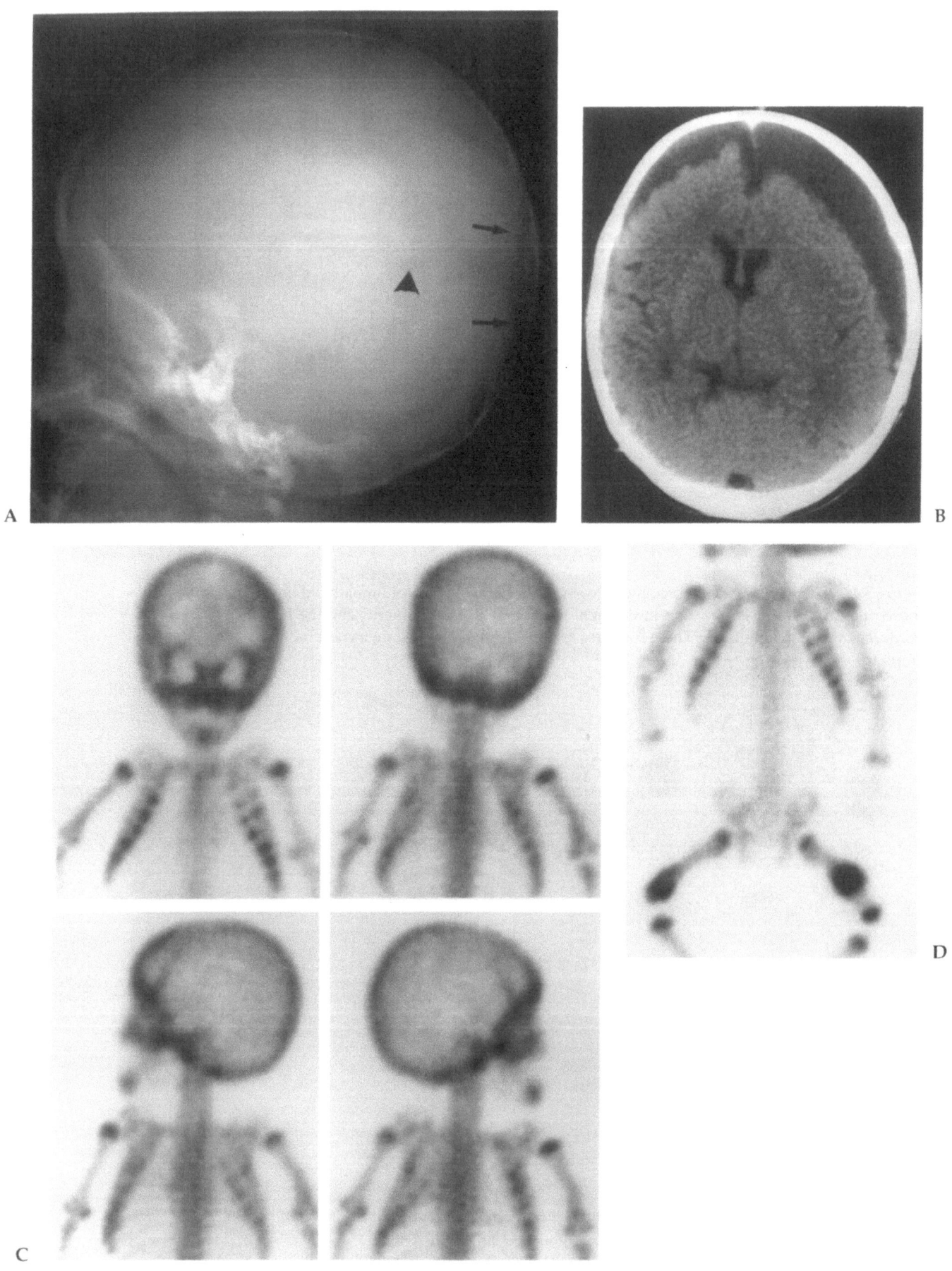

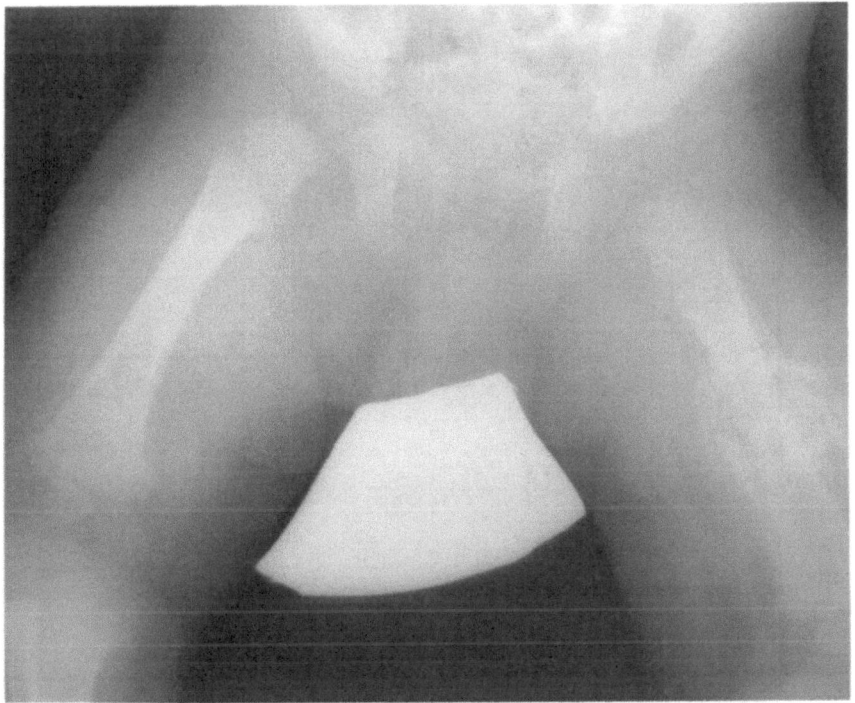

E

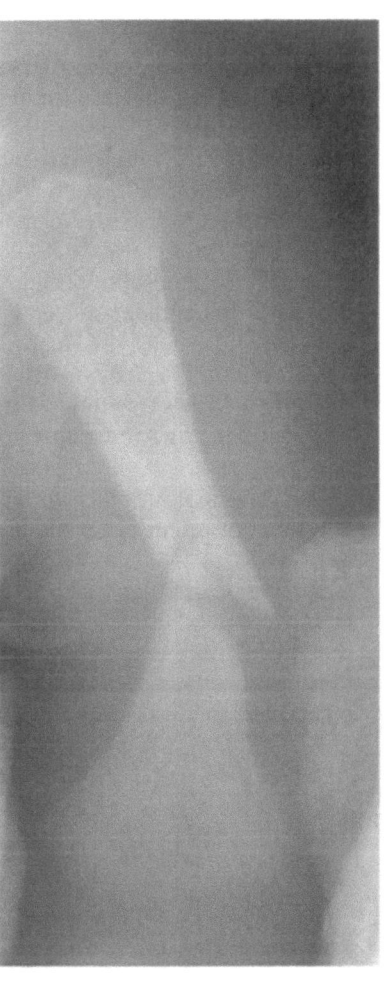

F

Figure 3.45. (*cont'd.*) Radiographic skeletal survey shows fractures of varying ages. There is a relatively new fracture in the distal right femur with periosteal reaction (E). A transverse left femoral diaphyseal fracture with exuberant periosteal reaction and callus is present (E). A more acute fracture of the right humeral diaphysis with medial angulation and dorsal displacement is demonstrated (F).

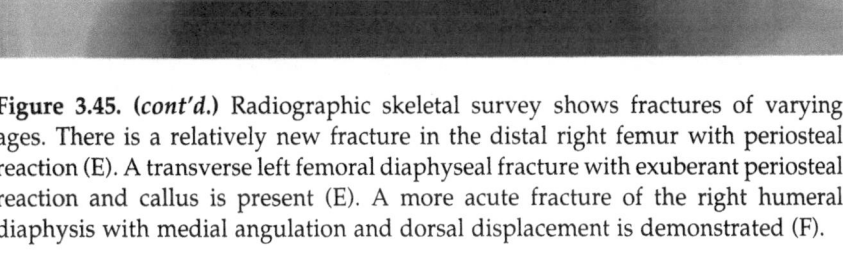

Figure 3.45. Child abuse. A lateral skull radiograph (A) reveals multiple skull fractures including diastatic parietal (arrowhead) and occipital (arrows) fractures in an 8-month-old boy. Computed tomography (B) shows bilateral low density extraaxial fluid collections consistent with old subdural hematomas. Skeletal scintigraphy does not demonstrate a skull fracture (C). Markedly increased ^{99m}Tc-MDP localization is demonstrated in the distal right femoral metadiaphysis and left femoral diaphysis (D). Diffusely increased localization of a lower intensity is present in the right humeral diaphysis.

Figure 3.46. Child abuse. A fracture involving the left glenoid is identified radiographically (A) and scintigraphically (B). It is best depicted with pinhole magnification (B, right panel). Multiple bilateral anterolateral rib fractures demonstrated by skeletal scintigraphy (B,C: left anterior oblique projection) are not identified on the chest radiograph. Bilateral femoral fractures with extensive callus are present (D). Fractures of the femoral diaphysis are typically associated with significant soft tissue swelling and limited range of motion. The exuberant callus that has formed in this child indicates that medical attention was not promptly sought and, in itself, serves as evidence of neglect. The femoral fractures are associated with marked ^{99m}Tc-MDP localization (E). Less prominently increased localization affecting the tibiae suggests radiographically occult tibial injuries.

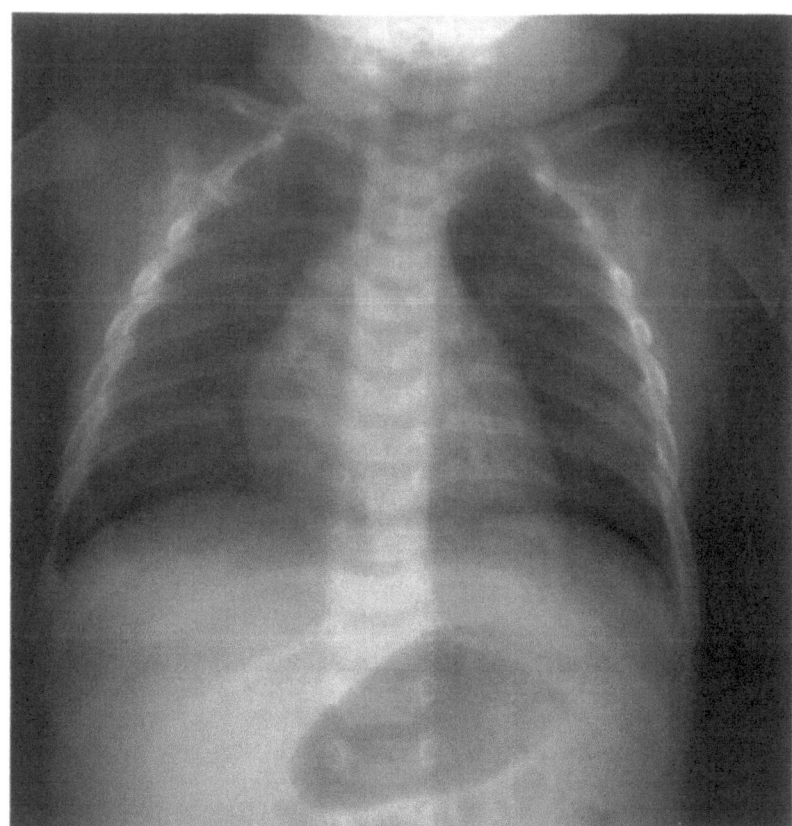

A

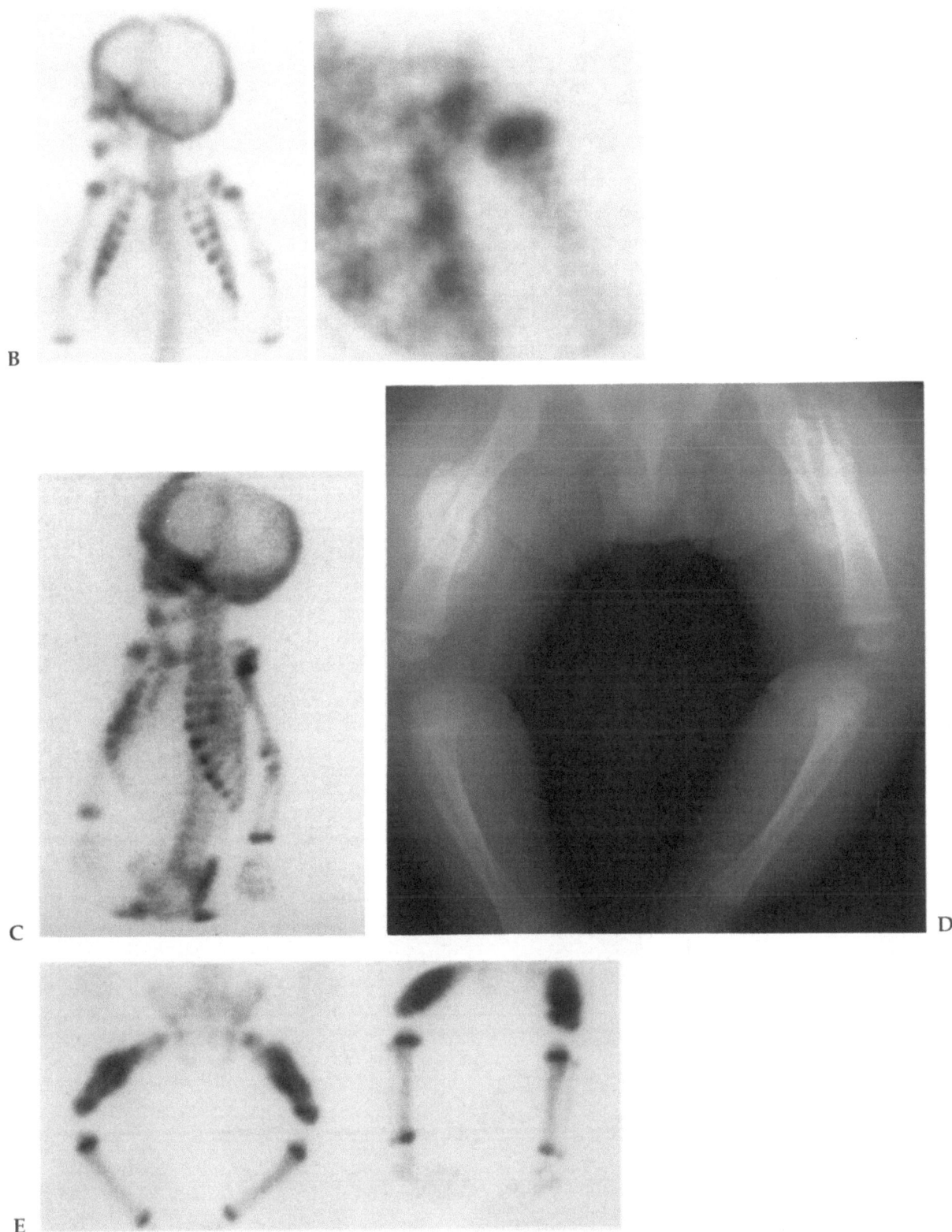

Figure 3.46 (*cont'd*). Caption is on facing page.

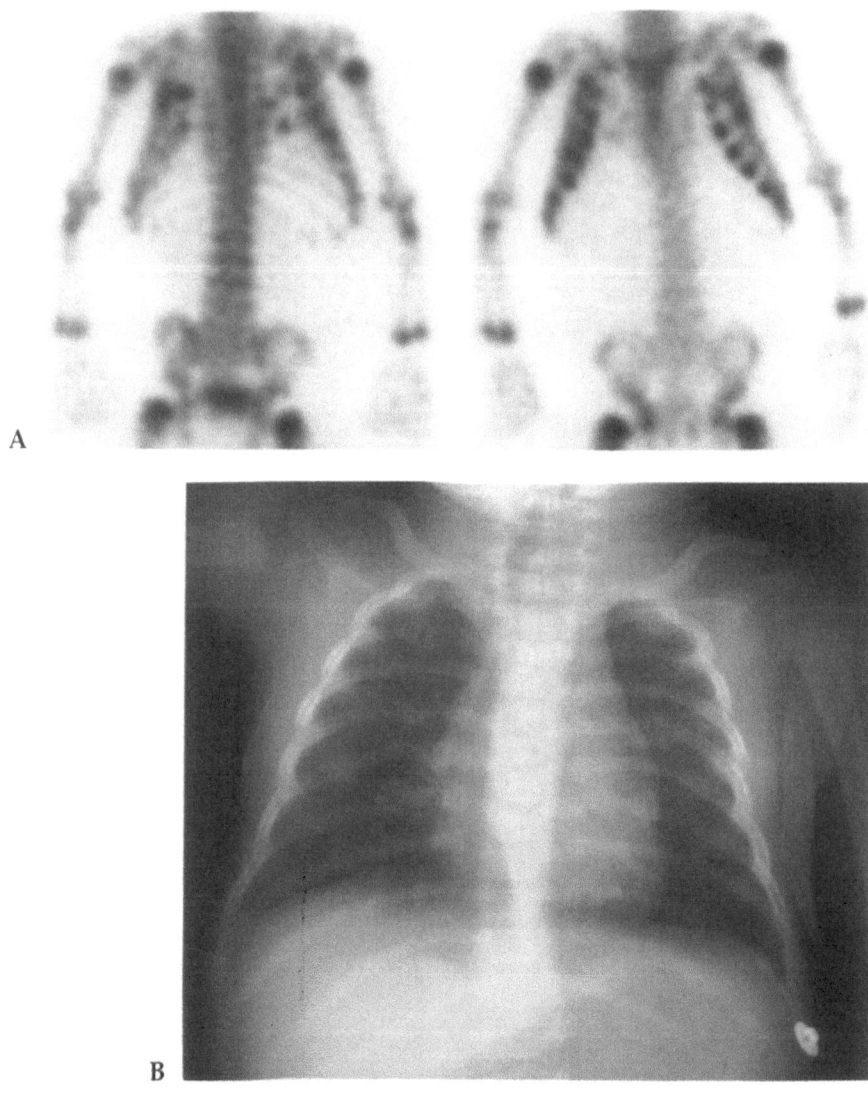

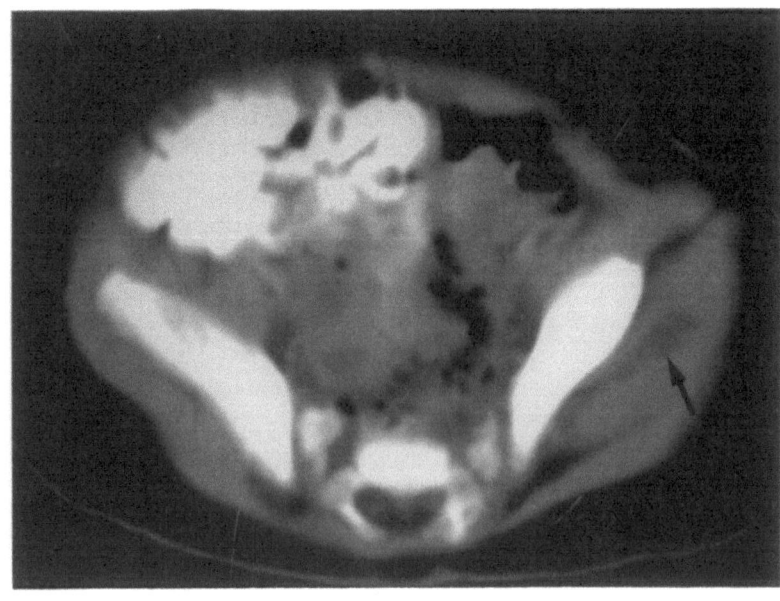

Figure 3.47. Child abuse. Skeletal scintigraphy reveals evidence of multiple posterior and lateral rib fractures (A). A chest radiograph also depicts multiple posterior rib fractures with variable amounts of callus suggesting that they are in different stages of healing (B). Abdominal CT of this 7-month-old girl shows a hematoma in the left gluteal musculature (C).

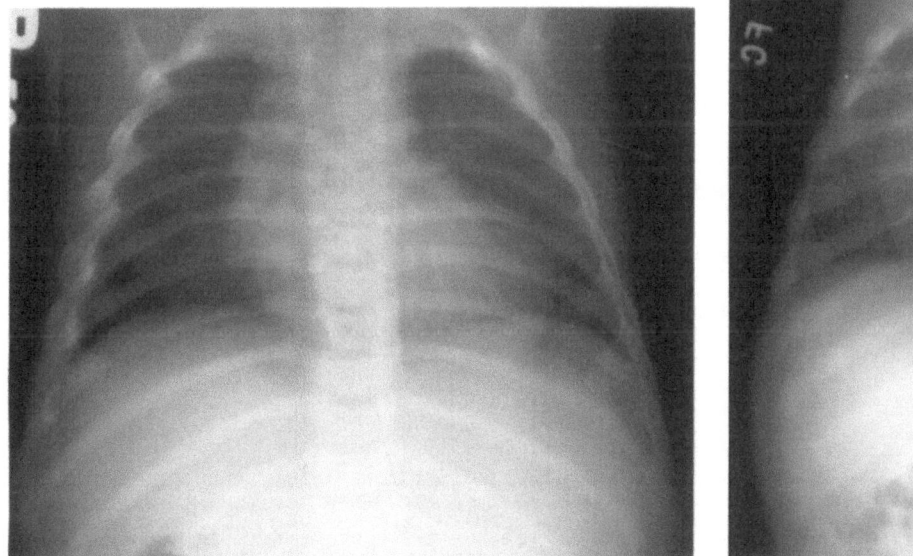
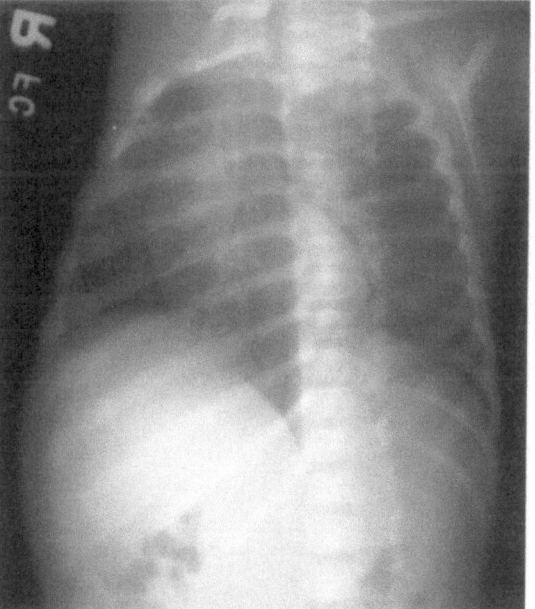

Figure 3.48. Child abuse. Skeletal scintigraphy (A) depicts sites of increased tracer localization in multiple right ribs. The right anterior oblique projection (lower left panel) and right lateral projection (lower right panel) assist in depicting the extent of injury to the anterolateral right third to eighth ribs. Callus associated with the right anterolateral rib fractures is identified radiographically (B,C).

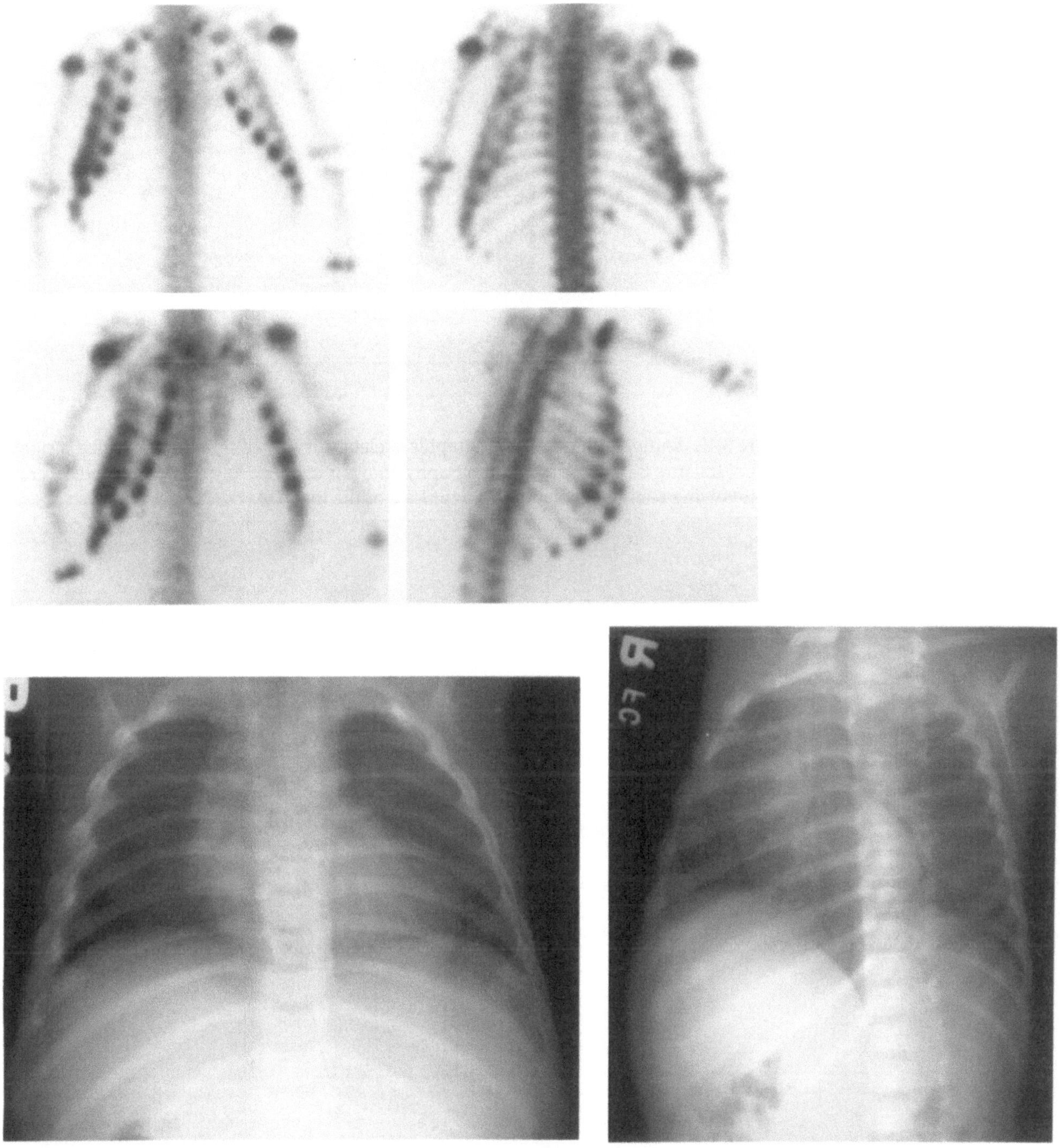

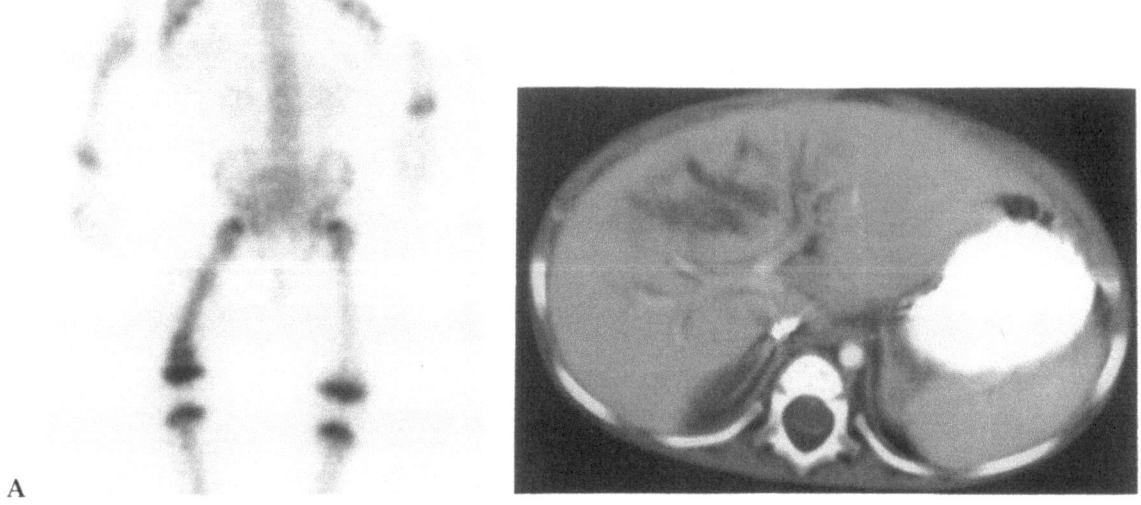

A   B

Figure 3.49. Radiographic and scintigraphic skeletal surveys of this child revealed a right femoral fracture (A). Computed tomography shows a complex low density stellate laceration involving a large portion of the right lobe of the liver (B).

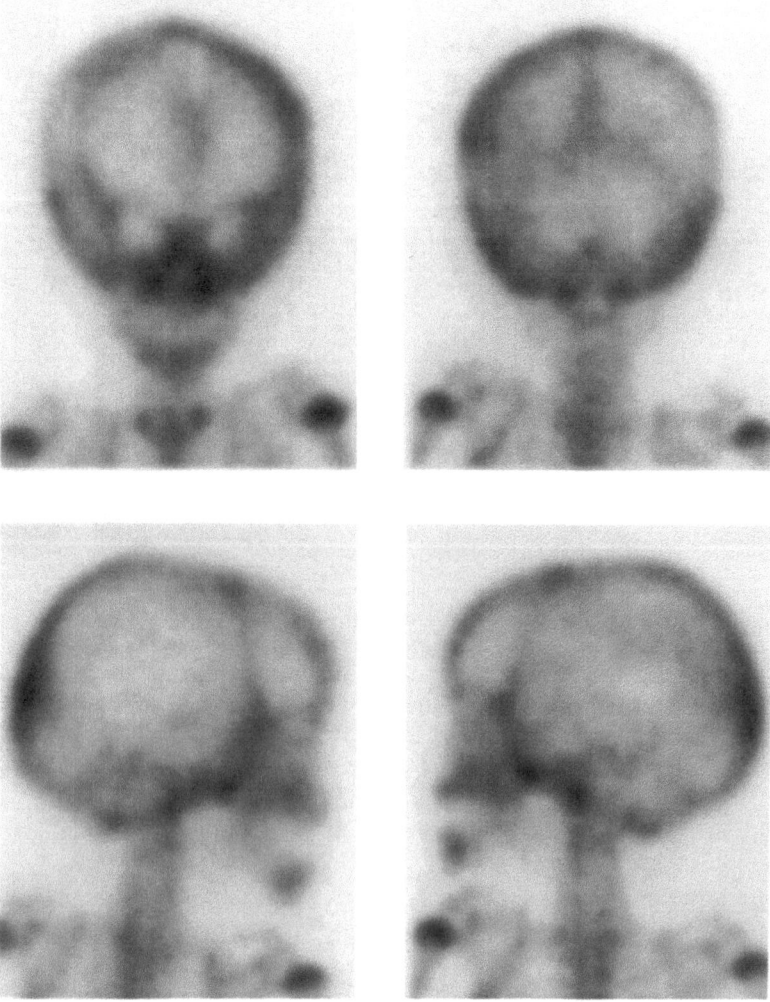

A

Figure 3.50. Child abuse. Asymmetric localization of ^{99m}Tc-MDP in the skull is noted (A). There is greater localization in the left than right temporal, parietal, and occipital bones (anterior, posterior, left and right lateral images).

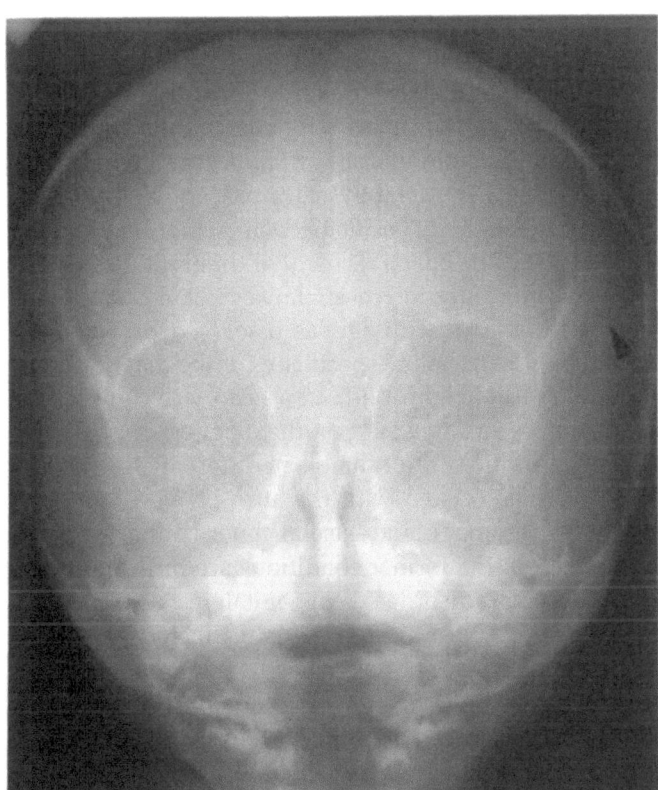

B

Figure 3.50. (*cont'd.*) Anteroposterior (B) and lateral (C) radiographs show a left parietal fracture (arrowhead and arrow). The fracture is confirmed and shown to be non-depressed with CT (D).

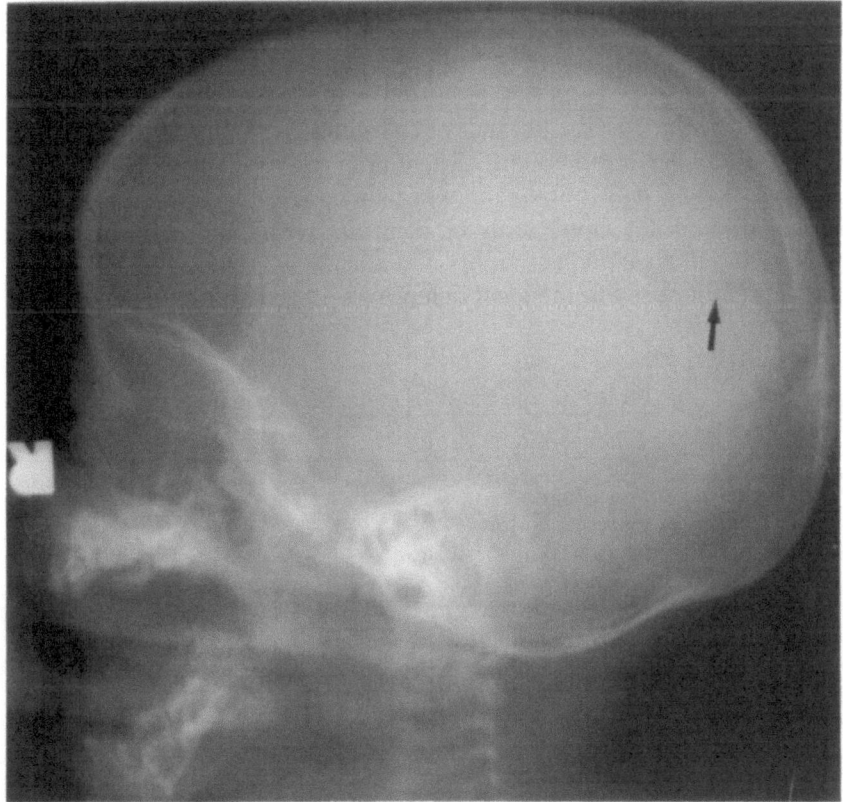

C

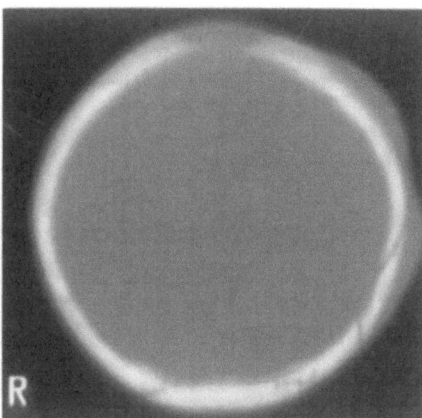

D

Injury Specificity and Differential Diagnosis

When approaching cases of suspected child abuse, imaging specialists are often questioned concerning the specificity of various injuries for child abuse. While no single type of injury is pathognomonic, certain injuries or patterns of injuries are highly specific for the diagnosis (Table 3.1). Metaphyseal, rib, scapular, spinous process, and sternal fractures carry the highest specificity. Demonstration of multiple fractures, particularly when they are bilateral, involve different anatomic regions, or are of different ages, significantly increases the suspicion of abuse.[41] The specificity of diaphyseal injuries varies with age, as discussed previously. Linear skull fractures are common but carry a low specificity for the diagnosis as they may occur with falls from a modest height. Without a history of significant trauma, depressed skull fractures more strongly suggest the diagnosis.[31]

Considerations regarding injury specificity are valuable in differentiating child abuse from other conditions that are associated with fractures or whose radiographic appearance simulates the appearance of the skeletal abnormalities seen in physically abused children. Included in the former conditions are birth trauma, osteogenesis imperfecta, neuromuscular disorders, congenital insensitivity to pain, and, in boys, Menkes' syndrome. Examples of the latter include disease states in which metaphyseal abnormalities are present, such as leukemia, rickets, congenital syphilis, scurvy, and Schmid-type metaphyseal chondrodysplasia, as well as conditions associated with prominent periosteal bone formation, such as the physiologic periosteal new bone formation seen in the first 2 to 8 months of life, infantile cortical hyperostosis (Caffey's disease), and hypervitaminosis A.[40,41,47]

Of the conditions associated with fracture, birth trauma and osteogenesis imperfecta warrant specific consideration. Birth trauma is associated with various fractures, most commonly clavicular or humeral fractures. Callus should be visible radiographically by 2 weeks of age; its absence implies that delivery was not causative.[40] Osteogenesis imperfecta (OI) is a group of disorders characterized by excessive bone fragility due to a disturbance of collagen formation. Clinical manifestations such as blue sclerae and abnormal dentition, and radiographic findings such as osteopenia, skeletal deformities, and wormian bones suggest the diagnosis in most cases.[47] Although OI should only be confused with child abuse in rare cases with mild to moderate osseous fragility and normal sclera (type IV OI), this distinction is frequently raised in the legal defense of alleged abuse.[41]

Table 3.1. Specificity of radiographic findings.

High specificity
   Metaphyseal lesions
   Posterior rib fractures
   Scapular fractures
   Spinous process fractures
   Sternal fractures
Moderate specificity*
   Multiple fractures, especially bilateral
   Fractures of different ages
   Epiphyseal separations
   Vertebral body fractures and subluxations
   Digital fractures
   Complex skull fractures
Common, but low specificity*
   Clavicular fractures
   Long bone shaft fractures
   Linear skull fractures

*Moderate- and low-specificity lesions become high when history of trauma is absent or inconsistent with injuries.
Reprinted from Kleinman,[39a] with permission.

Imaging Approach

Protocols for evaluating suspected victims of child abuse vary based on individual preferences and expertise. Certain points should be considered in developing an appropriate imaging strategy, however. First, a combined modality approach (scintigraphy and radiography) maximizes the detection of both individual victims and individual fractures. The importance of identifying individual victims is self-apparent. The significance of detecting individual fractures is that the social and legal outcomes of child abuse are related to the number, extent, and severity of lesions that are defined.[12,13,35,42] Second, scintigraphy has a greater sensitivity than radiographs for detecting skeletal trauma. In some cases, scintigraphy may provide the only evidence of skeletal trauma. In other cases, injuries that are not radiographically apparent at presentation become visible when a repeat radiographic survey is obtained 1 to 2 weeks later.[40,41] Skeletal scintigraphy lessens the need to perform a repeat radiographic study and the associated diagnostic delay and uncertainty. Scintigraphy is not so sensitive, however, that inconsequential, "day to day" trauma generally results in an abnormal study; in the setting of possible abuse, an abnormal study must be taken as evidence of significant trauma and closely correlated with the clinical history. Third, when fractures are detected, radiography is useful in estimating their age, in demonstrating displacement, and in excluding underlying pathology, such as osteogenesis imperfecta. Fourth, high-quality imaging, both radiographic and scintigraphic, must be performed and clinical diagnostic expertise must be available in any institution caring for abused children. Fifth, it must be emphasized that many abused children do not have evidence of skeletal trauma.[40,60] Further evaluation must never be deferred solely on the basis of normal radiographic and scintigraphic surveys.

Nonskeletal injuries associated with physical abuse are evaluated with anatomic cross-sectional studies, particularly CT (Figs. 3.45, 3.47, and 3.49). Although skeletal scintigraphy certainly cannot be relied on for this purpose, it should be carefully reviewed for manifestations of extraskeletal trauma. Craniocerebral trauma may be evidenced by the presence of radionuclide localization in a cephalohematoma, subdural hematoma, or cerebral contusion.[33] Increased renal localization of ^{99m}Tc-MDP has been related to renal contusion, traumatic myoglobinuria, and acute tubular necrosis in victims of child abuse.[33,82] Radionuclide localization in liver lacerations,[83] intestinal intramural hematomas, and muscular injury have also been observed in abused children.[33]

References

1. Albanese M, Pizzutillo PD, Family study of spondylolysis and spondylolisthesis. *J Pediatr Orthop* 1982;2:496–499.
2. Amato M, Totty WG, Gilula LA. Spondylolysis of the lumbar spine: demonstration of defects and laminal fragmentation. *Radiology* 1984;153:627–629.
3. Bellah RD, Summerville DA, Treves ST, et al. Low back pain in adolescent athletes: detection of stress injuries to the pars interarticularis with SPECT. *Radiology* 1991;180:509–512.
4. Birch JG, Herring JA, Maravilla KR. Splitting of the intervertebral disc in spondylolisthesis: a magnetic resonance imaging finding in 2 cases. *J Pediatr Orthop* 1986;6:609–611.
5. Blank S. Transverse tibial stress fractures: a special problem. *Am J Sports Med* 1981;9:322–325.
6. Blumberg K, Patterson RJ. The toddler's cuboid fracture. *Radiology* 1991;179:93–94.
7. Brodsky AE, Khalil MA. Talar compression syndrome. *Am J Sports Med* 1988;14:472–476.
8. Busch MT. Sports medicine. In: Morrisy RT, Weinstein SL, eds. *Lovell and Winter's Pediatric Orthopedics.* 4th ed. Philadelphia: Lippincott-Raven; 1996:1181–1228.

9. Carter DR. Mechanical loading histories and cortical bone remodelling. *Calcif Tissue Int* 1984;36:19–24.

10. Carty HM. Fractures caused by child abuse. *J Bone Joint Surg [Br]* 1993;75-B:849–857.

11. Cochrane GM. Osteitis pubis in athletes. *Br J Sports Med* 1971;5:233–235.

12. Conway JJ. Further comments on the role of the radionuclide skeletal survey in the diagnosis of the suspected abused child. *Radiology* 1983;148:574–575.

13. Conway JJ, Collins M, Tanz RR, et al. The role of bone scintigraphy in detecting child abuse. *Semin Nucl Med* 1993;23:321–333.

14. Dunbar JS. Obscure tibial fracture of infants—the toddler's fracture. *J Can Assoc Radiol* 1964;15:136–140.

15. Elliot S, Hutson MA, Wastie ML. Bone scintigraphy in the assessment of spondylolysis in patients attending a sports injury clinic. *Clin Radiol* 1988;39:269–272.

16. Fakharzadeh FF. Stress fracture of the finger in a bowler. *J Hand Surg [Am]* 1989;14:241–243.

17. Feldman KW, Brewer DK. Child abuse, cardiopulmonary resuscitation, and rib fractures. *Pediatrics* 1984;73:339–341.

18. Fernbach SK, Wilkinson RH. Avulsion injuries of the pelvis and proximal femur. *AJR* 1981;137:581–586.

19. Fredrickson BE, Baker D, McHolick WJ. The natural history of spondylolysis and spondylolisthesis. *J Bone Joint Surg [A]* 1984;66:699–707.

20. Freiberger R, Hersh A, Harrison M. Roentgen examination of the deformed foot. *Semin Roentgenol* 1970;5:341–353.

21. Fullerton LR, Snowdy HA. Femoral neck stress fractures. *Am J Sports Med* 1988;16:365–377.

22. Gelfand MJ, Ball WS, Oestreich AE, et al. Transient loss of femoral head Tc-99m diphosphonate uptake with prolonged maintenance of femoral head architecture. *Clin Nucl Med* 1983;8:347–354.

23. Gelfand MJ, Strife JL, Graham FJ, et al. Bone scintigraphy in slipped capital femoral epiphysis. *Clin Nucl Med* 1983;8:613–615.

24. Goldman AB, Pavlov H. Radionuclide bone scanning in subtalar coalitions: differential considerations. *AJR* 1982;138:427–432.

25. Grogan JP, Hemminghytt S, Williams AL, et al. Spondylolysis studied with computed tomography. *Radiology* 1982;145:737–742.

26. Hajek MR, Noble HB. Stress fractures of the femoral neck in joggers. *Am J Sports Med* 1982;10:112–116.

27. Hamilton WG. Foot and ankle injuries in dancers. *Clin Sports Med* 1988;1:143–173.

28. Hanson PG, Angevine M, Juhl JH. Osteitis pubis in sports activities. *Phys Sports Med* 1978;6:111–114.

29. Heinrichs EH, Senske BJ. Stress fracture of the ulnar diaphysis in athletes: case report and review of the literature. *South Dakota J Med* 1988;41:5–8.

30. Hershman EB, Mailly T. Stress fractures. *Clin Sports Med* 1990;1:183–214.

31. Hobbs CJ. Skull fracture and the diagnosis of abuse. *Arch Dis Child* 1984;59:246–252.

32. Holder LE, Michael RH. The specific scintigraphic pattern of "shin splints in the lower leg." *J Nucl Med* 1984;25:865–869.

33. Howard JL, Barron BJ, Smith GG. Bone scintigraphy in the evaluation of extraskeletal injuries from child abuse. *Radiographics* 1990;10:67–81.

34. Jackson DW, Wiltse LL, Cirincoine RJ. Spondylolysis in the female gymnast. *Clin Orthop* 1976;117:68–73.

35. Jaudes PK. Comparison of radiography and radionuclide bone scanning in the detection of child abuse. *Pediatrics* 1984;73:166–168.

36. Johnson DW, Farnum GN, Latchaw RE, et al. MR imaging of the pars interarticularis. *AJR* 1989;152:327–332.

37. Kaltsas DS. Stress fractures of the femoral neck in young adults. *J Bone Joint Surg [B]* 1981;63:33–37.

38. Kehl DK. Slipped capital femoral epiphysis. In: Morrisy RT, Weinstein SL, eds. *Lovell and Winter's Pediatric Orthopedics*. 4th ed. Philadelphia: Lippincott-Raven; 1996:993–1022.

39. Khoury MB, Kirks DR, Martines S, et al. Bilateral avulsion fractures of the anterior superior iliac spines in sprinters. *Skeletal Radiol* 1995;13:65–67.

39a. Kleinman PK. *Diagnostic Imaging of Child Abuse*. Baltimore: Williams & Wilkins; 1987.

40. Kleinman PK. Diagnostic imaging in infant abuse. *AJR* 1990;155:703–712.

41. Kleinman PK. Imaging of child abuse: an update. In: Kirks DR, ed. *Emergency Pediatric Radiology*. Reston, VA: American Roentgen Ray Society; 1995:189–195.

42. Kleinman PK, Blackbourne BD, Marks SC, et al. Radiologic contributions to the investigation and prosecution of cases of fatal infant abuse. *N Engl J Med* 1989;320:507–511.

43. Kleinman PK, Marks SC, Blackbourne B. The metaphyseal lesion in abused infants: a radiologic-histopathologic study. *AJR* 1986;146:895–905.

44. Kleinman PK, Marks SC, Richmond JM, et al. Inflicted skeletal injury: a postmortem radiologic-pathologic study in 31 infants. *AJR* 1995;165:647–650.

45. Lanyon LE. Functional strain as a determinant for bone remodelling. *Calcif Tissue Int* 1984;35:56–61.

46. Lanyon LE. Functional strain in bone tissue as an objective, and controlling stimulus for adaptive bone remodelling. *J Biomech* 1987;20:1083–1093.

47. Laor T, Jaramillo D, Oestrich A. Skeletal system. In: Kirks DR, ed. *Practical Pediatric Imaging. Diagnostic Radiology of Infants and Children*. 3rd ed. Philadelphia: Lippincott-Raven; 1997:327–510.

48. Lateur LM, Van Hoe LR, Van Ghillewe KV, et al. Subtalar coalition: diagnosis with the C sign on lateral radiographs of the ankle. *Radiology* 1994;193:847–851.

49. Lawson JP. Symptomatic radiographic variants in extremities. *Radiology* 1985;157:625–631.

50. Lonstein JE. Spondylolysis and spondylolisthesis. In: Morrisy RT, Weinstein SL, eds. *Lovell and Winter's Pediatric Orthopedics*. 4th ed. Philadelphia: Lippincott-Raven; 1996:717–737.

51. Lowe J, Schachner E, Hirschberg E, et al. Significance of bone scintigraphy in symptomatic spondylolysis. *Spine* 1984;9:653–655.

52. Lusins JO, Elting JJ, Cicoria AD, et al. SPECT evaluation of lumbar spondylolysis and spondylolisthesis. *Spine* 1994;19:608–612.

53. Maffuli N, King JB. Effects of physical activity on some components of the skeletal system. *Sports Med* 1992;13:393–407.

54. Martire JR. The role of nuclear medicine bone scans in evaluating pain in athletic injuries. *Clin Sports Med* 1987;6:713–737.

55. Matheson GO, Clement DB, McKenzie DC, et al. Scintigraphic uptake of ^{99m}Tc at nonpainful sites in athletes with stress fractures. The concept of bone strain. *Sports Med* 1987;4:65–75.

56. Matheson GO, Clement DB, McKenzie DC, et al. Stress fractures in athletes. A study of 320 cases. *Am J Sports Med* 1987;15:46–58.

57. Matin P. The appearance of bone scans following fractures, including immediate and long term studies. *J Nucl Med* 1979;20:1227–1231.

58. Matin P. Basic principles of nuclear medicine techniques for detection and evaluation of trauma and sports medicine injuries. *Semin Nucl Med* 1988;18:90–112.

59. McKee BW, Alexander WJ, Dunbar JS. Spondylolysis and spondylolisthesis in children: a review. *J Can Assoc Radiol* 1971;22:100–109.

60. Merten DF, Radkowski MA, Leonidas JC. The abused child: a radiological reappraisal. *Radiology* 1983;146:377–381.

61. Michael RH, Holder LE. The soleus syndrome. A cause of medial tibial stress (shin splints). *Am J Sports Med* 1985;13:87–94.

62. Miller JH, Sanderson RA. Scintigraphy of toddler's fracture. *J Nucl Med* 1988;29:2001–2003.

63. Morgan RC, Cranford AH. Surgical management of tarsal coalition in adolescent athletes. *Foot Ankle* 1986;7:183–193.

64. Mubarak SJ, Gould RN, Lee YF, et al. The medial tibial stress syndrome. *Am J Sports Med* 1982;10:201–205.

65. Noakes TD, Smith JA, Lindenberg G, et al. Pelvic stress fractures in long distance runners. *Am J Sports Med* 1985;13:120–123.

66. Orava S, Jormakka E, Hulkko A. Stress fractures in young athletes. *Acta Orthop Trauma Surg* 1981;98:271–274.

67. Ozonoff MB. *Pediatric Orthopedic Radiology*. 2nd ed. Philadelphia: W.B. Saunders; 1992.

68. Papanicolaou N, Wilkinson RH, Emans JB, et al. Bone scintigraphy and radiology in young athletes with low back pain. *AJR* 1985;145:1039–1044.

69. Pavlov H. Roentgen examination of groin and hip pain in the athlete. *Clin Sports Med* 1987;6:829–843.

70. Read MT. Single photon emission computed tomography (SPECT) scanning for adolescent back pain. A sine qua non? *Br J Sports Med* 1994;28:56–57.

71. Rettig AC, Shelbourne KD, McCarroll JR, et al. The natural history and treatment of delayed union stress fractures of the anterior cortex of the tibia. *Am J Sports Med* 1988;16:250–255.

72. Roach PJ, Cooper RA, Watson AS. Arm splints seen on bone scan in a volleyball player. *Clin Nucl Med* 1993;18:900–901.

73. Rosen PR, Micheli LJ, Treves ST. Early scintigraphic diagnosis of bone stress and fractures in athletic adolescents. *Pediatrics* 1982;70:11–15.

74. Rupani HD, Holder LE, Espinola DA, et al. Three-phase radionuclide bone imaging in sports medicine. *Radiology* 1985;156:187–196.

75. Sedlak AJ, Broadhurst DD. *Executive Summary of the Third National Incidence Study of Child Abuse and Neglect.* Washington, DC: Government Printing Office; 1996.

76. Sella EJ, Lawson JP, Ogden JA. The accessory navicular synchondrosis. *Clin Orthop* 1986;209:280–285.

77. Semon RL, Spengler D. Significance of lumbar spondylolysis in college football players. *Spine* 1981;6:172–174.

78. Smergel EM, Harcke T, Pizzutillo PD, et al. Use of bone scintigraphy in the management of slipped capital femoral epiphysis. *Clin Nucl Med* 1987;12:349–353.

79. Smith FW, Gilday DL, Ash JM, et al. Unsuspected costovertebral fractures demonstrated by bone scanning in the child abuse syndrome. *Pediatr Radiol* 1980;10:103–106.

80. Starshak RJ, Simons GW, Sty JR. Occult fracture of the calcaneus—another toddler's fracture. *Pediatr Radiol* 1984;14:37–40.

81. Stoskopf CA, Hernandez RJ, Kelikian A, et al. Evaluation of tarsal coalition by computed tomography. *J Pediatr Orthop* 1984;4:365–369.

82. Sty JR, Starshak RJ. The role of bone scintigraphy in the evaluation of the suspected abused child. *Radiology* 1983;146:369–375.

83. Sty JR, Wells RG. Child abuse: extraosseous abdominal bone imaging uptake. *Clin Nucl Med* 1994;19:1011.

84. Sty JR, Wells RG, Conway JJ. Spine pain in children. *Semin Nucl Med* 1993;23:296–320.

85. Sty JR, Wells RG, Starshak RJ, Gregg D. The musculoskeletal system. In: Sty J, Wells R, Starshak R, Gregg D, eds. *Diagnostic Imaging of Infants and Children.* Vol. 3. Gaithesburg: Aspen; 1992:233–405.

86. Sugimoto H, Ohsawa T. Ulnar collateral ligament in the growing elbow: MR imaging of normal development and throwing injuries. *Radiology* 1994;192:417–422.

87. Sullivan JA. The child's foot. In: Morrisy RT, Weinstein SL, eds. *Lovell and Winter's Pediatric Orthopedics.* 4th ed. Philadelphia: Lippincott-Raven; 1996:1077–1135.

88. Sundar M, Carty H. Avulsion fractures of the pelvis in children: a report of 32 fractures and their outcome. *Skeletal Radiol* 1994;23:85–90.

89. Taylor JA, Sartoris DJ, Huang GS, et al. Painful conditions affecting the first metatarsal sesamoid bones. *Radiographics* 1993;13:817–830.

90. Thomas SA, Rosenfield NS, Leventhal JM, et al. Long bone fractures in young children: distinguishing accidental injuries from child abuse. *Pediatrics* 1991;88:471–476.

91. Toridis TG. Stress analysis of the femur. *J Biomech* 1969;2:163–174.

91a. Treves ST, Connolly LP, Kirkpatrick JA, et al. Bone. In: Treves ST (ed) Pediatric Nuclear Medicine. 2nd ed. New York: Springer-Verlag 1995:233–301.

92. Tullos HS, Erwin WD, Woods GW, et al. Unusual lesions of the pitching arm. *Clin Orthop* 1972:88:169–182.

93. van den Oever M, Merrick MV, Scott JH. Bone scintigraphy in symptomatic spondylolysis. *J Bone Joint Surg [B]* 1987;69:453–456.

94. Veselko M, Smrkolj V. Avulsion of the anterior-superior iliac spine in athletes: case reports. *J Trauma* 1994;36:444–446.

95. Wechsler RJ, Schweitzer ME, Deely DM, et al. Tarsal coalition: depiction and characterization with CT and MR imaging. *Radiology* 1994;193:447–452.

96. Wilkinson RH, Hall JE. The sclerotic pedicle: tumor or pseudotumor. *Radiology* 1974;111:683–688.

97. Wiltse LL. The etiology of spondylolisthesis. *J Bone Joint Surg [A]* 1963;44:539–569.

98. Wolfgang GL. Stress fracture of the femoral neck in a patient with open femoral capital epiphyses. *J Bone Joint Surg [A]* 1977;59:680–681.

99. Wynne-Davies R, Scott JH. Inheritance and spondylolisthesis; a radiographic family survey. *J Bone Joint Surg [B]* 1979;61:301–305.

100. Zwas ST, Elkanovitch R, Frank G. Interpretation and classification of bone scintigraphic findings in stress fractures. *J Nucl Med* 1987;28:452–457.

4
Benign Conditions

This chapter reviews benign conditions of bone, in which skeletal scintigraphy plays an important role in diagnosis or follow-up. Conditions for which scintigraphy is not generally requested but whose frequency demands a familiarity on the part of pediatric nuclear medicine practitioners are also addressed.

Benign Bone-Forming Tumors

Osteoid Osteoma

Osteoid osteoma is a relatively common osseous lesion that is best considered a benign neoplasm, although a variety of possible etiologies, including inflammatory, traumatic, and vascular have been suggested.[55] Microscopically, osteoid osteoma consists of a central nidus that contains osteoid, osteoblasts, and vascular channels. The nidus, which is less than 1.5 cm in size, may be situated in cortical, medullary, or cancellous bone or in a subperiosteal location. It is often surrounded by dense reactive trabecular bone, particularly when cortical in location.

The majority of osteoid osteomas are located in the appendicular skeleton. Femoral and tibial locations account for more than 50% of all cases. In the long bones, these lesions are either diaphyseal or metaphyseal. Vertebral osteoid osteomas occur in the posterior elements and account for approximately 7% of cases.[55]

Osteoid osteomas are predominantly detected in adolescents and young adults. There is a male predominance. The tumor is rare in nonwhites. Pain, the most frequent presenting complaint, is believed to be related to a high concentration of prostaglandins[63] within the nidus. This hypothesis proposes that increased intralesional pressure due to a prostaglandin-mediated vasodilatation stimulates afferent nerve endings.[99] A classic symptom complex of nocturnal pain relieved by salicylates is present in a minority of patients.[55]

The typical radiographic appearance of a cortical osteoid osteoma is a radiolucency, corresponding to the nidus, with surrounding sclerosis and cortical thickening.[111] Cancellous osteoid osteomas incite a less intense sclerotic reaction that may be distant from the nidus. Cancellous osteoid osteomas often occur in an intraarticular location, particularly at the hip. Synovitis and joint fluid are often associated with such lesions. Other locations of cancellous osteoid osteomas include the small bones of the hands and feet and posterior elements of the spinal column. With vertebral lesions, the nidus is typically near or at the apex of a scoliotic curve. Subperiosteal osteoid osteomas, which are rare, excavate the cortex and produce minimal or no reactive sclerosis.[55]

Skeletal scintigraphy is essentially 100% sensitive for the detection of osteoid osteomas.[62] Whole body scintigraphy is particularly useful diagnostically when referred pain results in a radiographic examination missing an osteoid osteoma completely[116] and in cases where symptoms precede the development of a radiographic abnormality.[99] As the radiographic manifestations of diseases such as osteomyelitis, stress fracture, and osteosarcoma overlap with those of osteoid osteoma,[30] skeletal scintigraphy is also valuable when the classic findings are not present.

Prominent tracer delivery and early localization are often, but not invariably, noted on radionuclide angiography and tissue phase imaging (Fig. 4.1). The skeletal phase images typically show well-localized, focal, marked tracer localization in osteoid osteomas (Figs. 4.1–4.6). A characteristic pattern of intense localization in the nidus surrounded by less prominently increased localization in reactive bone has been described (Fig. 4.3).[41,42] This pattern is most commonly, although not uniformly, observed with lesions of the appendicular skeleton and is best demonstrated by pinhole magnification imaging.[91] Although not entirely specific for osteoid osteoma, the pattern is very highly suggestive of the diagnosis and is probably most closely associated with a cortical nidus. Single photon emission computed tomography (SPECT) is useful in localizing an osteoid osteoma in anatomically complex areas such as the spine (Fig. 4.4).

Thin section computed tomography (CT) is also useful in evaluating suspected osteoid osteomas that do not demonstrate the classic radiographic appearance and in delineating the nidus (Figs. 4.2–4.5). With CT, the nidus of an osteoid osteoma appears as a well-defined, oval or round, low-attenuation lesion that contains variable amounts of mineralization.[55] Magnetic resonance imaging (MRI) may also demonstrate the nidus (Fig. 4.6) but is generally less reliable than CT for this purpose. Due to the presence of extensive marrow and soft tissue edema, MRI may be suggestive of a more aggressive process.[2,40] As a whole-body examination is not practical with either CT or MRI, skeletal scintigraphy is the study of choice in cases where the location of a clinically suspected osteoid osteoma is uncertain.

Removal or ablation of the nidus provides pain relief. Surgically, this is accomplished with either en bloc resection of the nidus and adjacent reactive bone or with curettage of the nidus. Block resection can markedly weaken the strength of the bone in which the osteoid osteoma is located and may necessitate a bone graft to repair the operative defect. Curettage is much less likely to structurally weaken the affected bone, but may leave some of the nidus unexcised. This is an extremely important consideration as the nidus must be excised completely for pain relief.

Various scintigraphic techniques facilitate the localization of a nidus for curettage and ensure its complete excision, both of which are rendered difficult by the marked reactive bone formation commonly associated with an osteoid osteoma.[88,103,108,112] We favor intraoperative pinhole imaging with a mobile gamma camera. This technique most reliably ensures complete excision of the nidus (Figs. 4.5 and 4.6).

Prior to surgery, all patients undergo diagnostic skeletal scintigraphy, preferably within a few days of surgery. For intraoperative scintigraphy, radiopharmaceutical is administered 4 hours prior to surgery. After surgical exposure of the involved bone, a scintigraphic image is recorded using a mobile gamma camera fitted with a pinhole collimator and enclosed in a sterile drape. Using a computer display monitor, a ^{99m}Tc point source is superimposed over the nidus. After localizing the nidus in this way, the surgeon completes an attempt at its excision and an image is obtained to determine if the nidus has been excised in its entirety. When this image reveals residual tissue with avid tracer localization, further excision is carried out. This process is repeated until there is no remaining area of focally intense tracer localization. A second scintigraphic technique involves the use of a radiosensitive scintillation probe and imaging or autoradiography of the specimen.[34,120] A third scintigraphic method, in vitro imaging of the excised specimen without examination of the operative field,[48] can demonstrate that some of the nidus has been removed but can not confirm its complete excision.

Recently, nonoperative techniques designed to limit bone resection in patients with osteoid osteoma have been successfully applied. These include CT-guided percutaneous excision,[4,69,113] which is optimized with immediate scintigraphic confirmation of a nidus's complete removal,[92] and CT-guided radiofrequency electrode ablation.[94] Medical management with long-term use of nonsteroidal antiinflammatory agents is an alternative employed in cases where excision carries a significant risk of disability or would be highly complex.[53] This approach is supported by the concept that osteoid osteoma is a self-limited lesion that eventually heals. The 6 to 15 years that this healing process may require[38,75,119] is unacceptably long in many cases, however.

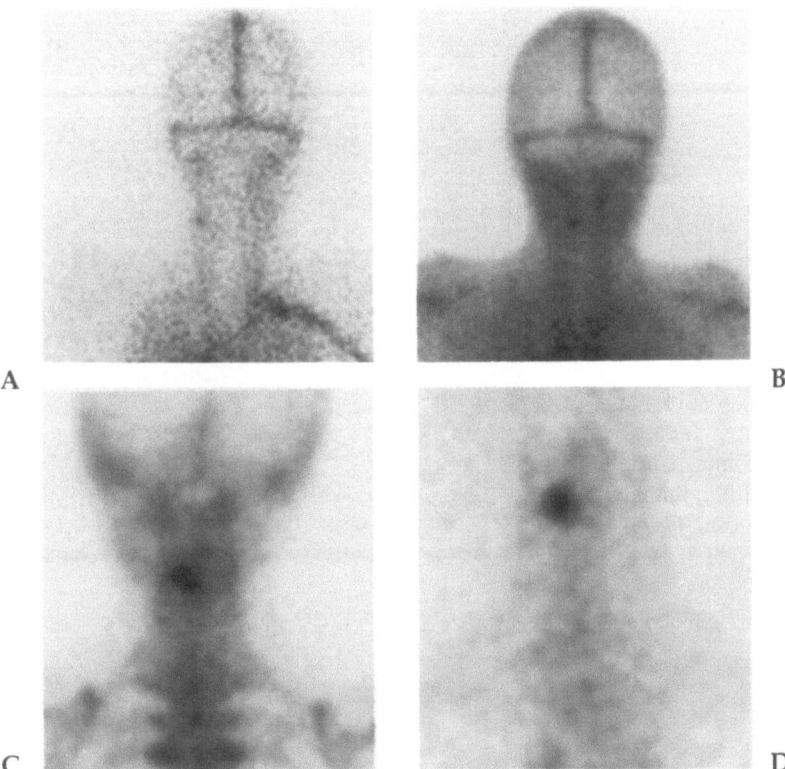

A B C D

Figure 4.1. Osteoid osteoma. Tracer delivery and early tracer localization is minimally increased in an osteoid osteoma of the left C4 pedicle as shown with posterior projections of radionuclide angiography (A) and tissue phase imaging (B). Posterior high-resolution (C) and pinhole magnification (D) skeletal phase imaging depict intensely increased tracer localization in the nidus.

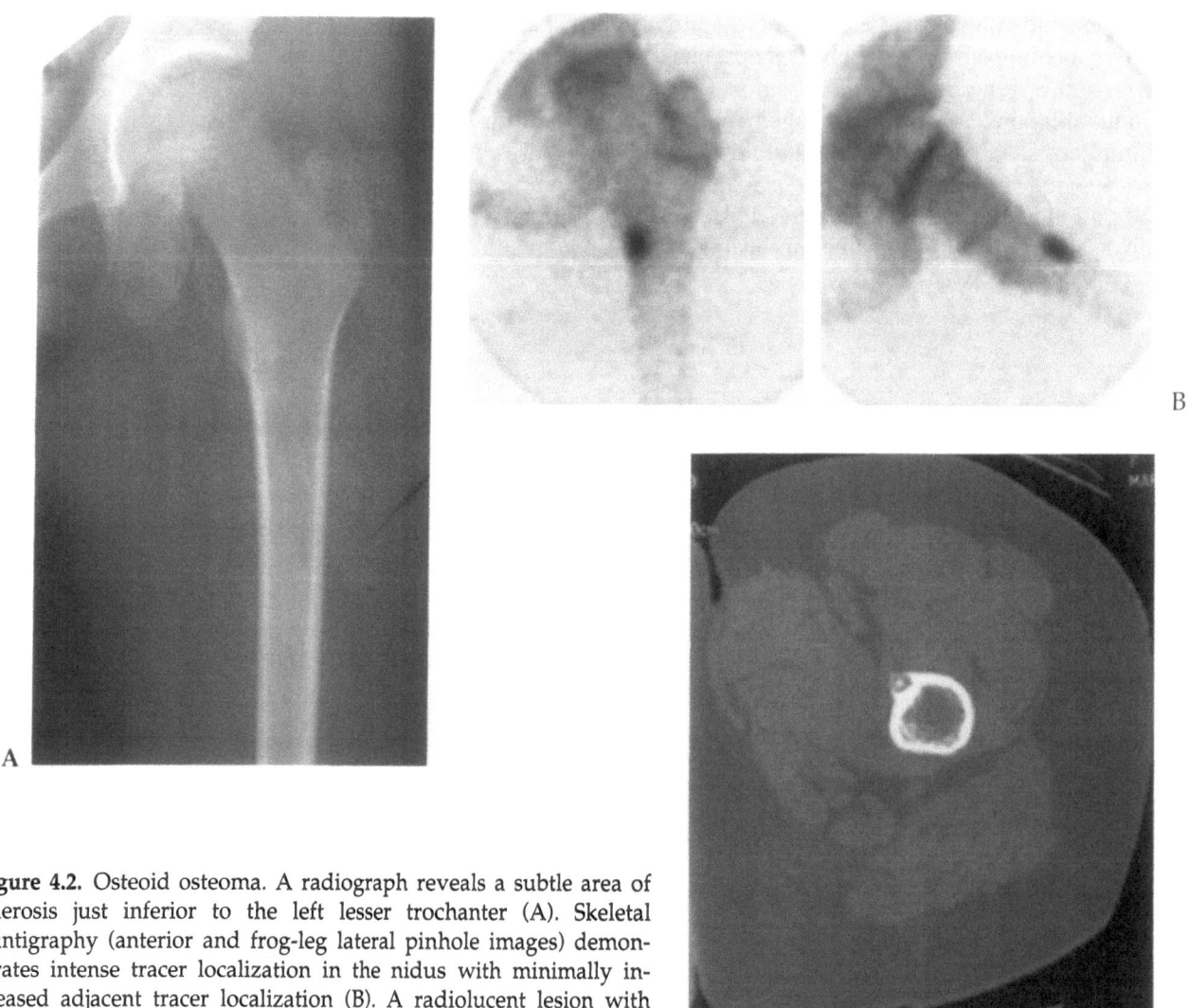

Figure 4.2. Osteoid osteoma. A radiograph reveals a subtle area of sclerosis just inferior to the left lesser trochanter (A). Skeletal scintigraphy (anterior and frog-leg lateral pinhole images) demonstrates intense tracer localization in the nidus with minimally increased adjacent tracer localization (B). A radiolucent lesion with central calcification is shown with CT (C).

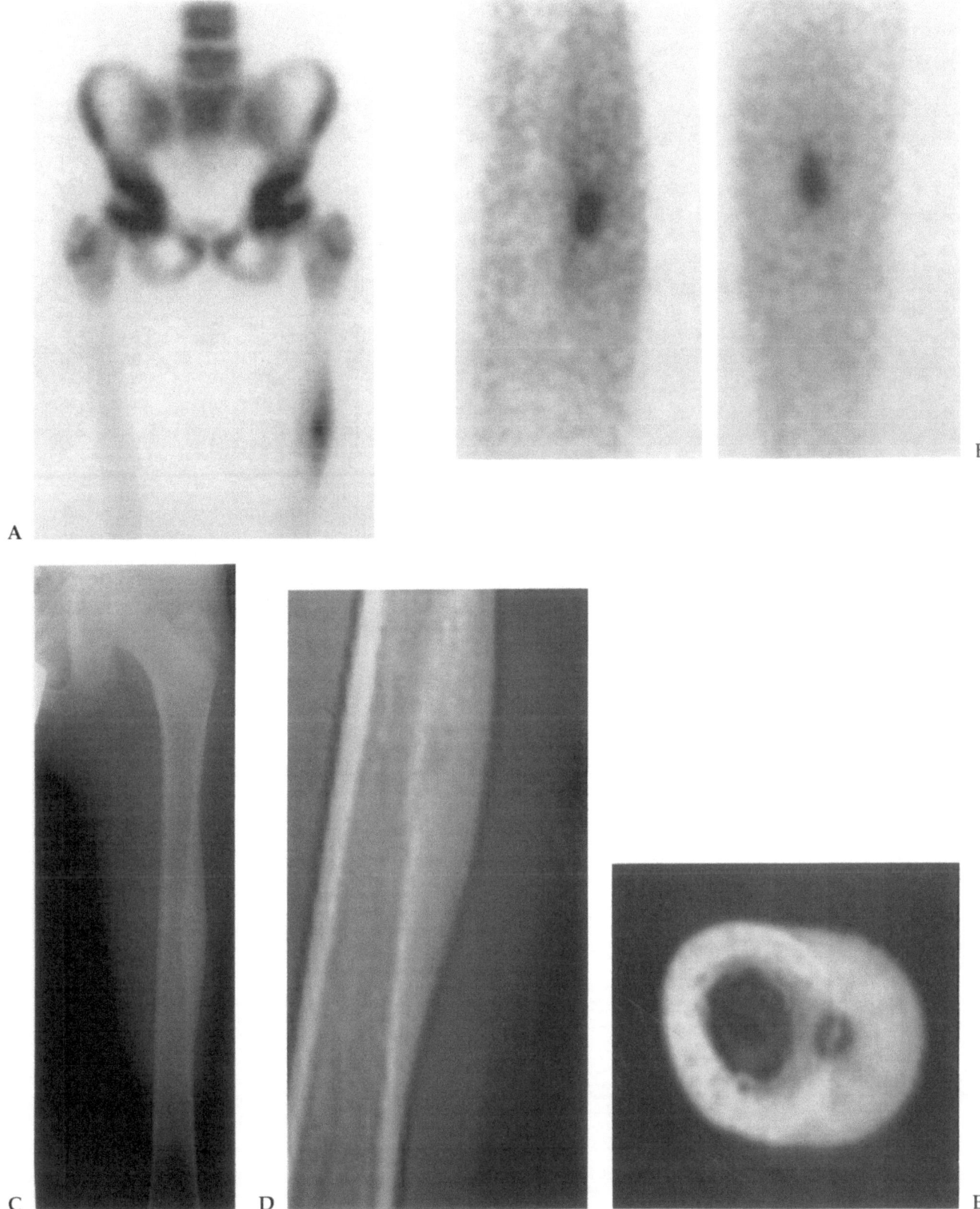

Figure 4.3. Osteoid osteoma. High-resolution planar (A) and pinhole scintigraphy (B, anterior and lateral projections) show markedly increased focal tracer localization in the nidus of an osteoid osteoma. This is surrounded by less prominently increased tracer localization in reactive bone. Extensive cortical thickening surrounding the radiolucent nidus is shown with a radiograph (C) and with a scout image obtained for CT (D). The nidus is depicted by CT (E).

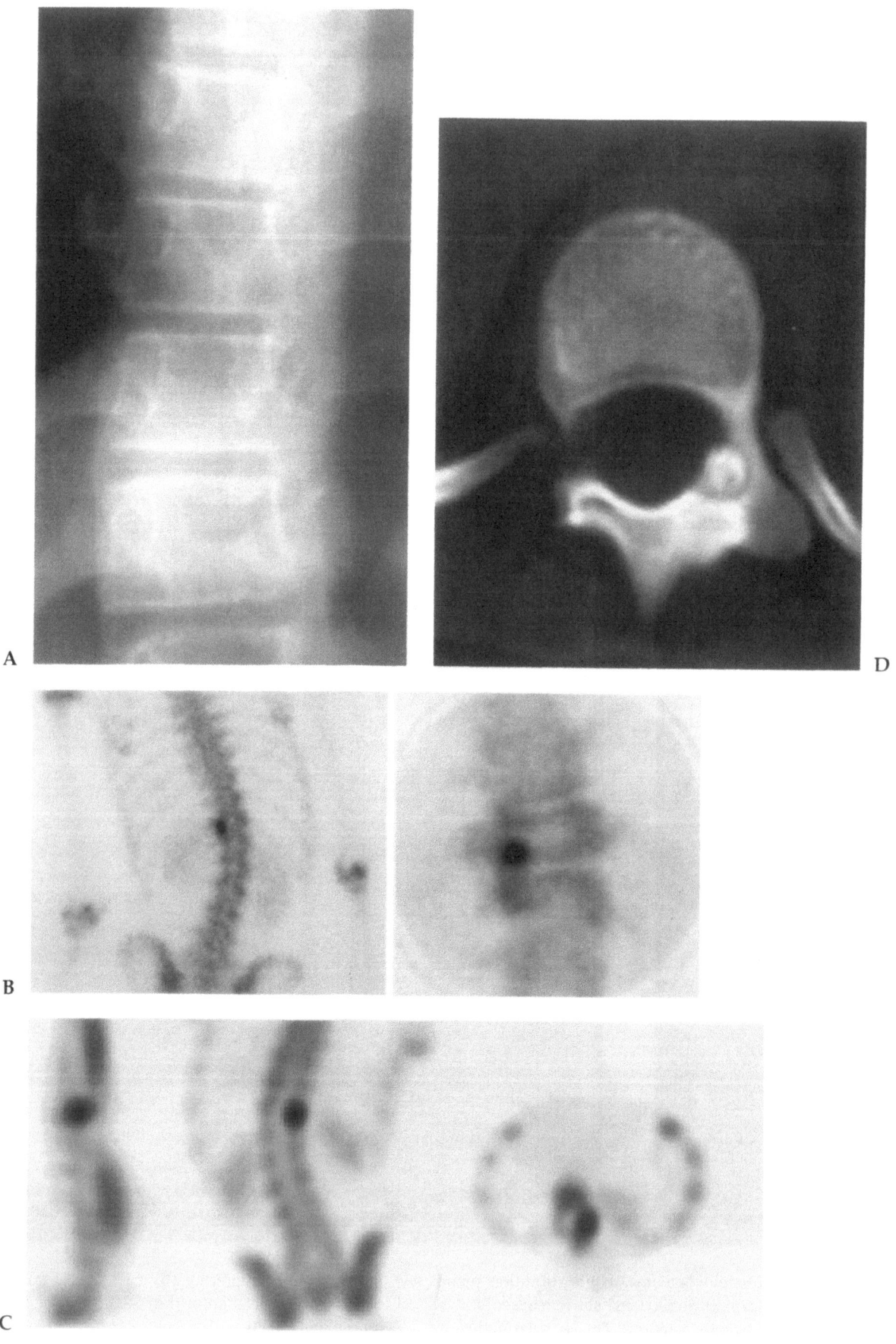

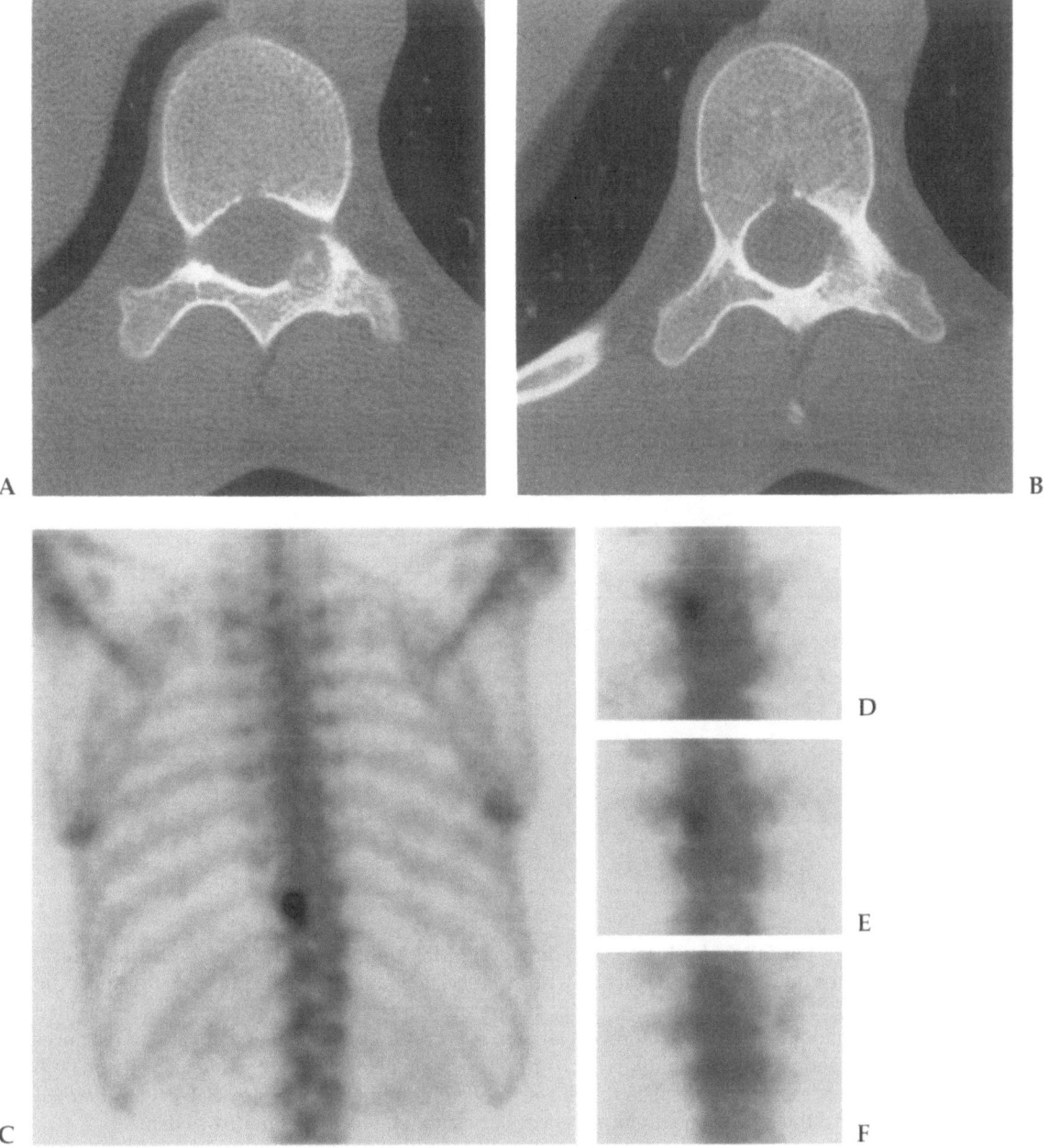

Figure 4.5. Osteoid osteoma. Computed tomography depicts calcification within the radiolucent nidus in the left pedicle of T10 (A) and adjacent sclerosis (B). Skeletal scintigraphy shows intense tracer localization in the nidus (C). Intraoperative pinhole scintigraphy also demonstrates focal tracer accumulation prior to attempted excision (D). Following an initial attempt at removal, focal tracer localization persisted (E). After further curettage, this was no longer present (F).

◀────

Figure 4.4. Osteoid osteoma. An anteroposterior radiograph of T8–T11 (A) of a child with a suspected osteoid osteoma demonstrates thoracic scoliosis convex to the right. An osteoid osteoma is not identified. High-resolution and pinhole magnification skeletal scintigraphy (B: posterior projections) demonstrate intense tracer localization at T11 in the nidus of an osteoid osteoma. Slightly increased adjacent tracer localization is shown with pinhole imaging. SPECT (C) shows the position of the nidus in the left pedicle of T11. Computed tomography (D) depicts the osteoid osteoma as a sclerotic lesion with an eccentrically positioned radiolucency.

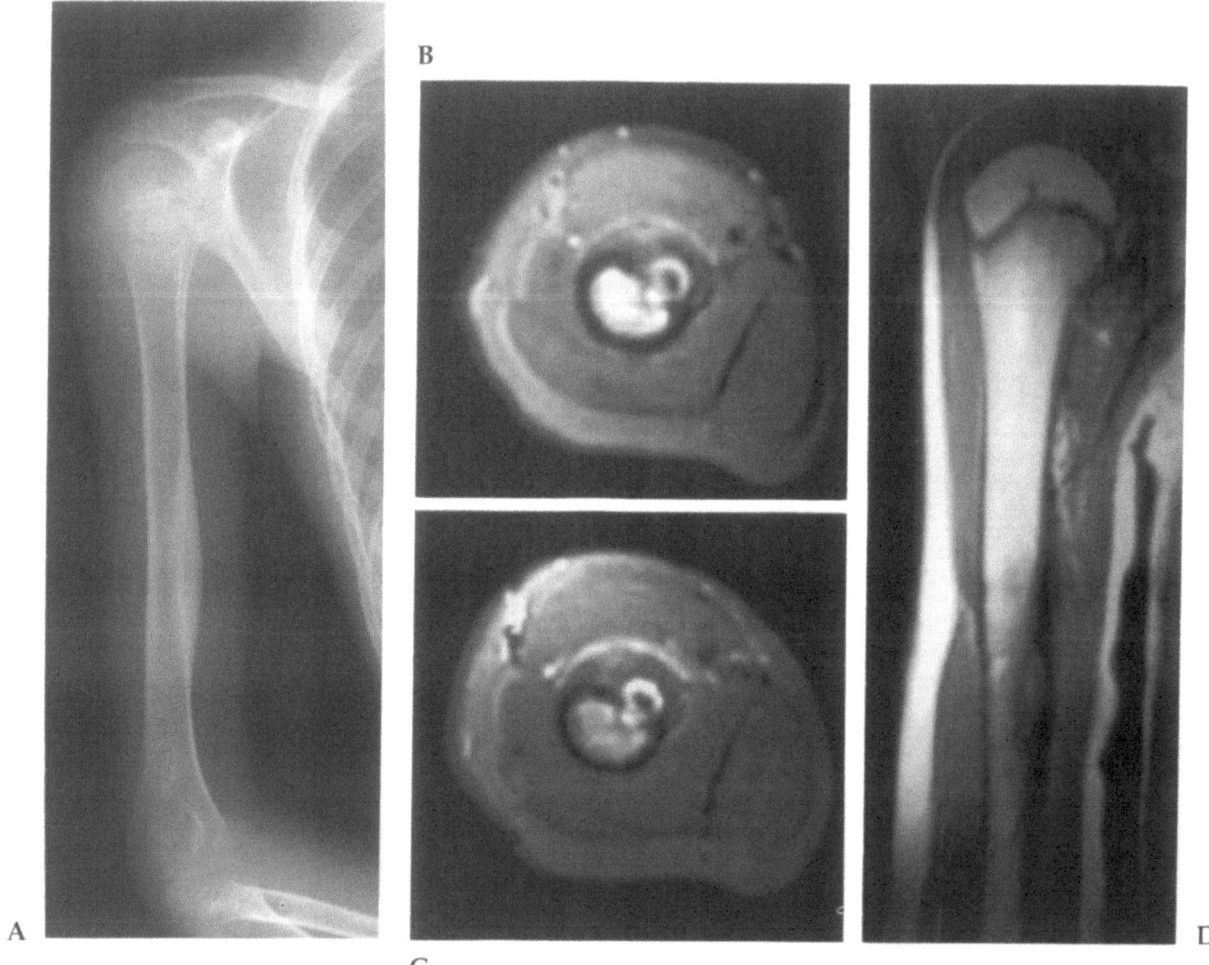

A

B

C

D

Figure 4.6. Osteoid osteoma. A radiograph of the right humerus (A) demonstrates thick, uninterrupted periosteal reaction with an associated radiolucency. Transaxial fast spin echo (FSE) T2-weighted images with fat saturation (B,C) and a coronal T1-weighted postgadolinium image (D) reveal an area of cortically based high T2 signal that enhances with gadolinium. The nidus, which appears as a small focus of low signal intensity on both sequences, is better depicted with the T2-weighted images. It is associated with marked cortical thickening and abnormal medullary signal indicative of marrow edema.

Osteoblastoma

Osteoblastoma is an uncommon lesion that is most often discovered in patients younger than 30 years of age. It is histologically similar to osteoid osteoma. A primary point of differentiation is size; the nidus of an osteoblastoma is larger than 1.5 cm. Osteoblastomas are most commonly located in the spine, particularly the posterior elements, and the long tubular bones. Some osteoblastomas are locally aggressive and there are rare cases of malignant change to osteosarcoma. Radiographically, an osteoblastoma may appear lytic, sclerotic, or demonstrate a mixed lytic-sclerotic pattern.[84,86,116] Scintigraphy can reveal intense tracer localization in an osteoblastoma, similar to that observed with osteoid osteoma (Fig. 4.7).

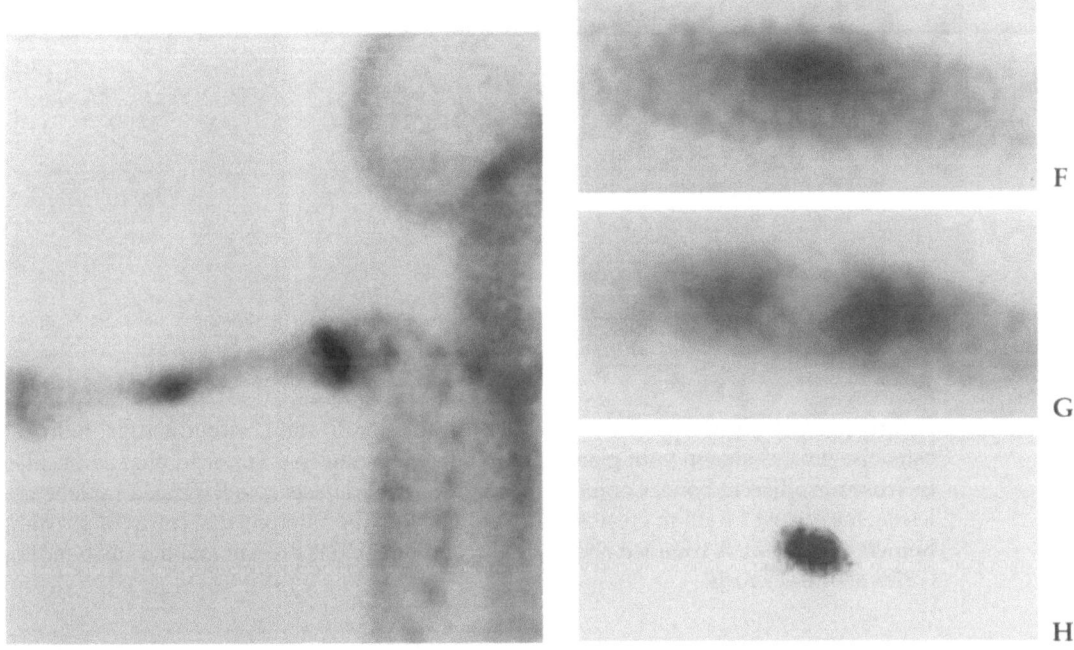

Figure 4.6 *(cont'd)*. Skeletal scintigraphy depicts focally intense tracer localization within the nidus and less prominently increased localization in adjacent reactive bone (E). Intraoperative pinhole scintigraphy shows the same pattern prior to excision (F). Immediately following excision, this is no longer present (G). The specimen shows intense tracer localization (H).

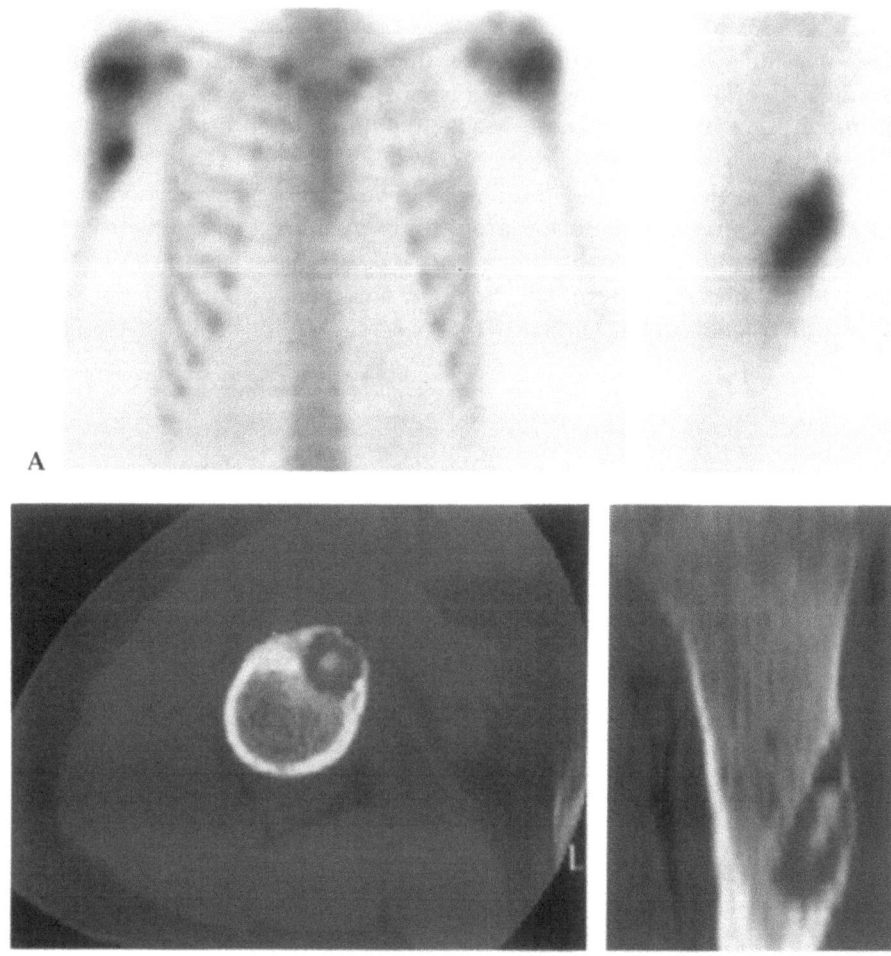

Figure 4.7. Osteoblastoma. There is intense tracer localization within a right humeral osteoblastoma as shown with planar and pinhole imaging (A). Tracer localization is also increased in adjacent bone. Computed tomography (B) depicts a well-defined radiolucent lesion, measuring 2.6 cm in greatest dimension, within the anteromedial cortex of the right humeral diaphysis. A rounded and sclerotic central region is present and the surrounding cortex shows sclerosis.

Benign Cortical Lesions

Fibrous Cortical Defect and Nonossifying Fibroma

Fibrous cortical defect and nonossifying fibroma are histologically similar cortical rests of fibrous tissue that are collectively referred to as benign cortical defects. These lesions are rarely identified in children prior to 18 months of age or in adults. The highest incidence is between the ages of 5 and 6 years. Benign cortical defects are present in 30% to 40% of children during development.[102] The vast majority are located in the lower extremities, particularly adjacent to the knee. The posteromedial distal femur is the most common location. Unilateral and bilateral benign cortical defects occur with equal frequency. The natural history is one of gradual healing through replacement by normal bone.[90]

Benign cortical defects are usually detected on radiographs performed to assess an unrelated complaint. Fibrous cortical defects appear radiographically as intracortical radiolucencies, often with sclerotic rims. They are typically 1 to 3 cm in diameter. Nonossifying fibromas, which represent persistence and enlargement of fibrous cortical defects, appear as eccentrically positioned, often multiloculated metaphyseal or metadiaphyseal radiolucencies.[78,109] The radiographic appearance of benign cortical defects is sufficiently characteristic that additional diagnostic imaging is rarely necessary.

Skeletal scintigraphy of benign cortical defects may reveal moderately increased tracer localization within the lesion (Fig. 4.8) or along its sclerotic margins (Fig. 4.9), although many produce little or no scintigraphic abnormality (Figs. 4.10 and 4.11). When markedly increased localization is present, pathologic fracture, cortical disruption, or associated bone stress should be considered (Fig. 4.12).[7,35]

The MRI appearance of benign cortical defects varies with the stage of healing. Decreased T2 signal due to collagen and hemosiderin deposition is frequently present. A peripheral zone of enhancement is typically seen on T1-weighted images following gadolinium.[89]

Multiple fibrous cortical defects occur in neurofibromatosis type I[64] and, in association with café-au-lait spots but without neurofibromas, in Jaffe-Campanacci syndrome.[105] Multiple fibrous cortical defects also occur in otherwise healthy children.

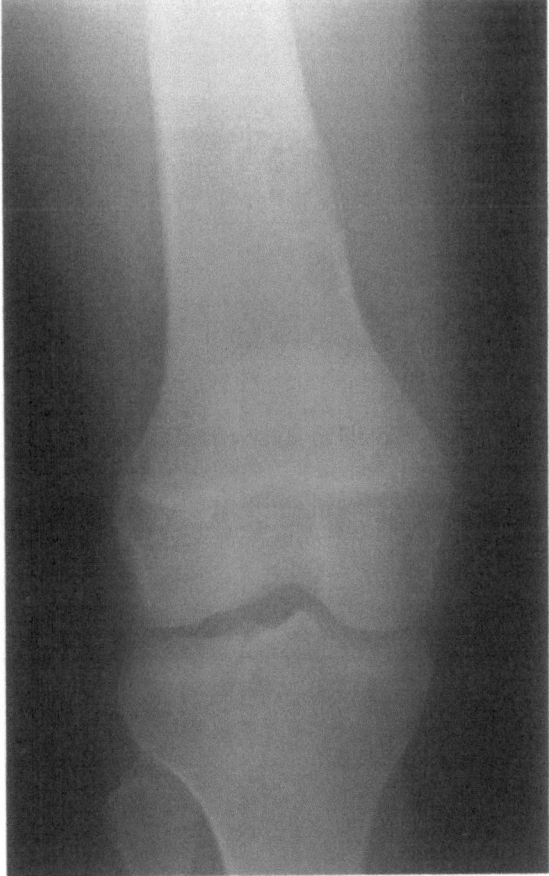

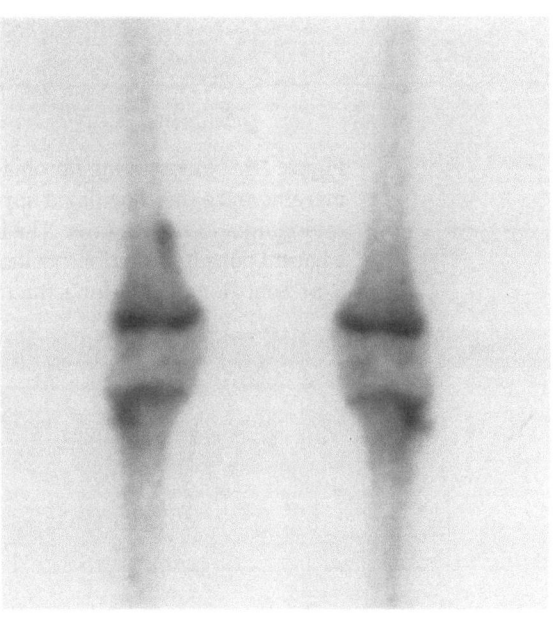

Figure 4.8. Nonossifying fibroma. A radiograph (A) depicts an eccentrically positioned multiloculated radiolucency with sclerotic margins in the distal right femoral metadiaphysis. The cortex appears thinned but not disrupted. Skeletal scintigraphy (B) shows increased tracer localization in the lesion.

A

B

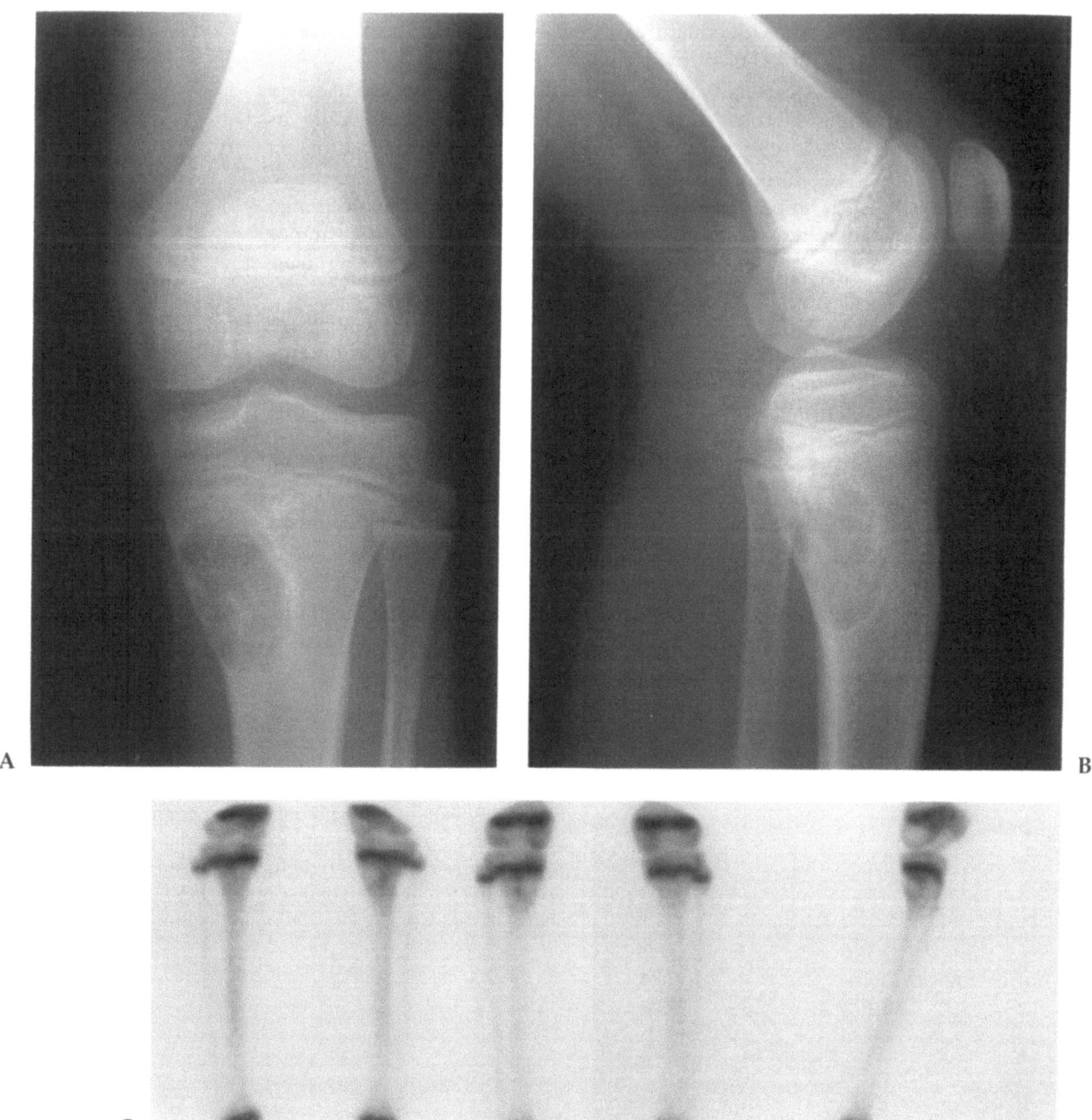

Figure 4.9. Nonossifying fibroma. A metadiaphyseal tibial radiolucent lesion with sclerotic margins and a multiloculated appearance is shown with anteroposterior (A) and lateral (B) radiographs of the left knee. The lesion has slightly decreased tracer localization relative to adjacent bone (C, anterior, posterior, and medial projections). Increased tracer localization is present along the lesion's inferior, medial, and posterior margins.

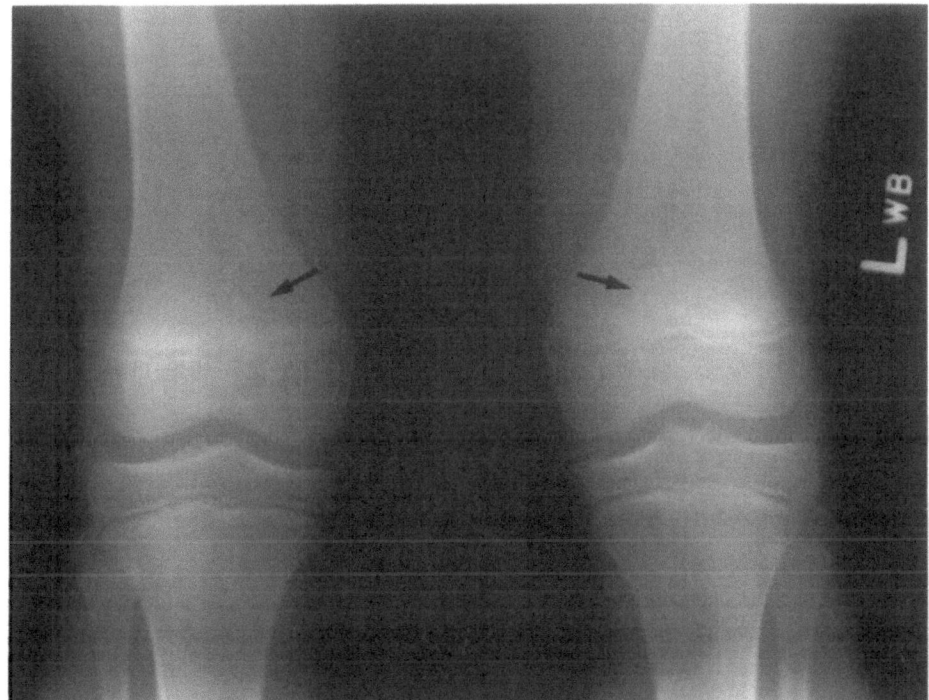

A

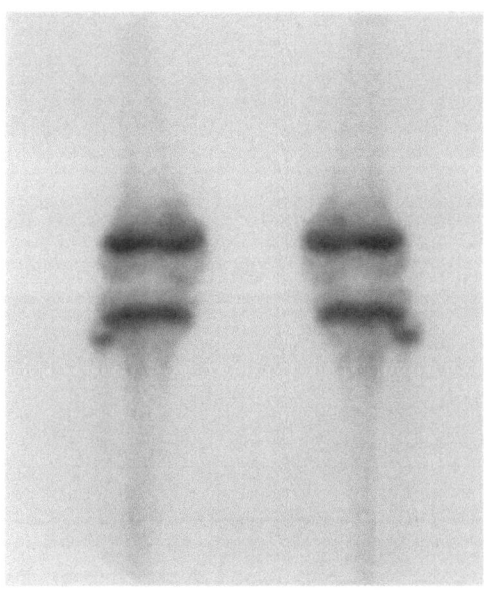

B

Figure 4.10. Fibrous cortical defects. A radiograph (A) reveals bilaterally symmetric radiolucencies with sclerotic rims in the distal femoral metaphyses (arrows). Skeletal scintigraphy (B) is essentially normal; it shows only a subtle degree of increased tracer localization corresponding to the fibrous cortical defects.

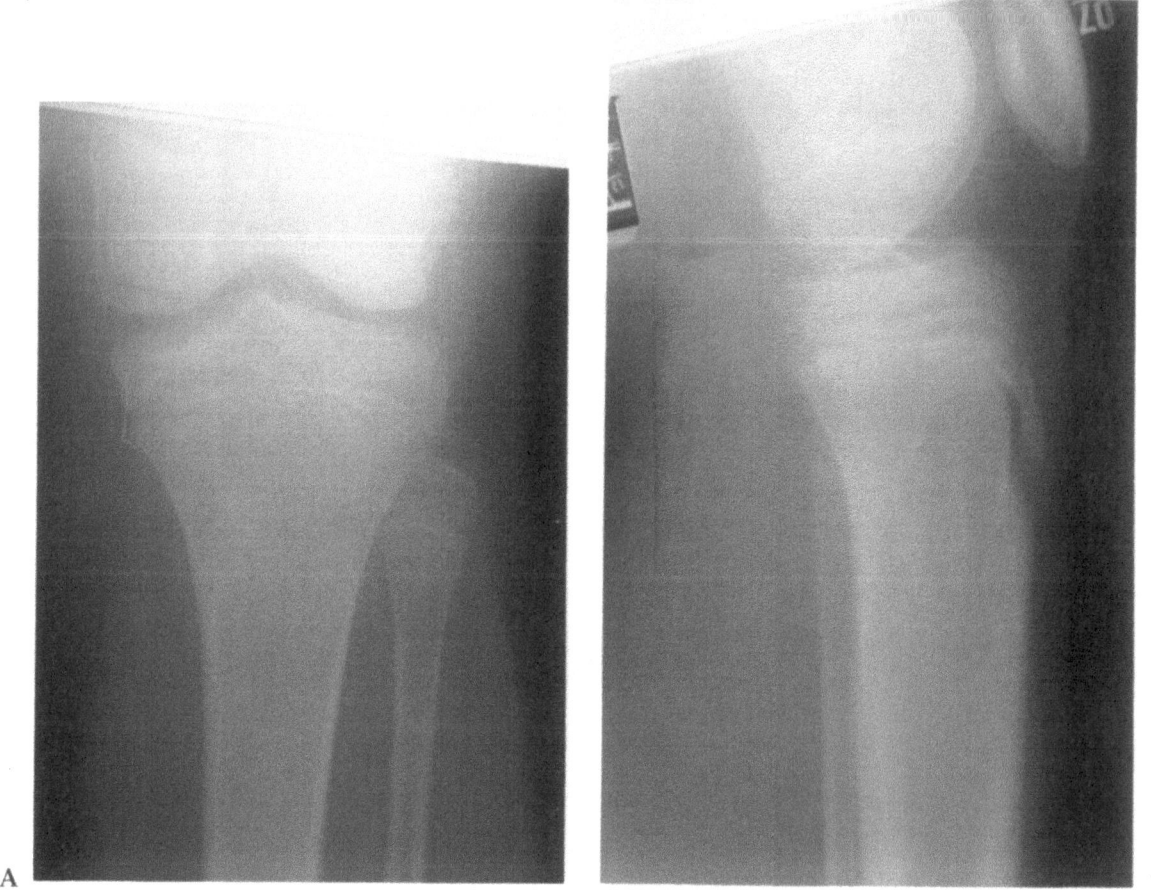

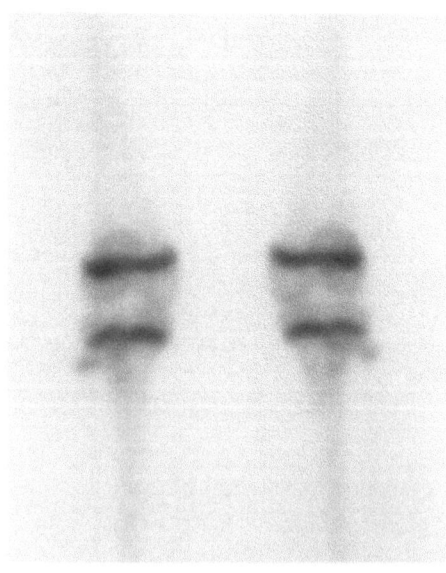

Figure 4.11. Nonossifying fibroma. Anteroposterior (A) and lateral (B) radiographs of the left knee demonstrate a radiolucent lesion with a sclerotic border in the metadiaphyseal tibia. The nonossifying fibroma is not convincingly demonstrated with skeletal scintigraphy (C, anterior projection).

Avulsive Cortical Irregularity

Avulsive cortical irregularity (distal femoral metaphyseal irregularity of child-hood, cortical desmoid) is a common radiographic finding in children between 3 and 17 years of age.[51] It occurs more frequently in boys and is often bilateral. The characteristic radiographic appearance is an area of irregular cortical margination along the posterior medial femoral condyle just superior to the adductor tubercle. Small cortical fragments may be demonstrated in the adjacent soft tissues. An adjacent benign cortical defect is often present.[59] Repetitive stress at the site of the attachment of the medial head of the gastrocnemius or adductor magnus muscles has been implicated as the etiology.[85,125]

The characteristic radiologic appearance and anatomic location of avulsive cortical irregularities along with patient age provide the diagnosis in the vast majority of cases. Biopsy, which may result in an erroneous diagnosis of osteosarcoma, should be avoided. In questionable cases or when acute symptoms are present, further imaging evaluation may prove beneficial. The first and simplest step is to obtain a radiograph of the contralateral extremity as avulsive cortical irregularities are often bilateral. A normal skeletal scintigram, which is typical with avulsive cortical irregularities, aids in confirming the diagnosis when there is a diagnostic uncertainty (Fig. 4.13).[10,57] Minimally increased tracer localization due to the avulsive etiology or an associated benign cortical defect does not exclude the diagnosis. Magnetic resonance imaging is useful in showing a rim of low signal at the origin of the medial head of the gastrocnemius and in revealing a contralateral radiographically occult avulsive cortical irregularity. Hypointense T1 and hyperintense T2 signal are visible with MRI, which may also reveal adjacent marrow edema.[125]

Figure 4.12. Nonossifying fibroma. A multilocular radiolucent lesion is present in the distal left tibial metadiaphysis (A, lateral radiograph).

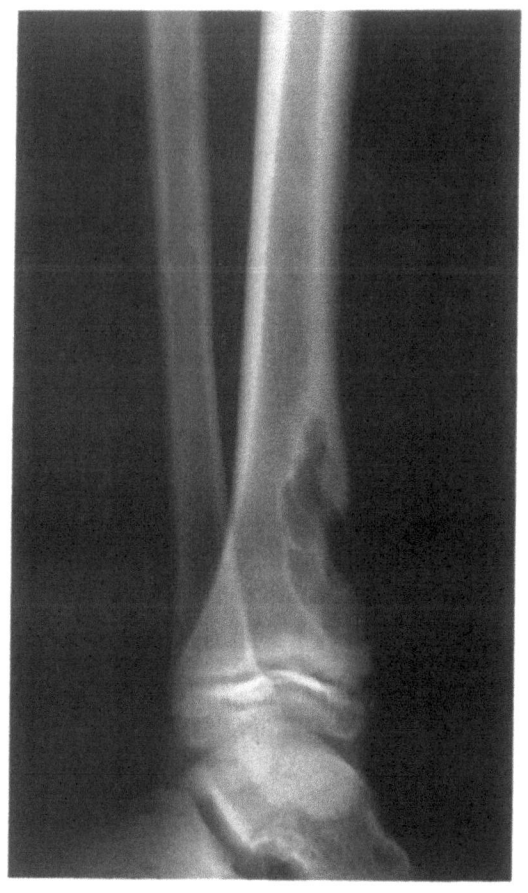

A

B

Figure 4.12 (*Cont.d*). Radionuclide angiography and tissue phase imaging show increased tracer delivery and localization (B, left panels).

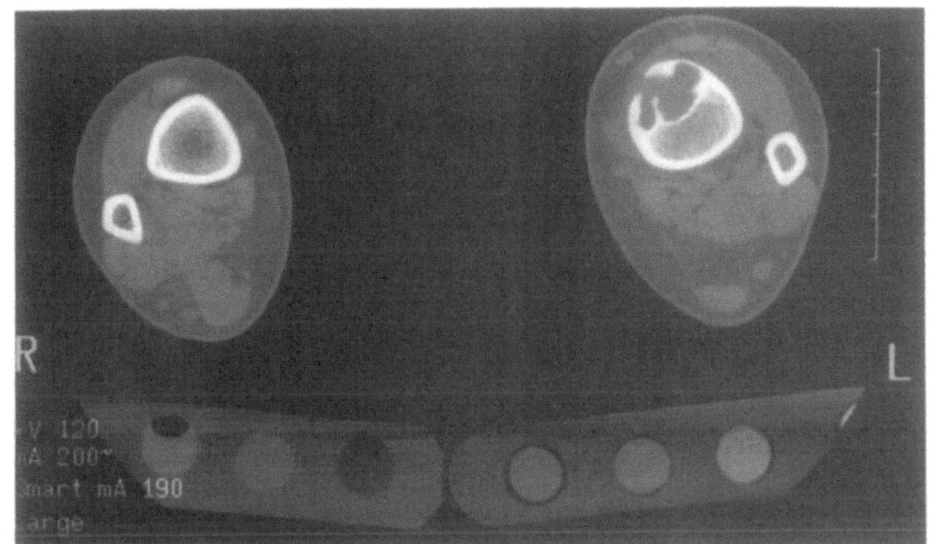

C

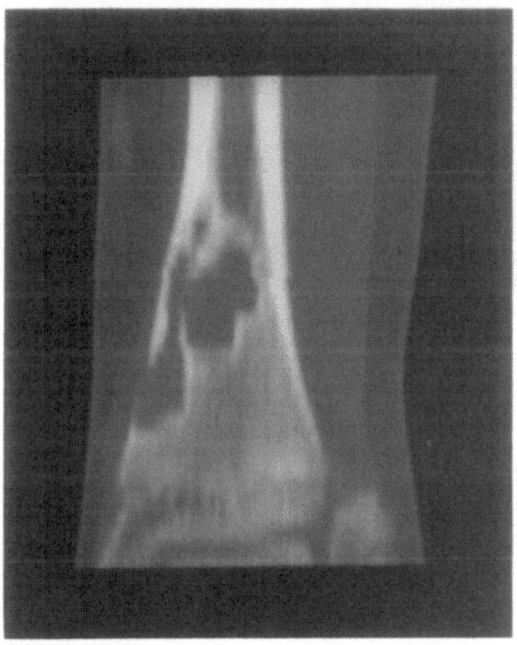

D

Figure 4.12 (*Cont.d*). Increased tracer localization is also shown by skeletal phase imaging (B, right panel). Computed tomography (C,D) demonstrates an area of cortical disruption.

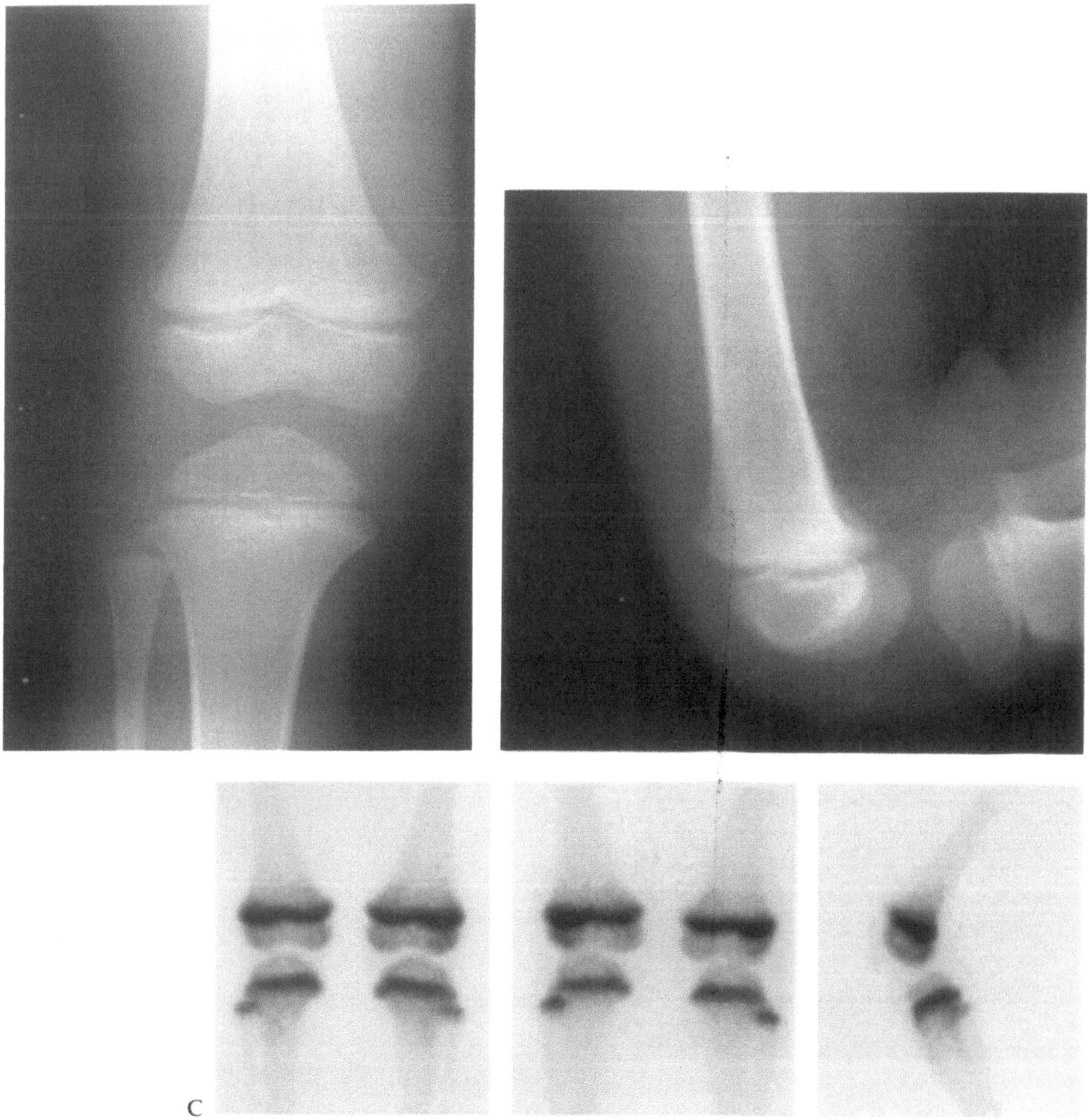

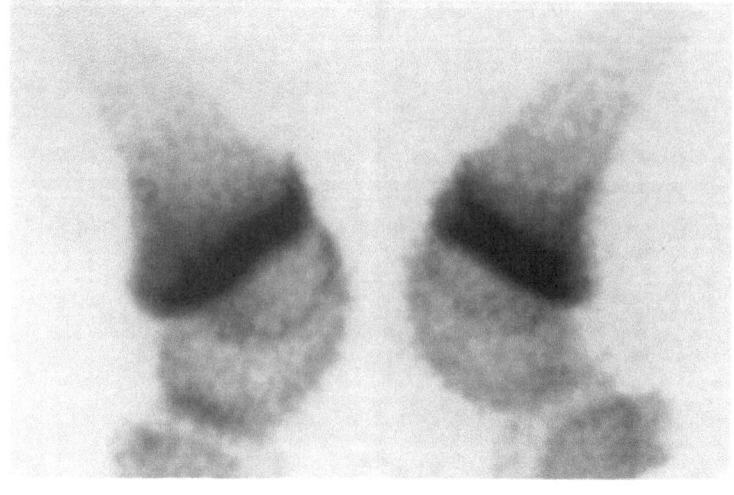

Figure 4.13. Avulsive cortical irregularity. Anteroposterior (A) and lateral (B) radiographs of the right femur reveal the distal femoral metaphysis to have a radiolucent appearance with spiculation of the cortical margin posteriorly. Anterior, posterior, and right medial projections from skeletal scintigraphy are normal (C). Medial pinhole images of the left (D) and right (E) distal femurs show a symmetric appearance to the distal femurs.

Cystic Lesions

Simple Bone Cyst

Simple bone cyst accounts for nearly 15% of all bone lesions. The presumed etiology is interstitial fluid stasis secondary to trauma or venous obstruction. The lesion is more commonly diagnosed in males than females. It consists of serosanguineous or serous fluid-filled cavities with thin fibrous linings. As many as 95% of simple bone cysts occur in the long bones. Proximal humeral and proximal femoral locations account for up to 75% to 85% of all cases. Simple bone cysts also occur in the pelvis (Fig. 4.14) and calcaneus.[59,78,109]

In the long bones, simple cysts arise in the metaphysis adjacent to the physis. As the bone grows, the physis grows away from the lesion, which comes to lie in a diaphyseal or metadiaphyseal location. The natural history of simple bone cysts varies. A simple bone cyst may heal spontaneously and be replaced with normal bone. Growth disturbances, limb-length discrepancy, and deformity can result with larger cysts. Pathologic fracture is a common complication. The lesions usually come to attention on radiographs obtained for an unrelated reason or after fracture.[59]

Prevention of pathologic fracture is the goal of treatment, when a simple bone cyst is detected as an incidental imaging finding. Larger lesions, those in weight-bearing sites, and those that persist into adulthood are typically treated with direct injection of corticosteroids into the cyst. Curettage and packing with autologous bone is required in a small percentage of cases.[104]

Simple bone cysts have a characteristic radiographic appearance that makes biopsy unnecessary for diagnosis in all but a few cases. They appear as expansile thin walled intramedullary radiolucencies surrounded by intact thin cortex. Although expanded, the transverse width of the affected bone tends to be no greater than that of its physis. Osseous ridges in the cyst wall impart a multiloculated appearance to some simple bone cysts. A periosteal reaction is not present unless a fracture has occurred. With fracture, a cortical fragment is occasionally identified in the dependent portion of the cyst ("fallen fragment sign"), where it "falls" unimpeded by the internal architecture or thin fluid of the cyst.[87] Additional imaging of simple bone cysts is rarely required. The MRI signal characteristics and CT attenuation values suggest a fluid-filled structure. Following gadolinium administration, the walls of the lesion and internal septations enhance.[9,59] The presence of septations belies the term *unicameral* that is often affixed to this lesion. Fluid-fluid levels are occasionally seen with CT and MRI.[9,114]

Skeletal scintigraphy is not performed as part of the standard evaluation of these lesions. Due to their relative frequency, some come to attention on a skeletal scintigram performed for an unrelated indication. Depending on the size and location of the cyst, scintigraphy may be normal, reveal minimally increased radionuclide localization around the periphery of the cyst or focally decreased localization without such a surrounding rim. With associated fracture or bone stress, more intense focal or diffuse tracer localization is typically present.[109] Pinhole imaging assists in showing decreased localization associated with simple bone cysts.

Aneurysmal Bone Cyst

An aneurysmal bone cyst is an expansile lytic lesion that contains thin-walled, blood-containing cavities. Aneurysmal bone cysts are believed to develop in normal bone secondary to venous obstruction or arteriovenous fistulization following trauma. Approximately 30% of aneurysmal bone cysts develop in association with a preexisting lesion, presumably due to a tumor-induced vascular anomaly. Com-

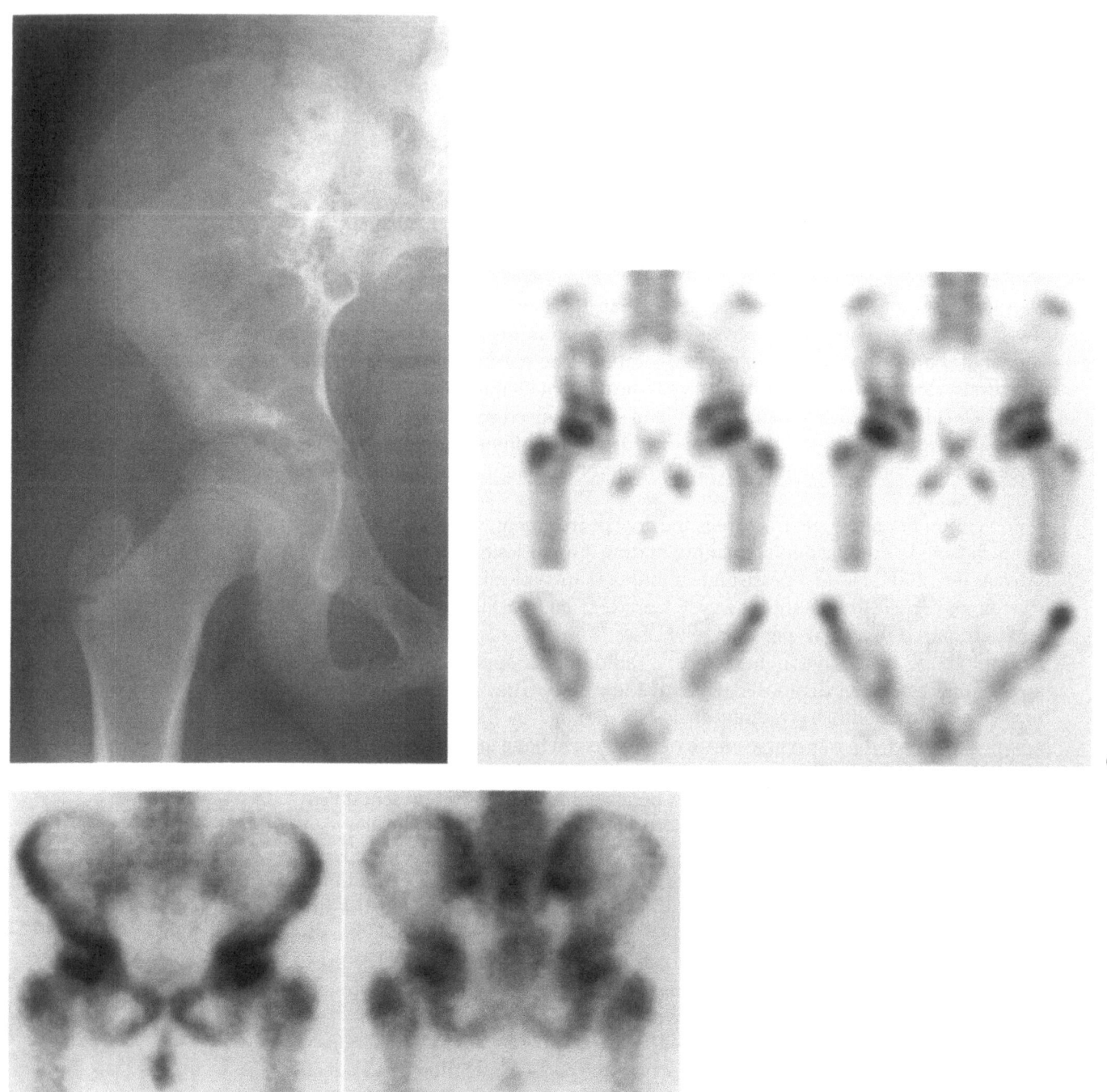

Figure 4.14. Simple bone cyst. A pelvic radiograph (A) shows a multiloculated radiolucency adjacent to the right sacroiliac joint. Anterior (left panel) and posterior images (B) demonstrate slightly greater ^{99m}Tc-MDP localization in the right ilium adjacent to the sacroiliac joint. An area of decreased tracer localization corresponding to the cyst is shown with SPECT (C).

mon precursor lesions include giant cell tumor, chondroblastoma, osteoblastoma, nonossifying fibroma, simple bone cyst, fibrous dysplasia, Langerhans cell histiocytosis, and osteosarcoma.[56]

Aneurysmal bone cysts are found slightly more frequently in females than males. Excluding those that develop in preexisting lesions, more than 80% are seen in the first two decades of life. They are rarely encountered in children prior to the age of 5 years. Essentially any portion of the skeleton may be affected. The long bones harbor more than 50% of all aneurysmal bone cysts. The spine and pelvis are other common locations. The most common clinical manifestations are pain and swelling. Neurologic findings may be present with vertebral lesions.[56,109]

Therapy of aneurysmal bone cysts has most commonly consisted of biopsy, to identify any associated lesion, followed by curettage and bone graft packing or surgical excision. Recurrence rates that approach or exceed 40% with these techniques have resulted in other approaches being attempted. Promising results have been obtained with intralesional liquid nitrogen,[68] and with selective arterial embolization.[22]

Aneurysmal bone cysts of the long bones usually appear as eccentric, lytic, expansile, occasionally trabeculated lesions (Fig. 4.15). Most are metaphyseal in location. A small percentage are diaphyseal. The transverse width of this lesion often exceeds the width of the adjacent physis. Periosteal elevation may be present and the cortex can appear thinned or absent.[56] Spinal and pelvic aneurysmal bone cysts are typically lytic expansile lesions. Involvement of the posterior elements, often extending into the vertebral body, is characteristic of spinal lesions (Fig. 4.16). Multiple fluid-fluid levels are commonly seen with MRI and CT (Figs. 4.16 and 4.17). Septa, which enhance following gadolinium administration, are well demonstrated with MRI.[45]

With skeletal scintigraphy, angiographic and tissue phase images usually depict increased tracer delivery and prominent early tracer localization (Fig. 4.15). Skeletal phase images typically show peripherally increased tracer localization with a more central area of decreased localization (Figs. 4.15 and 4.17). Diffusely increased or diffusely decreased localization are associated with some lesions. Aneurysmal bone cysts demonstrate an extended pattern of radionuclide localization beyond their true limits in a small percentage of cases. Skeletal scintigraphy does not differentiate an aneurysmal bone cyst that is associated with another lesion from one that is not, except presumptively in cases where metastatic lesions are detected.[43,109]

Figure 4.15. Aneurysmal bone cyst. A radiograph (A) shows eccentric radiolucent expansion of the distal left femoral diaphysis.

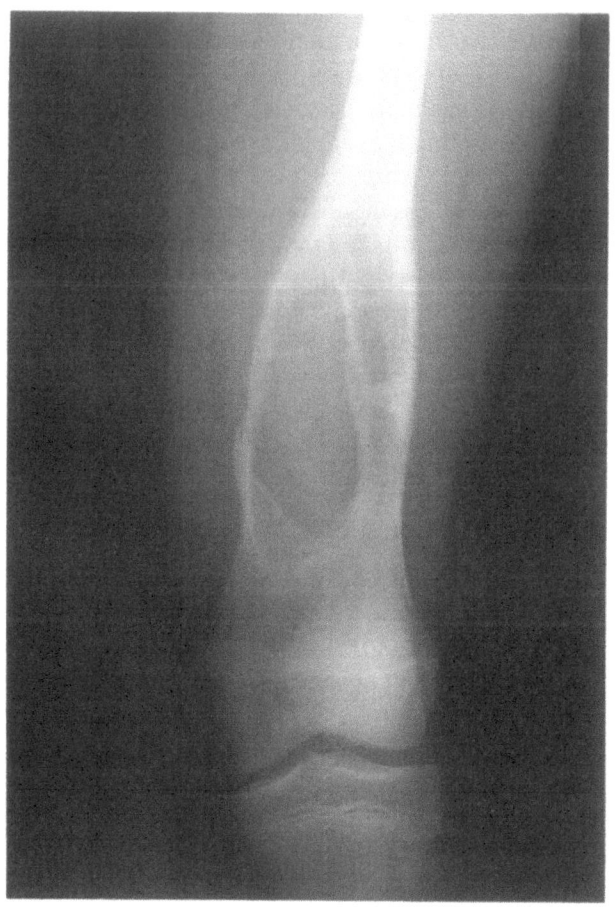

A

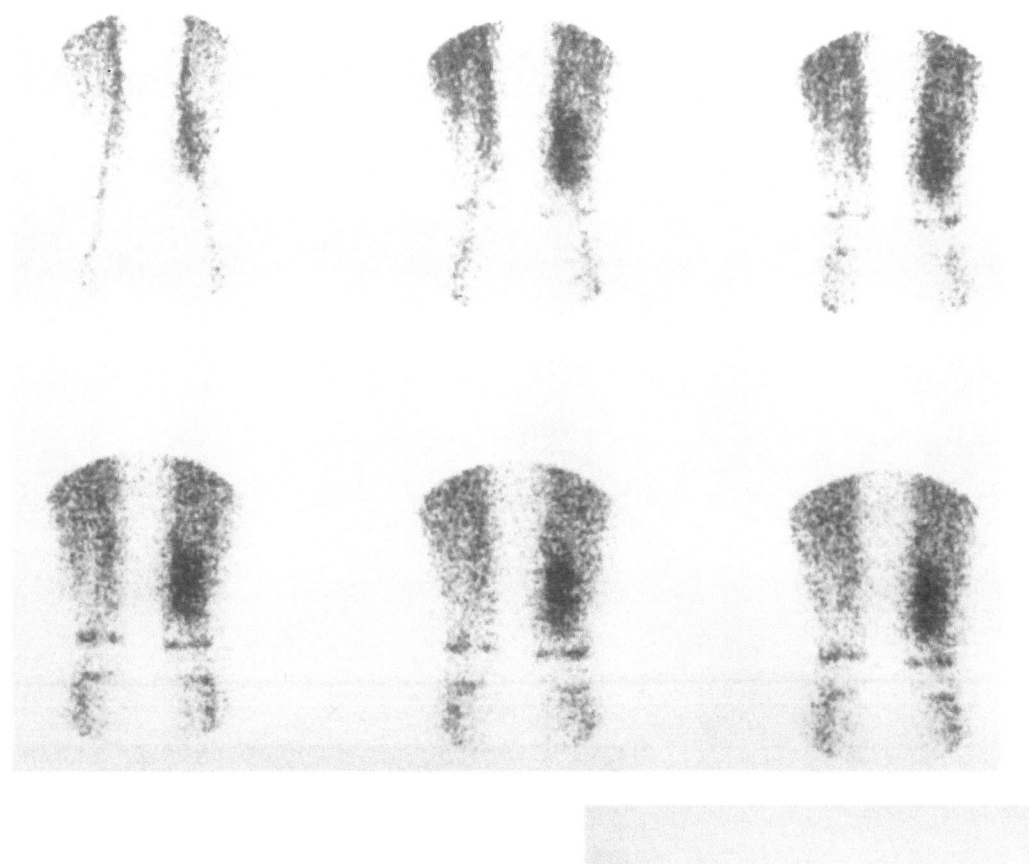

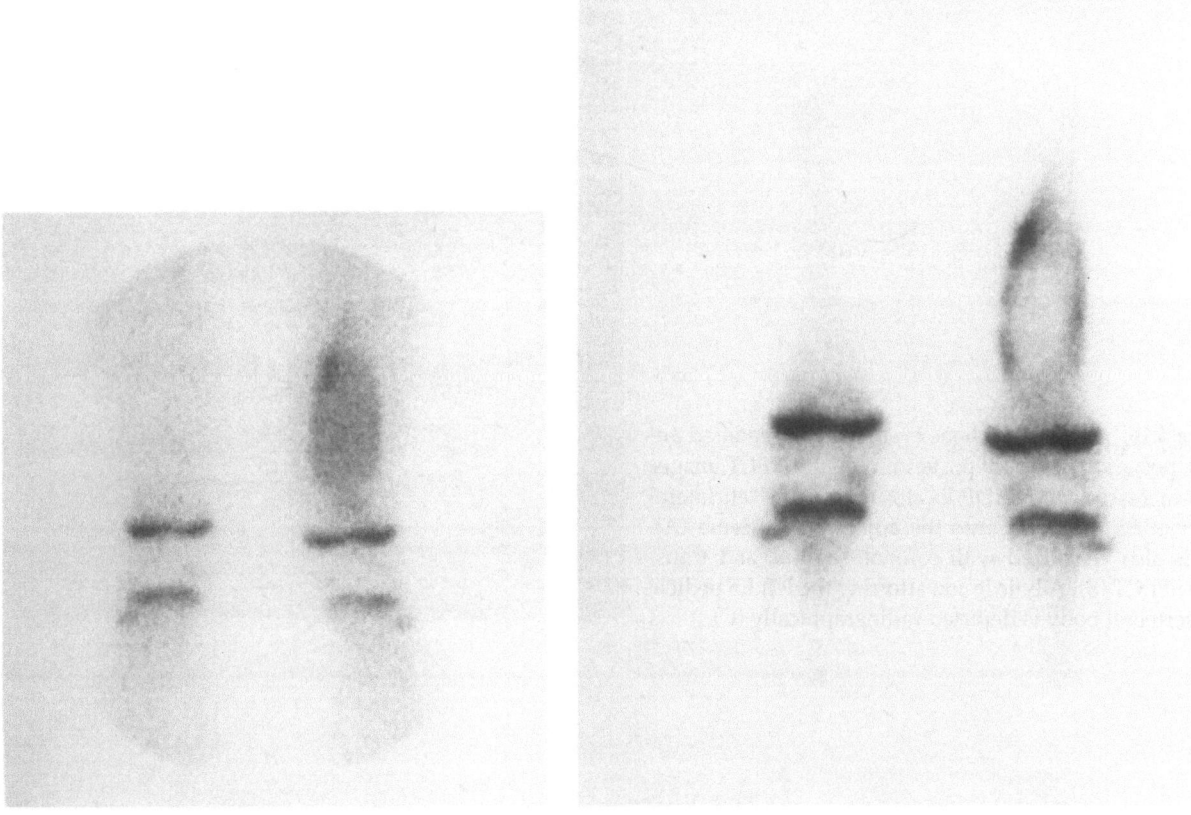

Figure 4.15 (*Cont.d*). Radionuclide angiography (B) demonstrates increased tracer delivery and tissue phase imaging (C) shows prominent tracer localization to the entire lesion. Skeletal phase imaging (D) shows increased tracer localization along the lesion's periphery and centrally decreased tracer localization. (Case courtesy of Drs. J. Sty and R.G. Wells, Children's Hospital of Wisconsin. Reprinted from Treves, 113a with permission.)

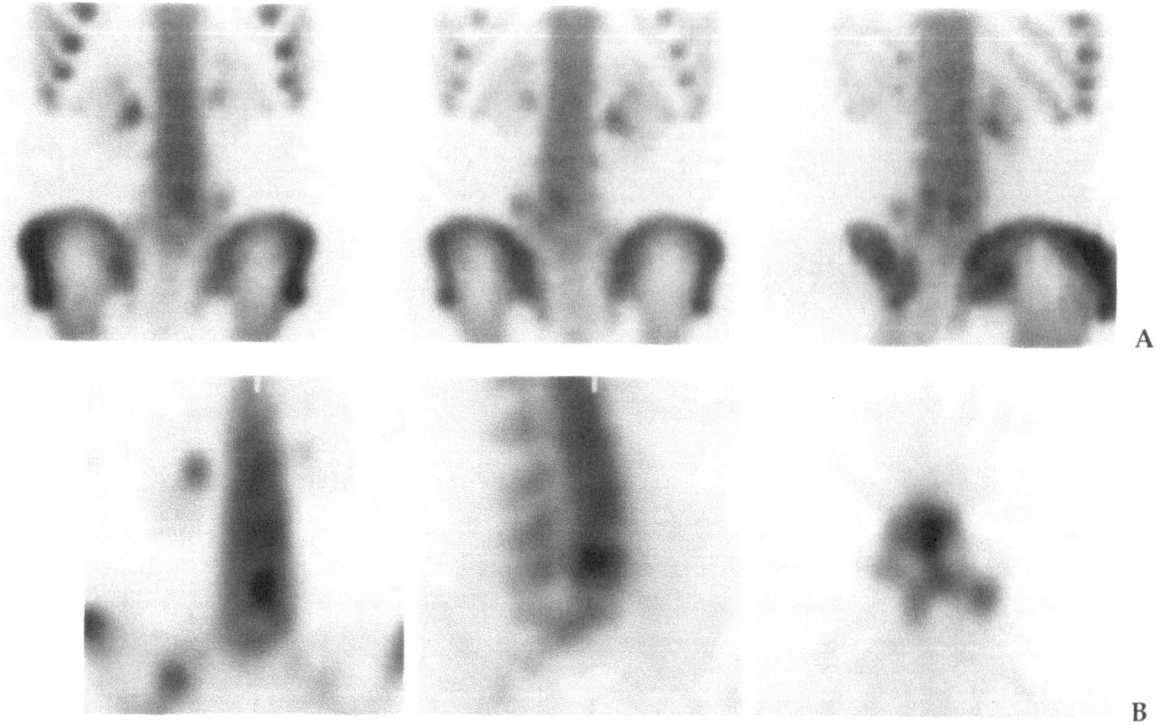

A

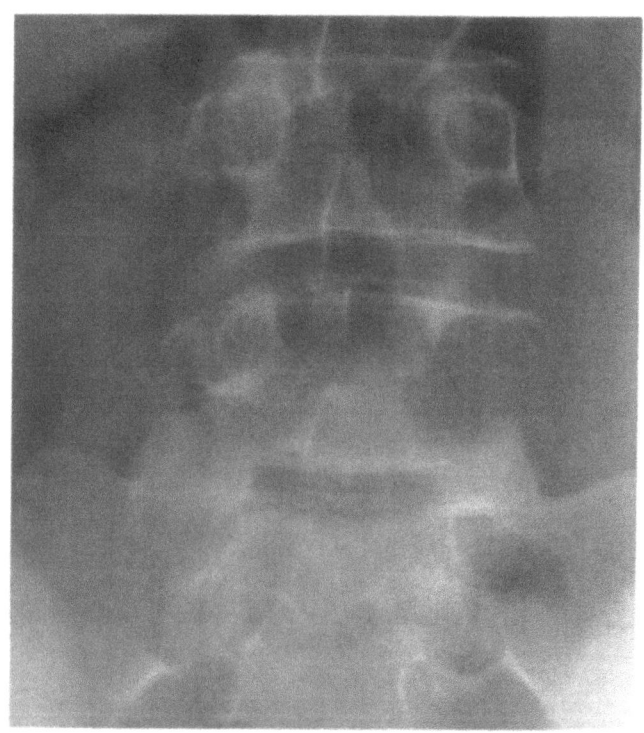

B

Figure 4.16. Aneurysmal bone cyst. Volume rendered anterior, posterior, and right posterior oblique SPECT images show increased ^{99m}Tc-MDP localization in the left lateral aspect of L5 extending into the adjacent soft tissue (A). This is also visualized with coronal, sagittal, and transverse SPECT (B). A lytic lesion affecting the left L5 pedicle and vertebral body is depicted radiographically (C).

C

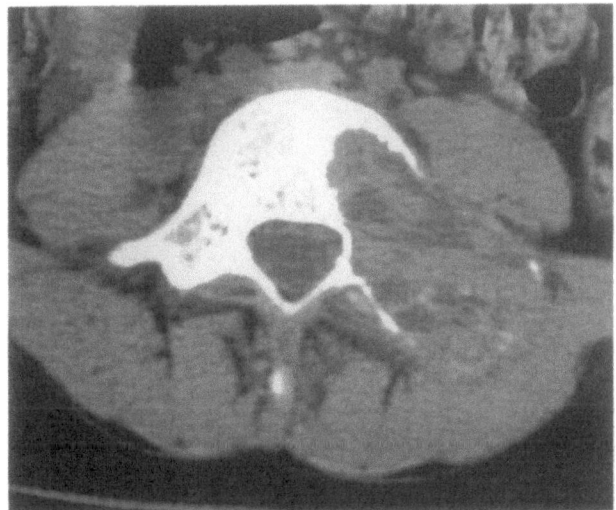

D

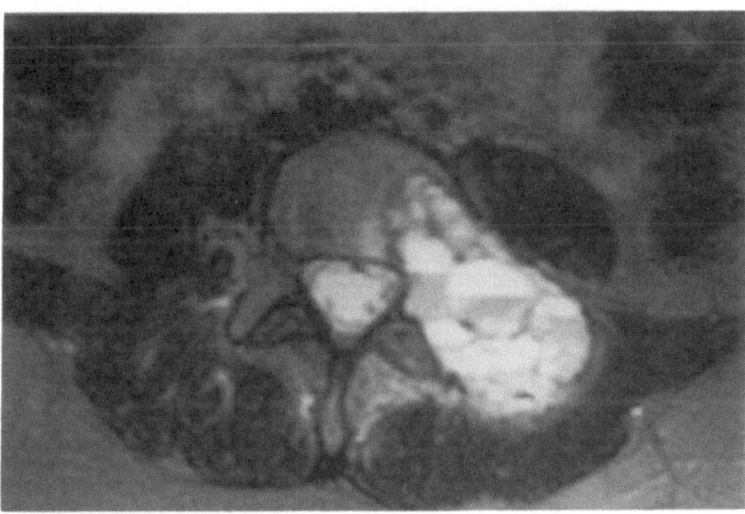

E

Figure 4.16 (*Cont.d*). Computed tomography (D) and MRI (E) show an expansile lytic mass that is centered in the left pedicle of L5 and extends into the L5 vertebral body. Multiple fluid-fluid levels are present within the mass.

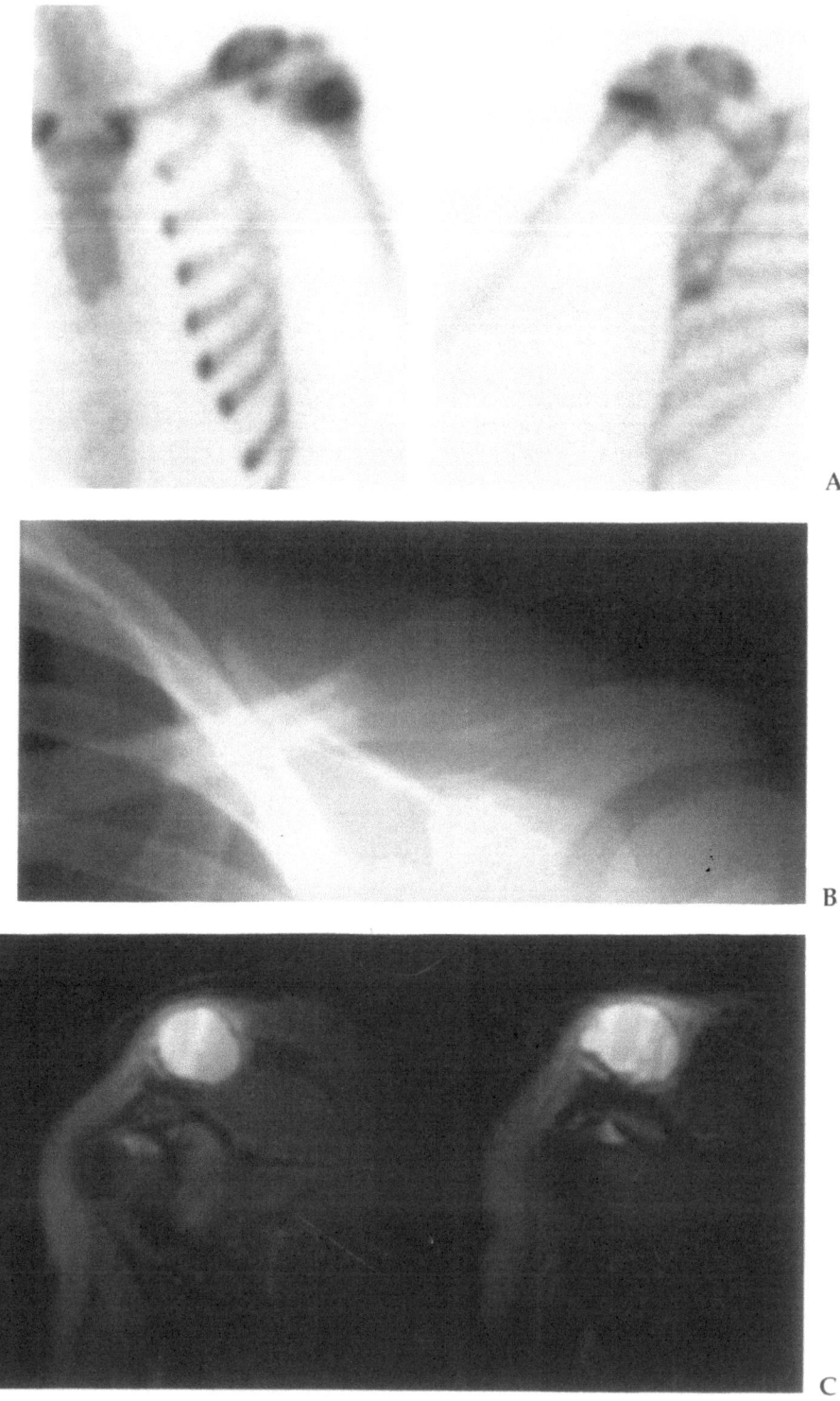

A

B

C

Figure 4.17. Aneurysmal bone cyst. Skeletal scintigraphy (anterior and posterior projections) depicts increased tracer localization along the periphery of an expansile lesion affecting the left clavicle (A). Lytic expansion of the distal left clavicle is shown radiographically (B). Magnetic resonance imaging shows multiple fluid-fluid levels (C).

Benign Cartilaginous Tumors

Osteochondroma

An osteochondroma (exostosis) consists of normal bone with cortex and a marrow cavity. The lesion is covered by a cartilaginous cap that ossifies with skeletal maturity.[44,109] Osteochondromas are derived from cartilage that separates from a physis, proliferates autonomously, undergoes enchondral ossification, and grows perpendicular to the physis from which it originated.[72] Growth of these lesions may continue into the third decade of life. Most osteochondromas occur sporadically as solitary lesions (Figs. 4.18–4.20). Occasionally, an osteochondroma results from physeal damage secondary to radiation therapy[61] or trauma. A solitary osteochondroma carries a small risk of malignant transformation, estimated as less than 2%.[49]

Approximately 80% of osteochondromas are discovered in individuals younger than 20 years of age.[84] There is a slight male predominance.[37] These lesions are most frequently found in the metaphyses of long bones, particularly the femur, tibia, and humerus. Approximately 40% are located about the knee.[37] They are occasionally found in other sites, including the small bones of the hands and feet, the pelvis, calvaria, scapula, and spine, where they involve the posterior elements. The presenting complaint is typically a firm, slowly growing, painless mass located near a joint. A less frequent presentation is pain due to irritation of adjacent muscles or neurovascular bundle, fracture, or inflammation of an overlying bursa. Surgical removal is indicated when the lesions are symptomatic or when there are signs suggestive of malignant transformation.

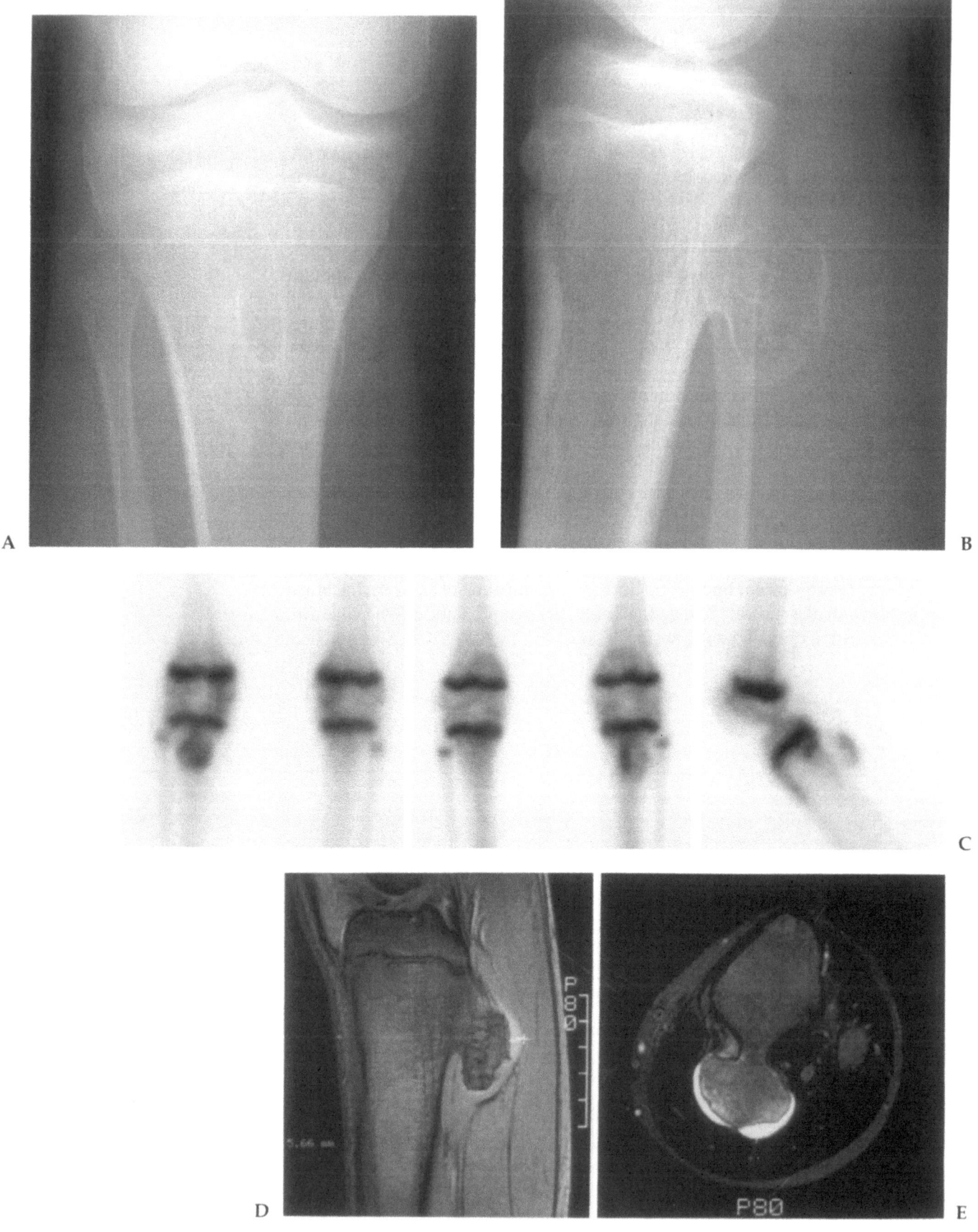

Figure 4.18. Anteroposterior (A) and lateral (B) radiographs of the right tibia demonstrate an osteochondroma. Increased ⁹⁹ᵐTc-MDP localization overlying the right metadiaphyseal tibia on anterior and posterior images, is shown to correspond to the periphery of the osteochondroma with a medial projection (C). Sagittal gradient recall echo imaging (D) and a transaxial T2-weighted image (E) show an approximately 5.7 mm thick cartilaginous cap that corresponds to the site of ⁹⁹ᵐTc-MDP localization.

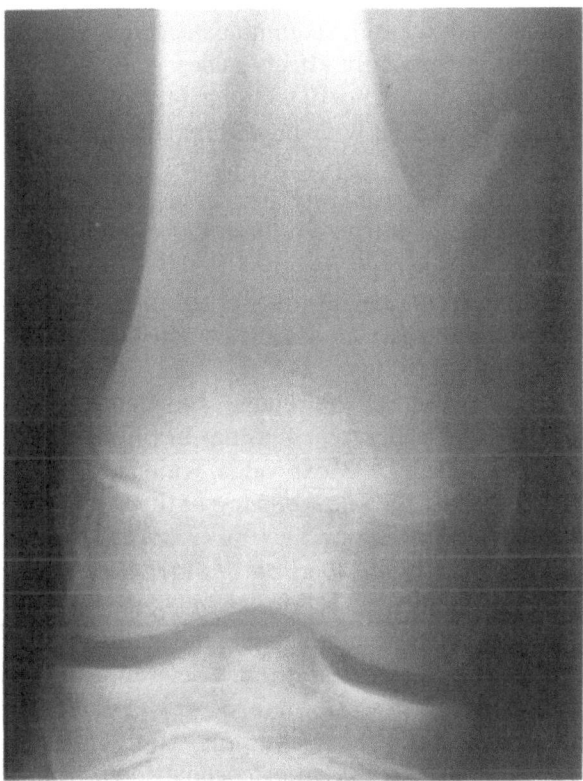

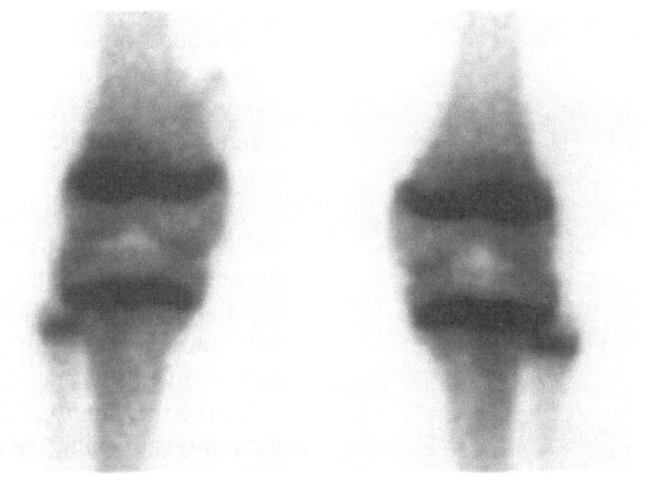

Figure 4.19. Osteochondroma. An osteochondroma of the right distal femur is depicted radiographically. Note that the long axis of the lesion is directed proximally from the adjacent physis (A). Skeletal scintigraphy shows tracer localization of a similar intensity to that in adjacent bone (B).

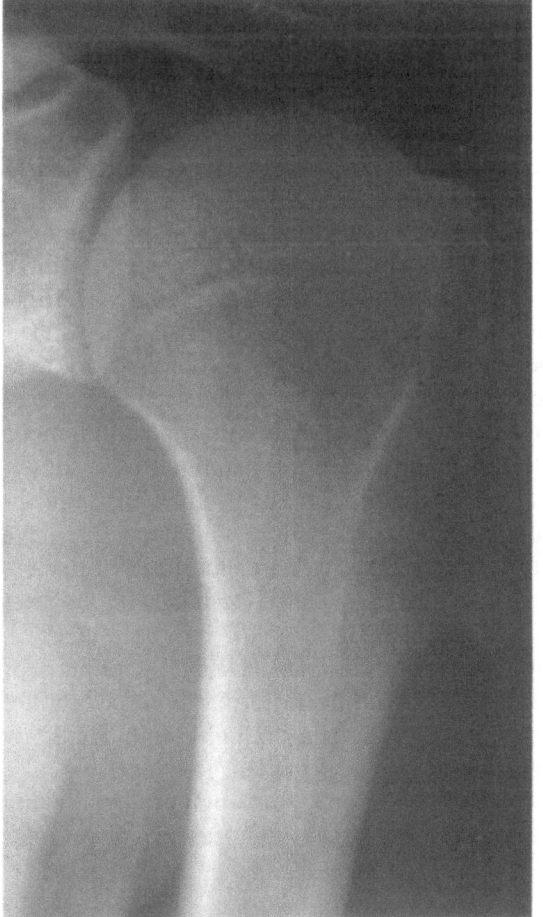

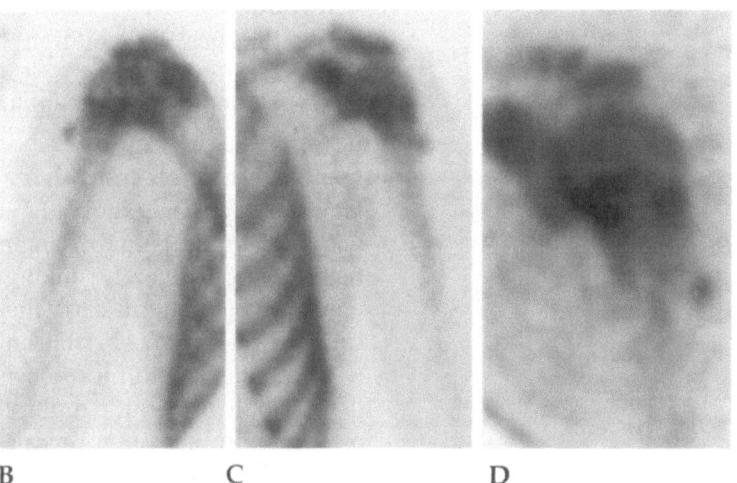

Figure 4.20. A radiograph shows an osteochondroma of the proximal left humerus (A). Posterior (B) and anterior (C) planar images and an anterior pinhole image (D) show mildly increased tracer localization in the right humeral osteochondroma.

Multiple osteochondromas occur in the setting of multiple hereditary exostoses (osteochondromatosis, diaphyseal aclasis), the most common skeletal dysplasia. This autosomal dominant disorder predominantly affects males. It is typically diagnosed by age 2 years.[59] Estimates of the incidence of malignant transformation (predominantly to chondrosarcoma) in patients with hereditary multiple exostoses range from 5%[86] to 30%.[37]

A solitary osteochondroma appears radiographically as a sessile or pedunculated osseous excrescence. Its cortex and medullary cavity are continuous with those of adjacent bone. An overlying lucency corresponding to the cartilaginous cap may be visible. Radiographic clues to malignant transformation include an indistinct bony margin particularly near the cap, an associated soft tissue mass, and an area of lucency within the osteochondroma.[31,59]

Marked modeling abnormalities, including shortening, broadening, and metaphyseal flaring are the most striking radiographic findings in children with hereditary multiple exostoses (Figs. 4.21–4.23).[44,109] Coxa valga, widened femoral metaphyses, valgus deformity of the tibia at the knee, bowing of the radius and ulna, and ulnar shortening are particularly common.

When a solitary lesion thought to be an osteochondroma is identified, additional imaging can be useful to establish continuity of cortex and marrow from the affected bone into the lesion, evaluate a lesion's relationship to the neurovascular bundle, assess the possibility of malignant transformation, and determine if multiple lesions are present.

Demonstration of cortical continuity with CT[37] or, more importantly, marrow continuity with MRI[60] is valuable in differentiating an osteochondroma from a periosteal osteosarcoma, a lesion that may appear similar radiographically. Impingement on a neurovascular bundle can be demonstrated with either CT or MRI.[100] In children, the cartilaginous cap, which is most accurately evaluated with MRI (Fig. 4.18),[37] may normally approach 3 cm in thickness. Assessment of its thickness in children tends not to be useful[46] for identifying those osteochondromas at greatest risk of malignant transformation. Enhancement patterns following gadolinium administration provide insight into the histopathology of an osteochondroma in an adult patient. Peripheral enhancement, which correlates with fibrovascular tissue covering the nonenhancing cartilaginous cap, suggests benignity. Curvilinear septal enhancement is associated with low-grade chondrosarcomas. Inhomogeneous or homogeneous enhancement is suggestive of a high-grade chondrosarcoma.[32] It is not clear that these enhancement patterns carry the same significance in children, however, as normal cartilage may show variable enhancement during childhood.

In a patient with an osteochondroma, the primary role of scintigraphy is to demonstrate or exclude multiple lesions (Figs. 4.21–4.24). Skeletal scintigraphy of osteochondromas often reveals increased tracer localization in the cartilaginous cap. The remainder of the lesion typically shows tracer localization that is similar to that of adjacent normal bone. Scintigraphy has not proven useful in distinguishing lesions that have undergone malignant transformation from those that have not. Various criteria for this determination, including tracer localization that increases over time, persistent increased localization relative to normal bone after skeletal maturity, and increased localization relative to an internal standard, such as the sacroiliac joint, have not proved valid. A normal skeletal scintigram or one showing localization in the lesion equal to that in normal bone, while not completely excluding malignant transformation,[46] makes it highly unlikely, however.[86] Three-phase skeletal scintigraphy may reveal evidence of local vascular changes related to an osteochondroma. A radionuclide angiogram showing asymmetric arterial perfusion or venous stasis suggests the presence of vascular compression.[100]

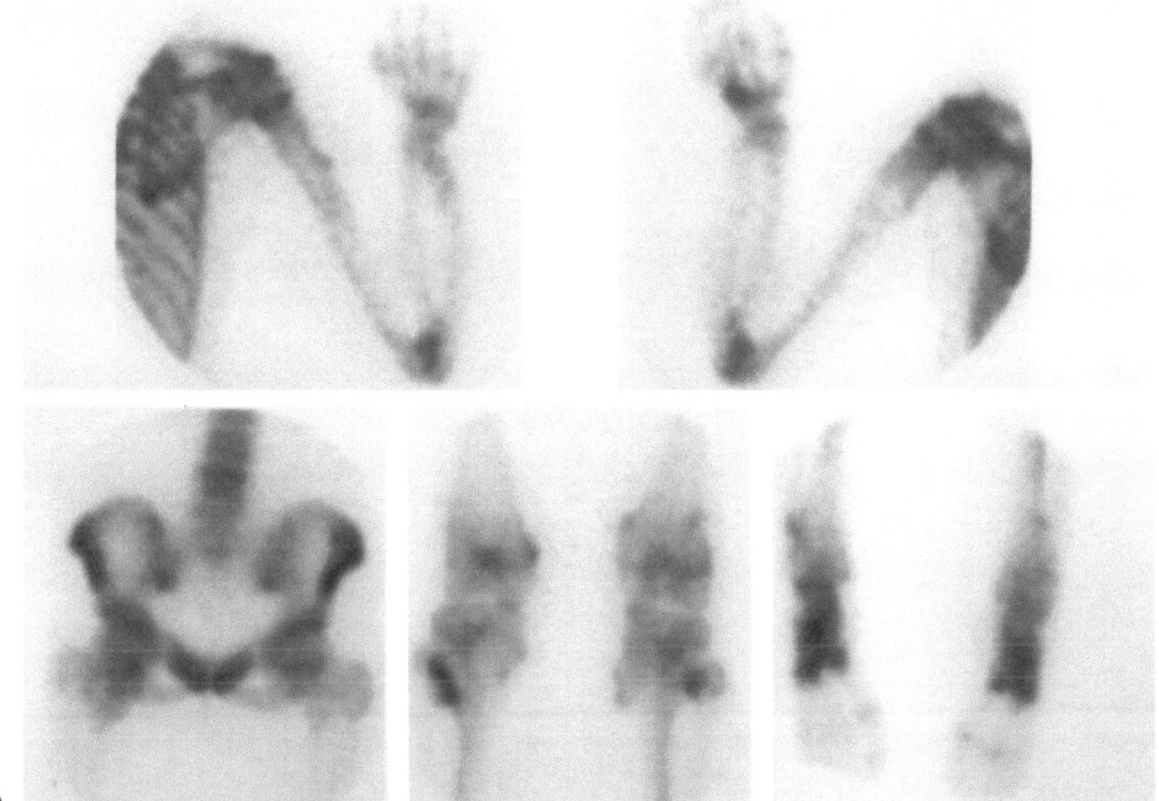

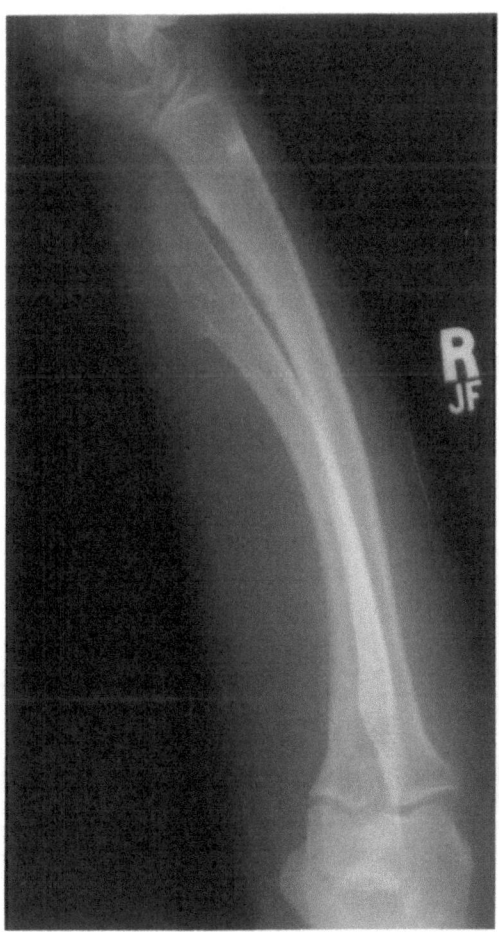

Figure 4.21. Hereditary multiple exostoses. Skeletal scintigraphy (A, upper row: posterior projections; lower row: anterior projections) depicts extensive abnormalities of tracer localization and bone modeling. The long bones of the upper and lower extremities, the hands, the right scapula, and the pelvis are affected. A correlative radiograph of the right forearm depicts bowing deformity and ulnar shortening (B).

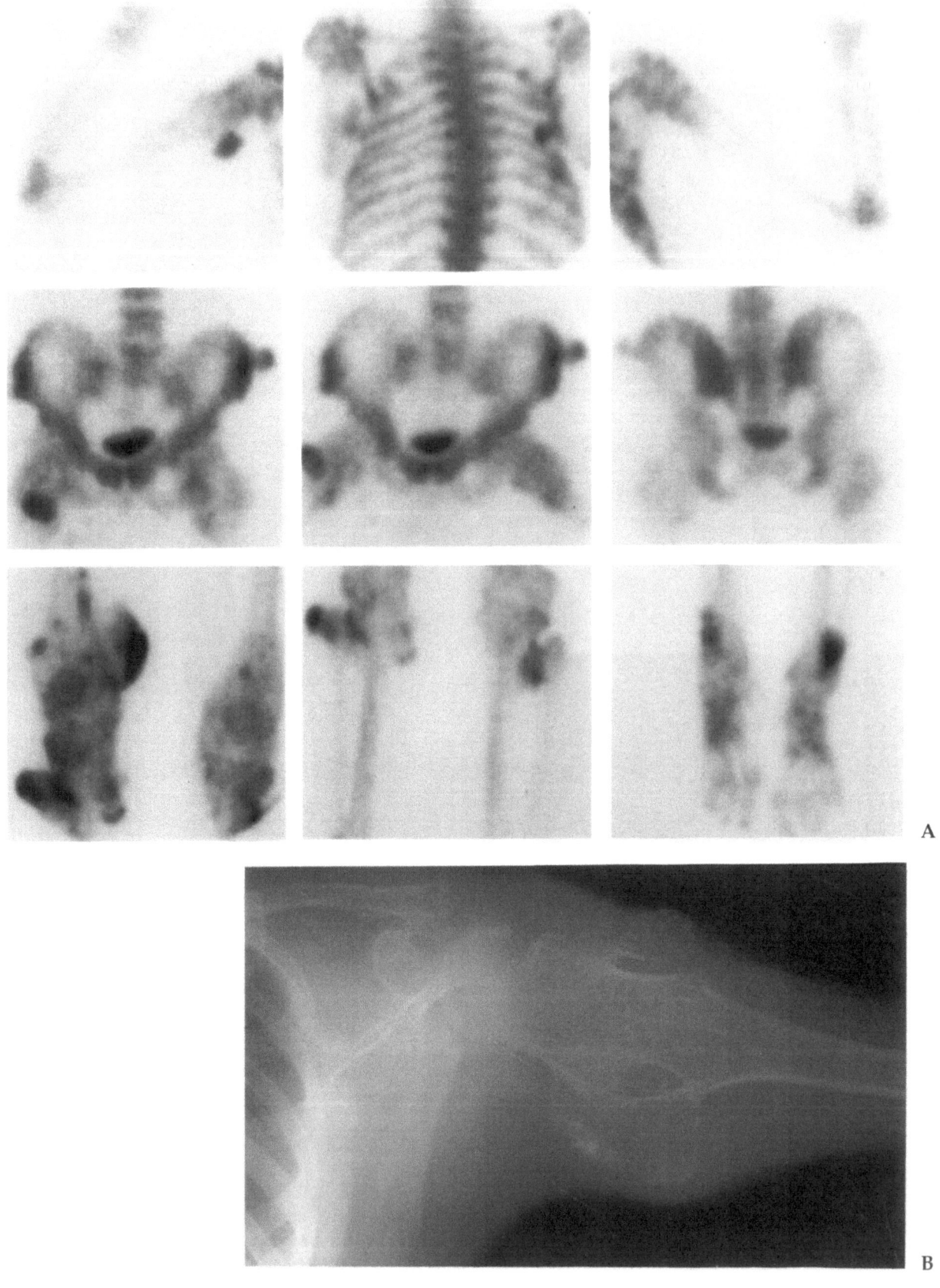

Figure 4.22. (A) and (B) Caption on p. 167.

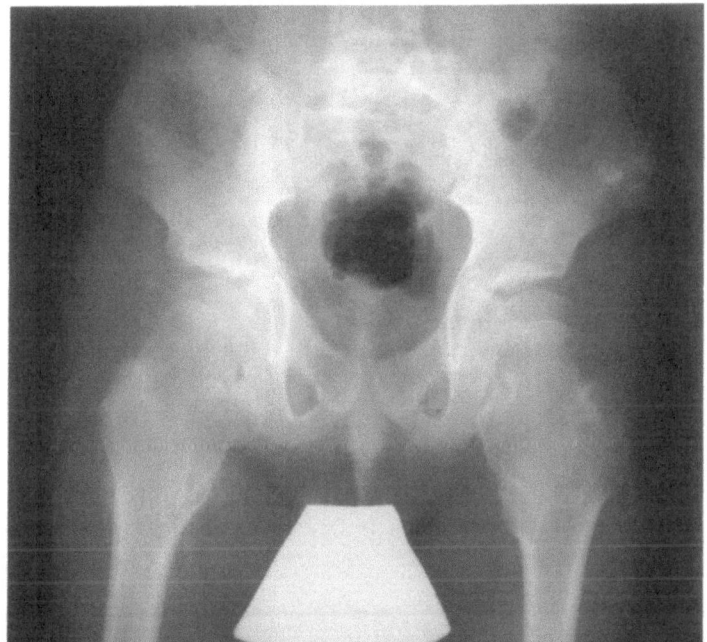

C

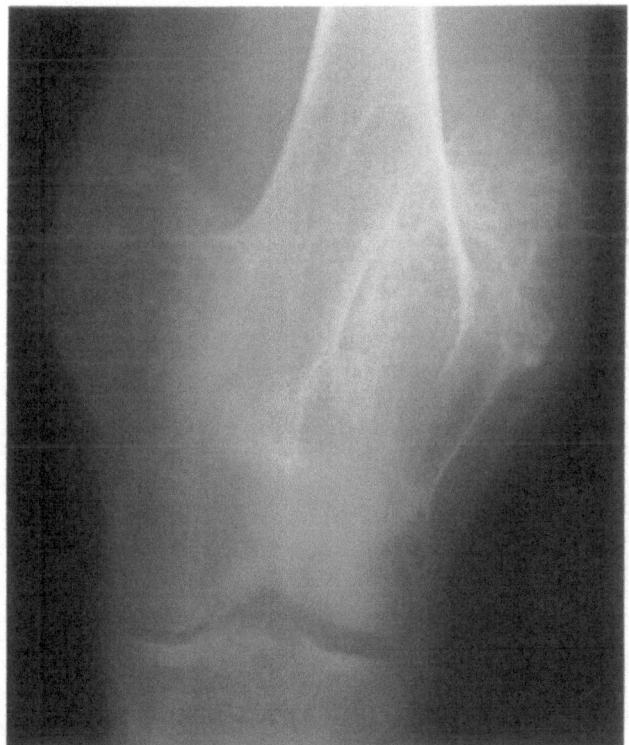

D

Figure 4.22. Hereditary multiple exostoses. Skeletal scintigraphy (A) demonstrates extensive deformities and abnormalities of tracer localization. (Upper extremity and thorax: posterior projections; pelvis; anterior, frog-leg, and posterior projections; lower extremities: anterior projections.) Correlative radiographs of the left shoulder (B), pelvis (C), and right knee (D) depict osteochondromas and bone deformity.

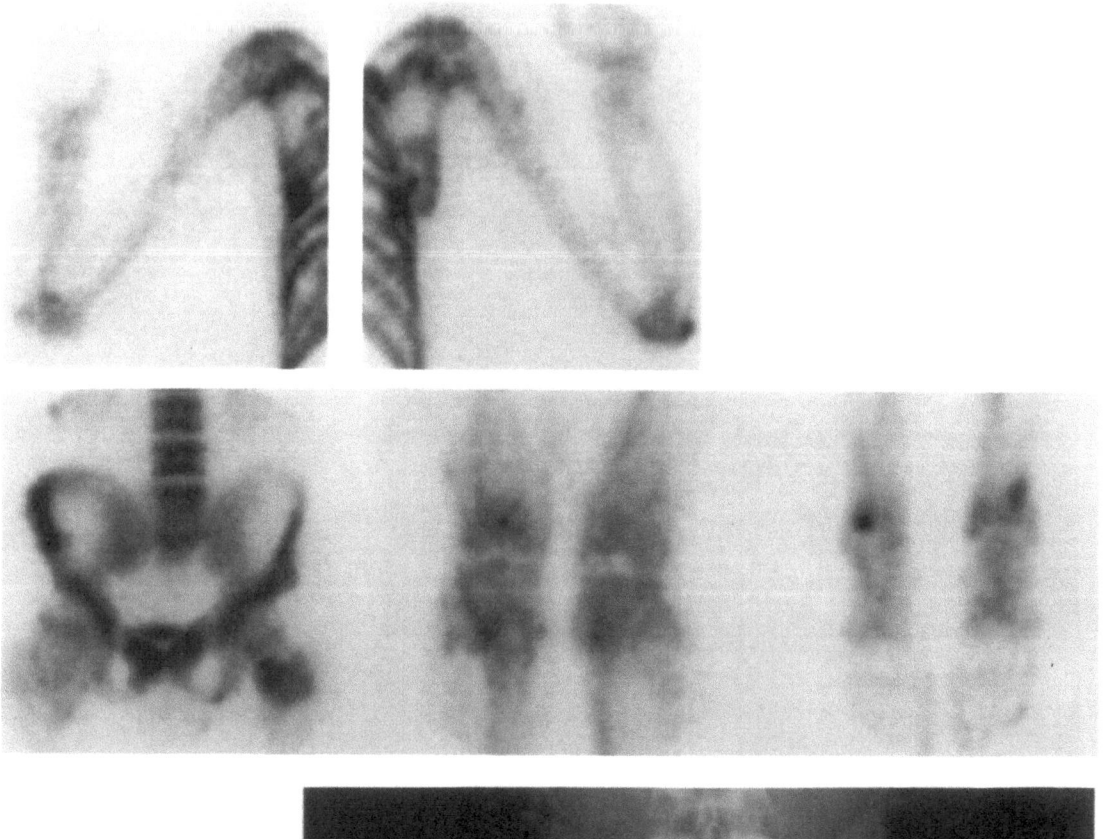

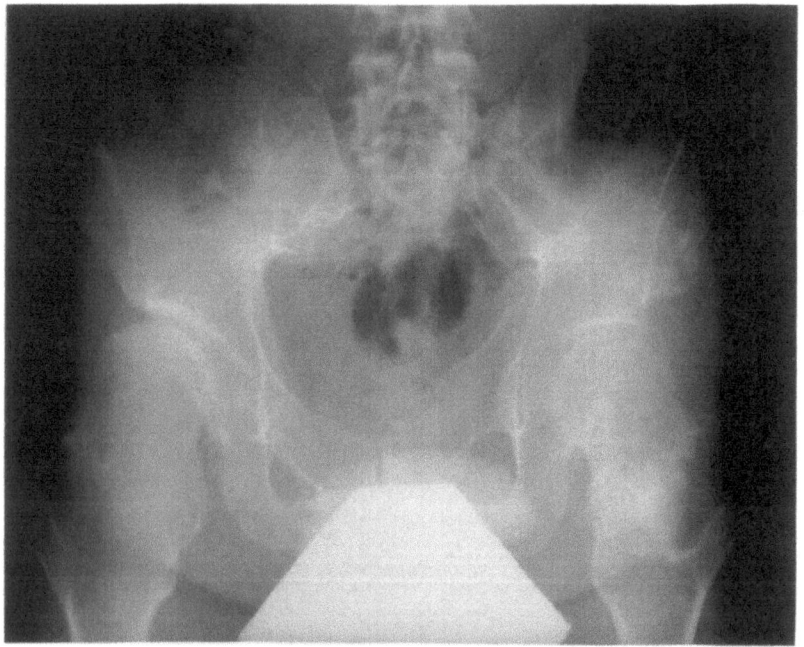

Figure 4.23. Hereditary multiple exostoses. Skeletal scintigraphy shows multiple sites of abnormal tracer localization affecting the long bones of the upper and lower extremities, the scapulae, ribs, and pelvis (A). Correlative radiographs of the pelvis (B), left proximal femur (C), and knees (D) demonstrate multiple exostoses and associated deformity.

Figure 4.23 (*cont'd.*)

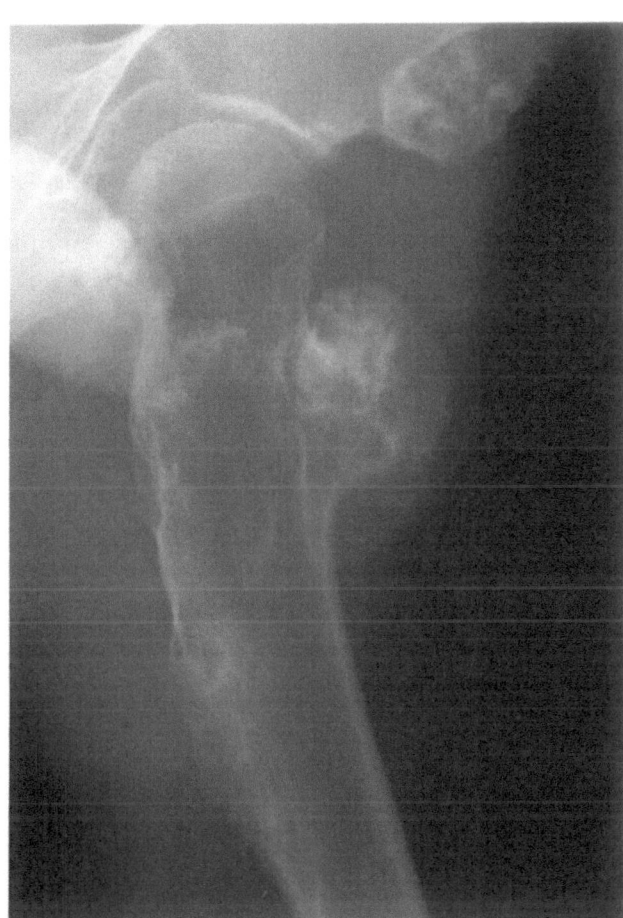

C

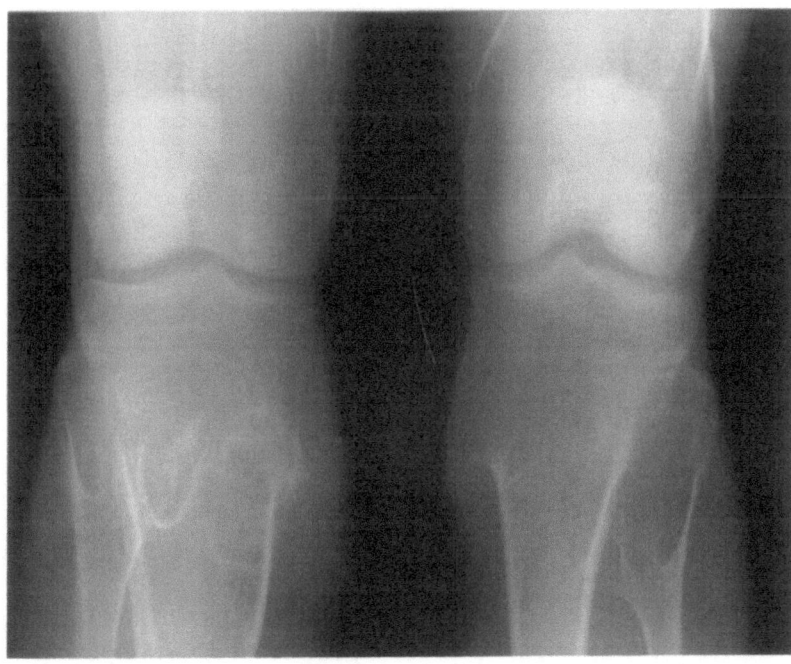

D

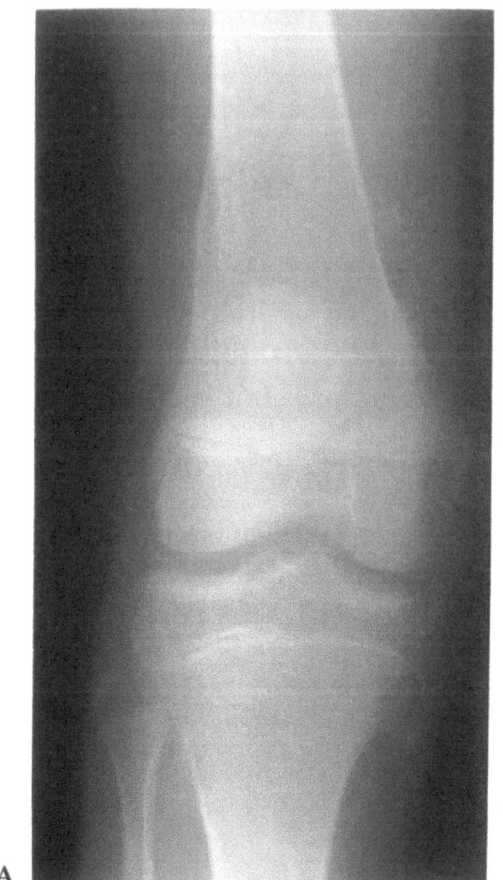

A

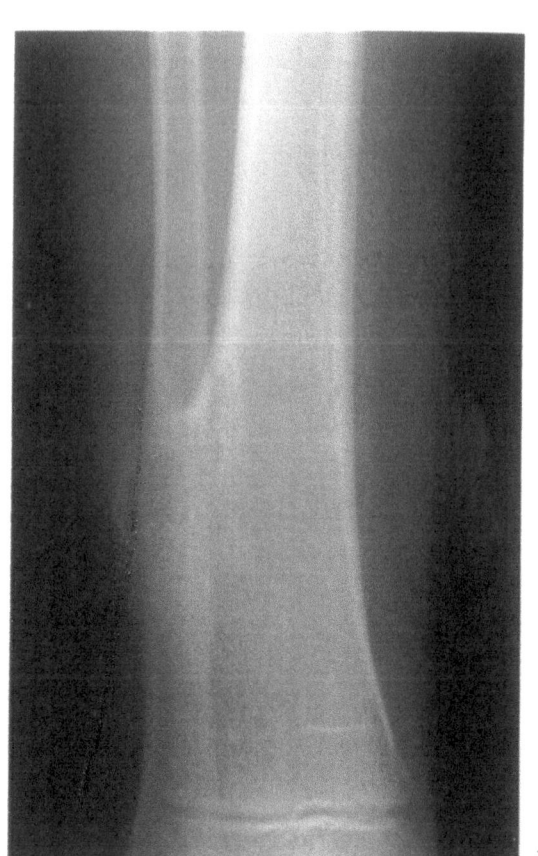

B

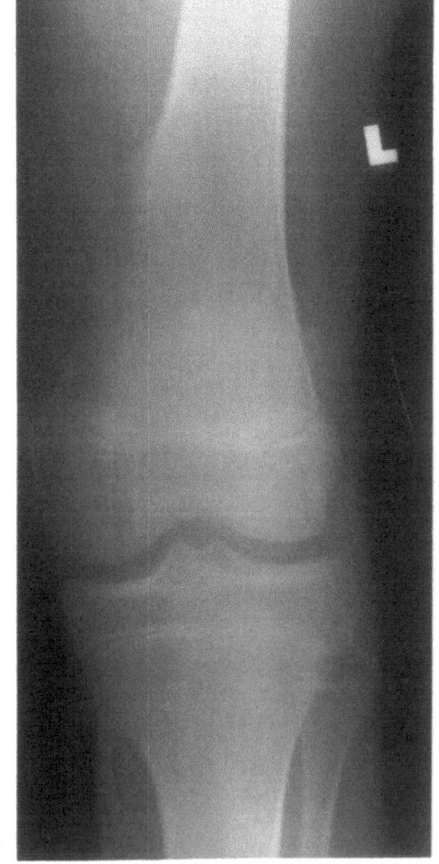

C

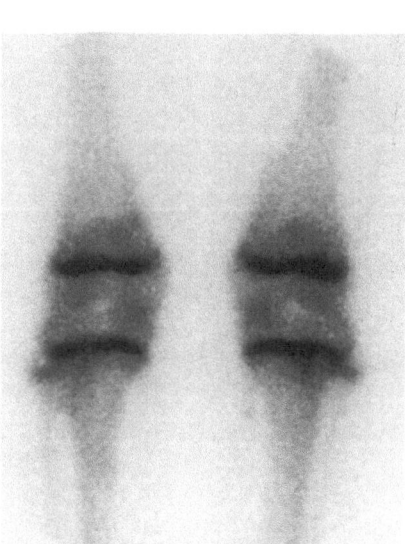

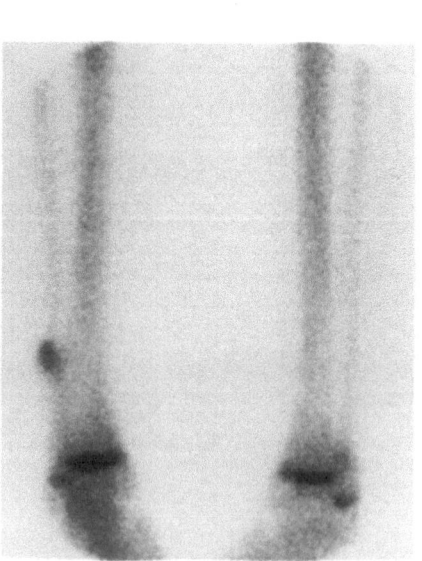

D

Enchondroma

An enchondroma is a benign tumor composed of mature hyaline cartilage surrounded by lamellar enchondral bone.[37] It most likely arises from actively proliferating physeal cartilage that does not undergo normal ossification.[59,72] The physis grows away from this unossified cartilaginous rest.

Enchondromas are detected throughout life with a peak incidence during the third decade.[37] The lesion occurs with equal frequency in males and females. Any bone preformed in cartilage can be affected. The most common locations are the small tubular bones of the hand and feet, the femur, and the humerus.[44] In the long bones, the lesions are usually metaphyseal or metadiaphyseal, commonly diaphyseal, and rarely epiphyseal or metaepiphyseal.[37] Enchondromas are usually detected after pathologic fracture or with radiographs obtained to assess an unrelated problem. When the radiographic findings are characteristic, no specific treatment is required.

Enchondromatosis (Ollier's disease) is an uncommon skeletal dysplasia characterized by multiple proliferating cartilaginous masses that are mostly enchondromas.[37] The lesions are often bilateral, although one side tends to predominate. Skeletal involvement can be widespread. Enchondromatosis affects the long bones, small tubular bones, and the flat bones. This dysplasia is significant due to associated angular and shortening deformities, pathologic fractures, and a risk of malignant transformation, usually to chondrosarcoma.[84,86] This complication has been estimated to occur in as many as one third to one half of patients.[44] Maffucci syndrome is a rare mesodermal dysplasia in which enchondromatosis is associated with soft tissue hemangiomas.

Enchondromas appear radiographically as expansile radiolucent lesions. The margins often appear lobulated. A thin sclerotic border is variably present. Endosteal scalloping is commonly observed.[37] Punctate, flocculent, or ring-like calcifications are often visible in enchondromas of older children and adults[59] but not in enchondromas of young children. Periosteal reaction is absent unless pathologic fracture has occurred.[37]

While radiographs are usually diagnostic for enchondroma, additional imaging may be requested to aid in confirming the diagnosis, assess cortical integrity, evaluate local extent of involvement, determine if malignant transformation has occurred, and demonstrate multiple lesions.

Figure 4.24. Variability of tracer localization in multiple osteochondromas. Osteochondromas of the right distal femur and proximal tibia (A), right distal tibia (B), and left distal femur and proximal tibia (C) are demonstrated radiographically. The right distal tibial lesion is associated with increased ^{99m}Tc-MDP localization, while the other lesions are not (D).

Computed tomography, by detecting mineralization that is not apparent on radiographs, can increase the level of confidence for differentiating this lesion from other radiolucent lesions, but does not assist in excluding malignant transformation. Cortical integrity can be assessed with CT or MRI. Optimal demonstration of the extent of the nonmineralized component of an enchondroma is provided by MRI. The MRI signal and enhancement characteristics of enchondromas are nonspecific. It has been suggested that benign enchondromas usually have a more homogeneous appearance than do chondrosarcomas on unenhanced MR images.[37] Following gadolinium administration, enchondromas demonstrate enhancing scalloped margins and curvilinear septa ("ring and arc pattern"). This pattern is indistinguishable from that seen with low-grade chondrosarcoma.[1]

Enchondromas typically are associated with increased tracer localization due to hyperemia, enchondral ossification, or adjacent reactive bone formation (Fig. 4.25). These lesions may, however, show either normal or decreased tracer localization. Skeletal scintigraphy does not distinguish those lesions that have undergone malignant transformation from those that have not. Skeletal scintigraphy is used to determine if multiple lesions are present (Fig. 4.25) and to assess the extent of involvement in children with enchondromatosis (Fig. 4.26).

Technetium-99mm–labeled red blood cell imaging can aid in depicting the cavernous hemangiomas of Maffucci syndrome.[115]

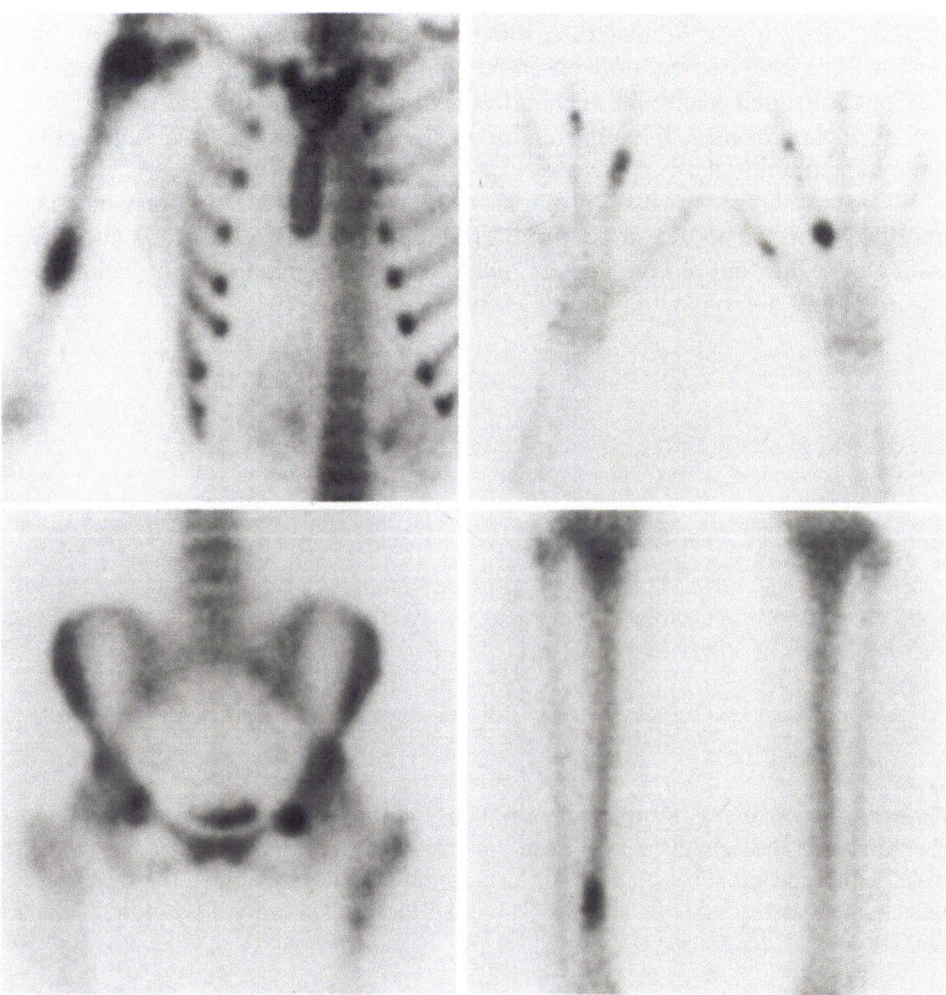

A

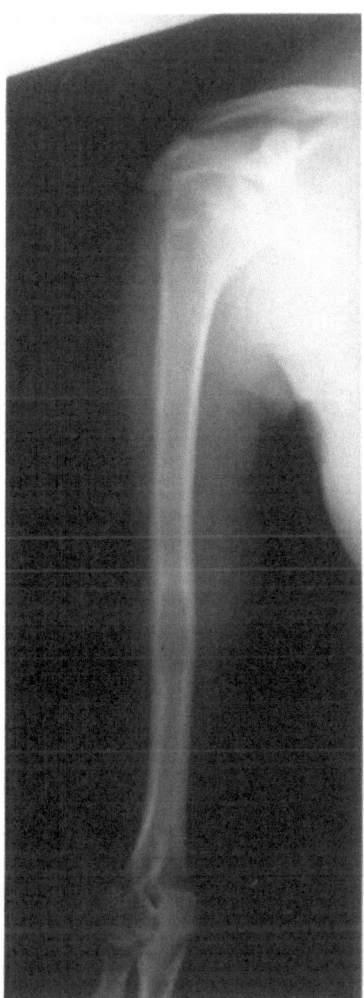

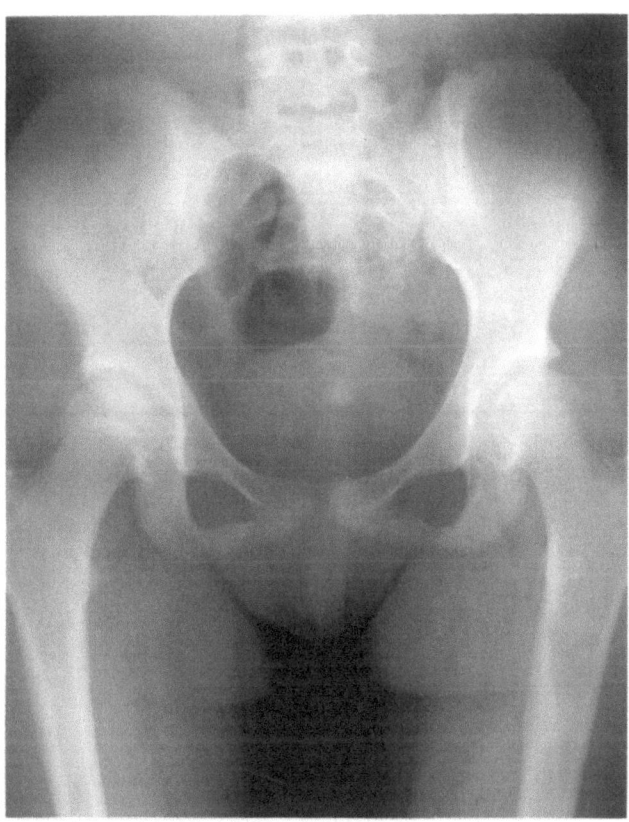

B   C

Figure 4.25. Multiple enchondromas. Areas of increased tracer localization are present in the right humerus, sternal manubrium, multiple phalanges of the hands, the left acetabulum, the left femur, and the right tibia (A). Correlative radiographs demonstrate radiolucent lesions of the right humerus (B), as well as the left acetabulum and femur (C).

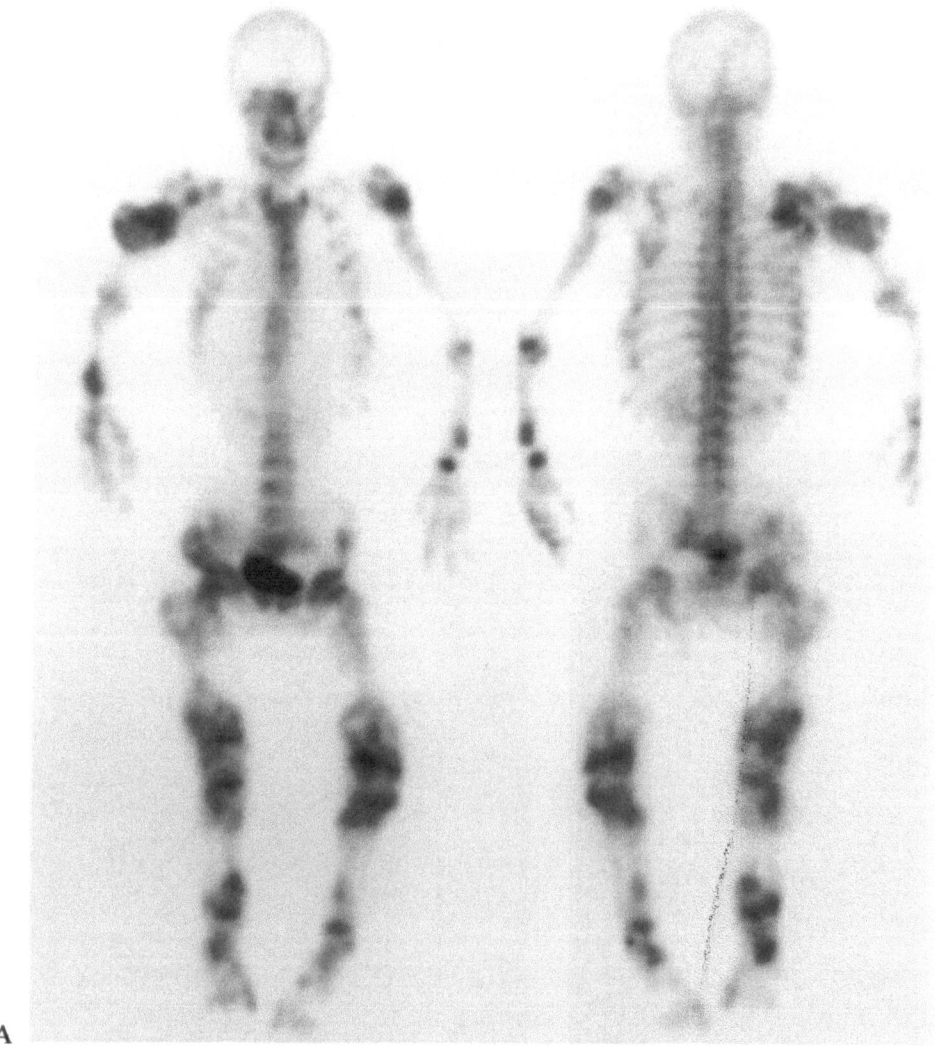

Figure 4.26. Enchondromatosis. Whole-body skeletal scintigraphy in the anterior and posterior projections defines the extent of skeletal involvement (A). The scintigraphic and radiographic abnormalities of the right proximal femur (B,C), the knees (D,E), and left forearm (F,G) are correlated.

A

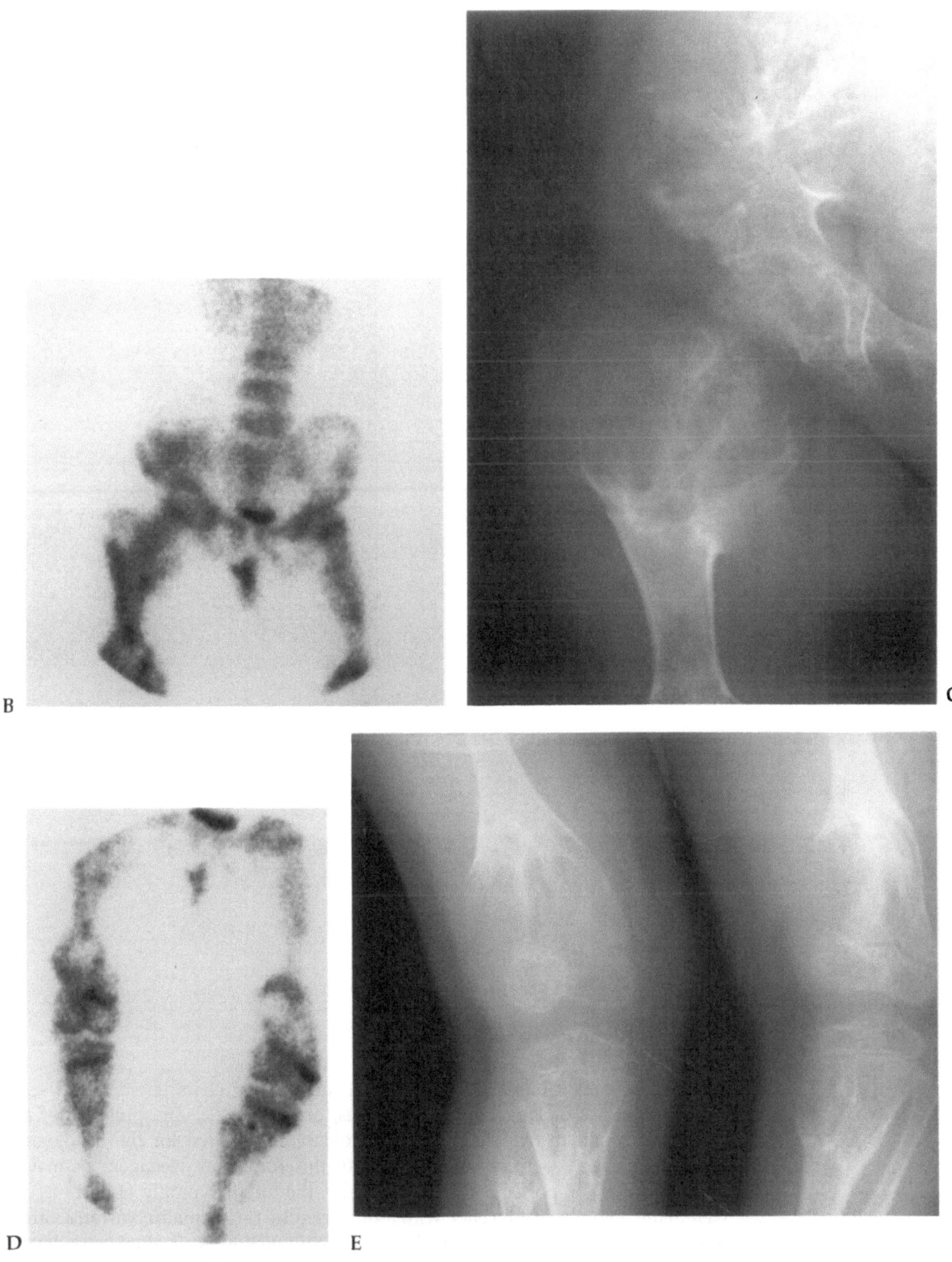

B

C

D

E

Figure 4.26 (*cont'd*). Caption is on p. 174.

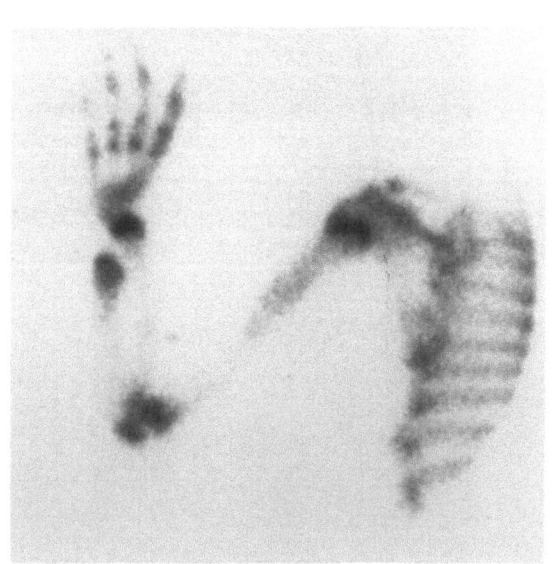

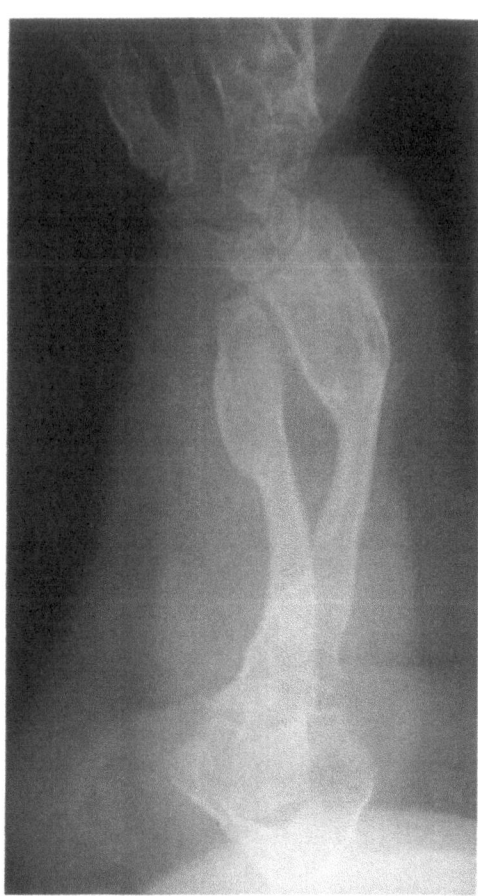

F

G

Figure 4.26 (*cont'd*). Caption is on p. 174.

Chondroblastoma

Chondroblastoma (Codman tumor), a rare benign tumor, characteristically arises in the epiphyses of long bones, apophyses, or the patella. The presence of a distinctive round to oval cell, the chondroblast, is required for the histologic diagnosis. Seventy percent of patients with this tumor are teenagers. A male predominance is reported.[37] Radiographically, the tumor typically appears as a well-defined epiphyseal lucency with a thin sclerotic rim. Chondroblastomas are reported to invariably demonstrate increased radionuclide localization on skeletal scintigraphy (Fig. 4.27). An extended pattern of increased localization frequently occurs.[44] Although scintigraphy has no significant role in the evaluation of chondroblastoma per se, it may be the first study to detect an abnormality in patients with this tumor. Additionally, since the radiologic differential diagnosis includes Langerhans cell histiocytosis, scintigraphy may be used during the diagnostic evaluation to exclude the presence of other skeletal lesions prior to biopsy and curettage.

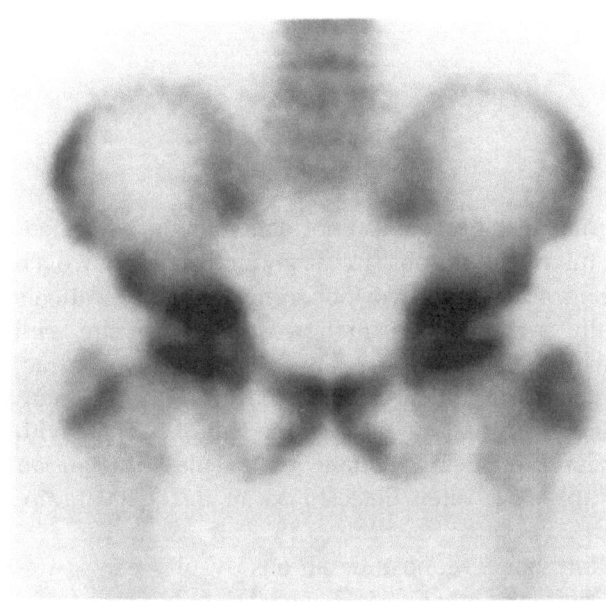

A

Figure 4.27. Chondroblastoma. There is increased tracer localization in the left greater trochanter (A). This is better depicted with pinhole magnification (B). A radiolucent lesion is present in the left greater trochanter (C).

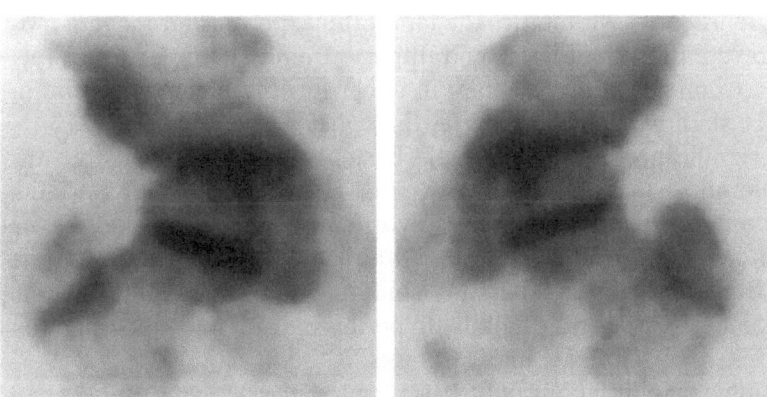

B

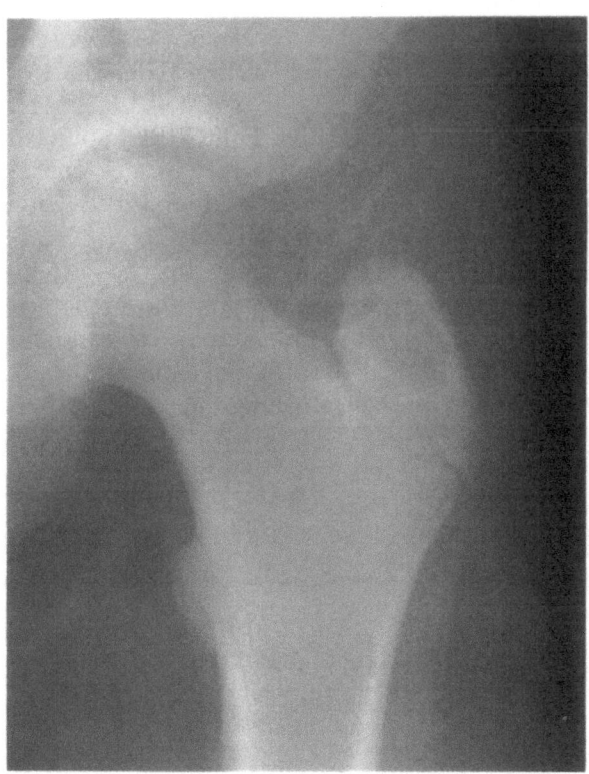

C

Fibrous Lesions

Fibrous Dysplasia

Fibrous dysplasia is a mesodermal developmental abnormality in which the medullary space is replaced with a mixture of fibrous stroma and trabeculae of woven bone. It occurs in monostotic (Fig. 4.28) and polyostotic forms (Fig. 4.29). Patients with fibrous dysplasia typically present in the first two decades of life with nonspecific symptoms that include pain, tenderness, and limp. Pathologic fracture, bowing deformity, leg length discrepancy, and facial asymmetry occur, particularly with polyostotic involvement. One third to one half of patients with polyostotic fibrous dysplasia have pigmented cutaneous macules (café-au-lait spots). Monostotic fibrous dysplasia is often detected as an incidental radiographic finding.[54,73]

Fibrous dysplasia involves any bone. Monostotic fibrous dysplasia most frequently affects the ribs, femur, tibia, and craniofacial bones. The polyostotic form, which is one sixth as common as the monostotic form, is typically unilateral or, when bilateral, markedly asymmetric. The femur, tibia, pelvis, and foot are most commonly involved. Rib, craniofacial, and upper extremity lesions are also relatively common. Craniofacial involvement in either form is characterized by involvement of the skull base and the sinuses (Figs. 4.29 and 4.30).[54]

The clinical significance of fibrous dysplasia stems from pathologic fractures and bowing deformities that may occur with either form and from the association between endocrine dysfunction and the polyostotic variant. Precocious sexual development occurs in 20% to 30% of girls with the polyostotic form (McCune-Albright syndrome). Other endocrine abnormalities, including Cushing syndrome, acromegaly, diabetes mellitus, hyperthyroidism, and hyperparathyroidism have been reported in about 5% of cases.[54,109]

The radiographic manifestations of fibrous dysplasia are variable. Mild expansion of a bone by an ill-defined homogeneous radiolucency with poorly structured trabeculations is the most characteristic appearance (Fig. 4.28). The lesions are often described as flame-shaped and of a ground-glass appearance. A thick sclerotic margin is frequently present.[54] Coxa vara ("shepherd's crook") deformity of the proximal femur is a characteristic abnormality.

The extent of local involvement can be assessed with CT and MRI. Lesions of fibrous dysplasia usually demonstrate low signal on T1-weighted images. The T2 signal characteristics are quite variable due to a heterogeneous composition to the lesions, with true cysts or fluid-fluid levels being present in some.[117]

The primary role of skeletal scintigraphy is to determine the presence, extent, and distribution of multiple lesions. Fibrous dysplasia typically shows marked skeletal tracer localization. This reflects the presence of immature woven bone and associated abnormal ossification. Rarely, fibrous dysplasia demonstrates only slightly increased radionuclide localization on skeletal scintigraphy.[39,57]

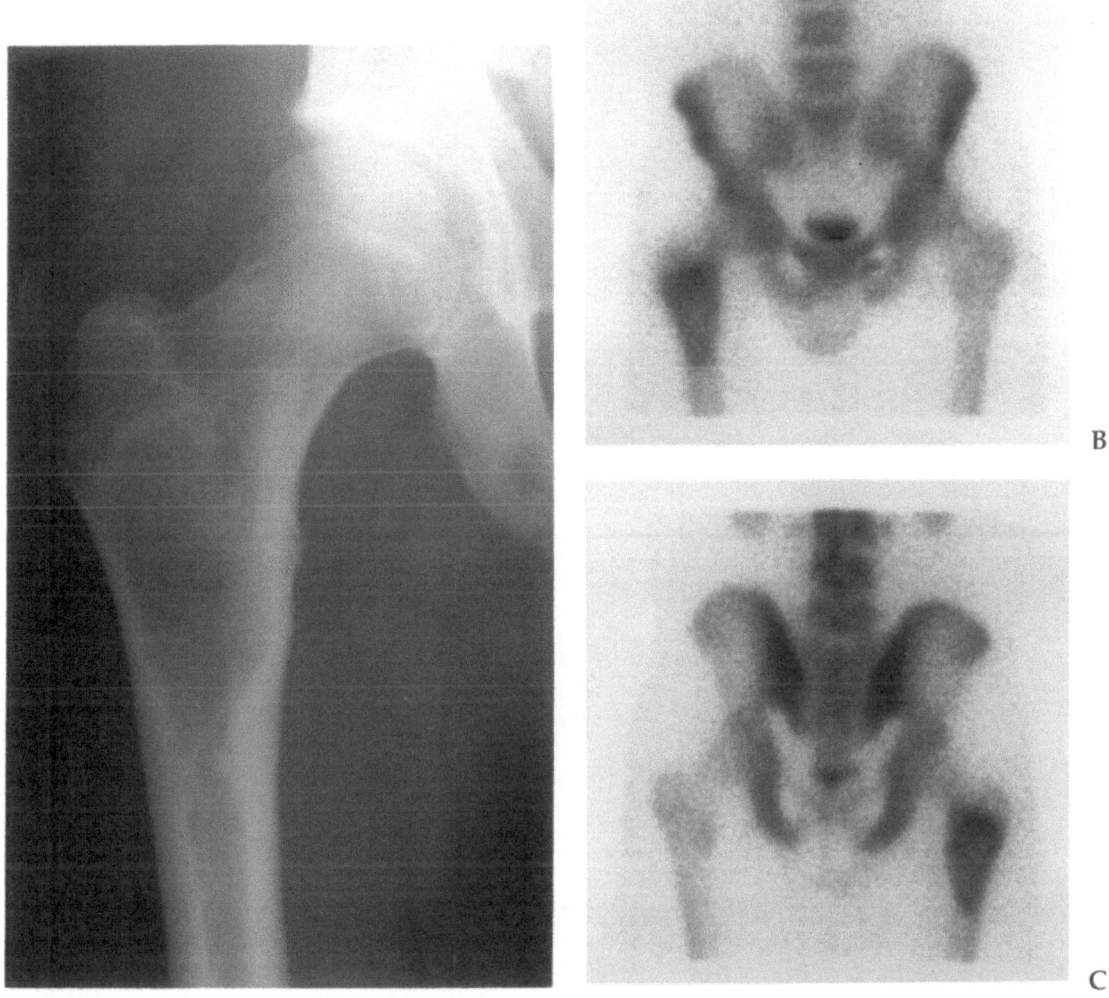

Figure 4.28. Fibrous dysplasia. A radiograph reveals a ground-glass radiolucency of the right femur with thinning of the endosteal cortex (A). Skeletal scintigraphy in the anterior (B) and posterior (C) projections demonstrates increased tracer localization along the lesion's periphery. This is most pronounced superiorly.

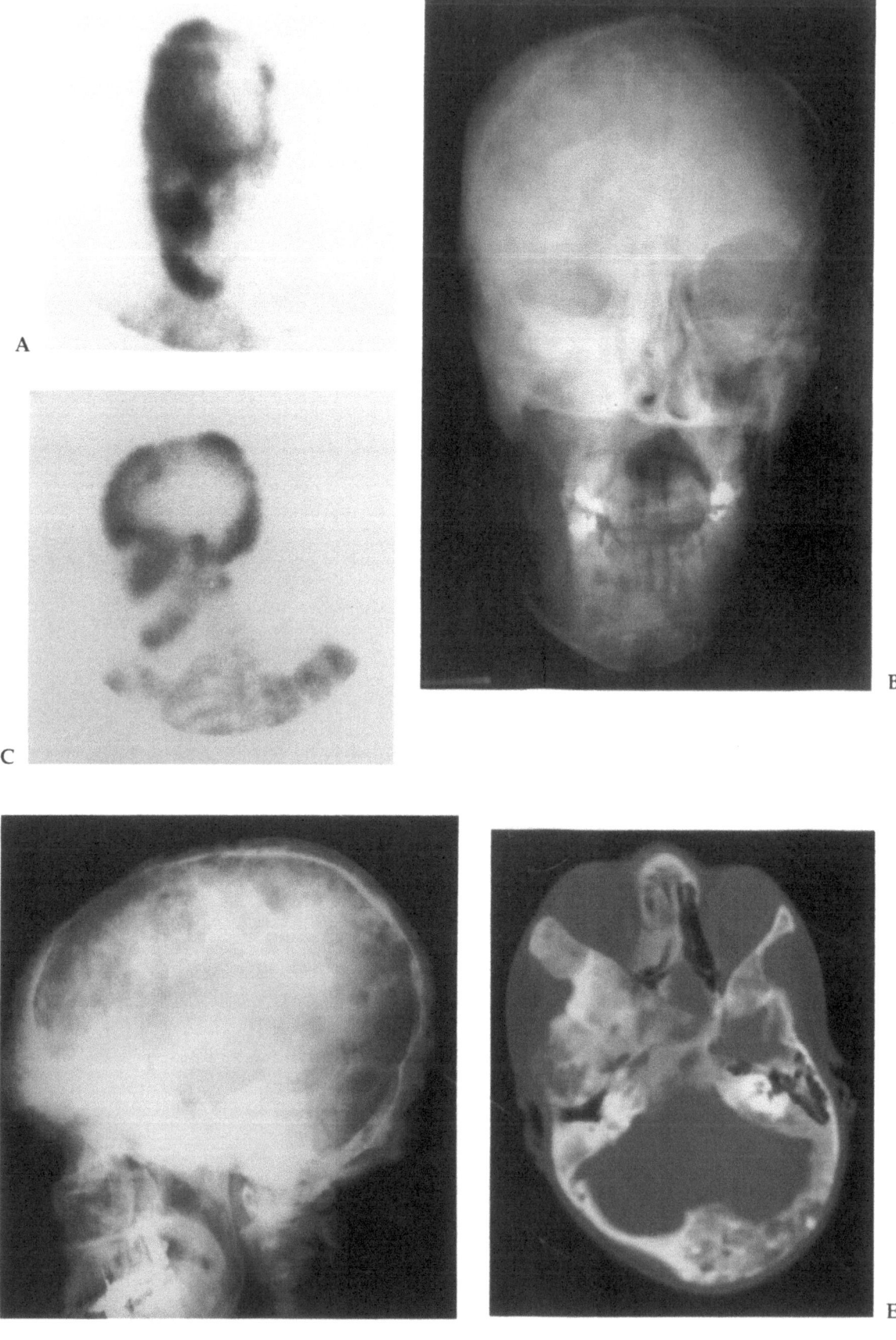

Figure 4.29. Polyostotic fibrous dysplasia. Areas of increased tracer localization within the skull demonstrated with an anterior skeletal scintigram (A) correlate with extensive radiographic abnormality depicted on the anteroposterior skull radiograph (B). This is also illustrated by correlation of lateral scintigraphic (C) and radiographic images (D). A selected transaxial CT image of the skull base shows marked osseous expansion sparing the right occiput (E).

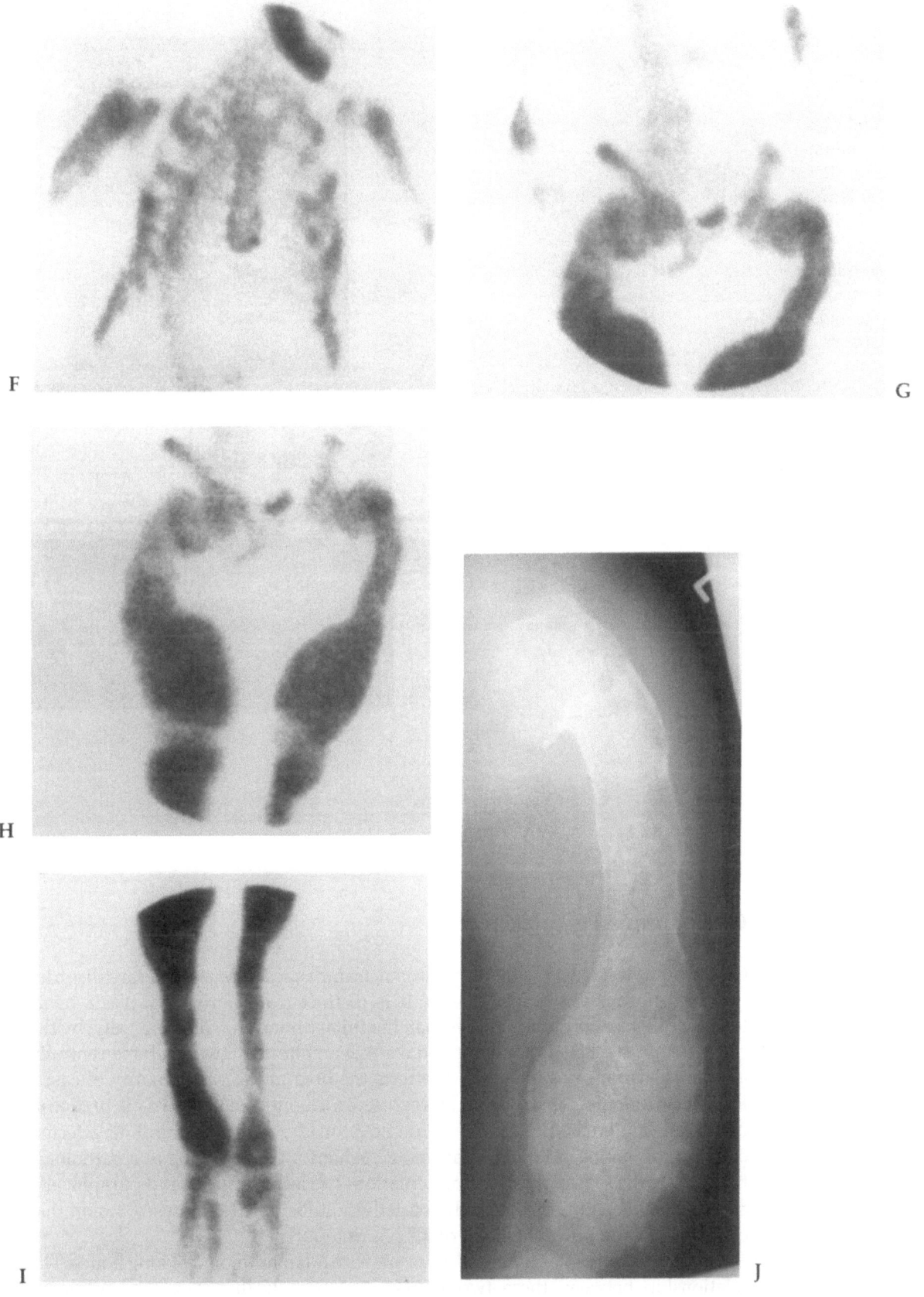

Figure 4.29 (*cont'd*). Anterior scintigraphic images of the thorax (F), pelvis (G), thighs (H), and calves and feet (I) depict diffuse skeletal involvement in this 17-year-old girl. A radiograph of the left femur provides a radiographic correlate (J).

Figure 4.30. Polyostotic fibrous dysplasia: craniofacial involvement. Correlative scintigraphic and T1-weighted, gadolinium-enhanced images show increased tracer localization and extensive heterogeneous signal abnormality associated with bony expansion of the frontal, sphenoid, and maxillary bones.

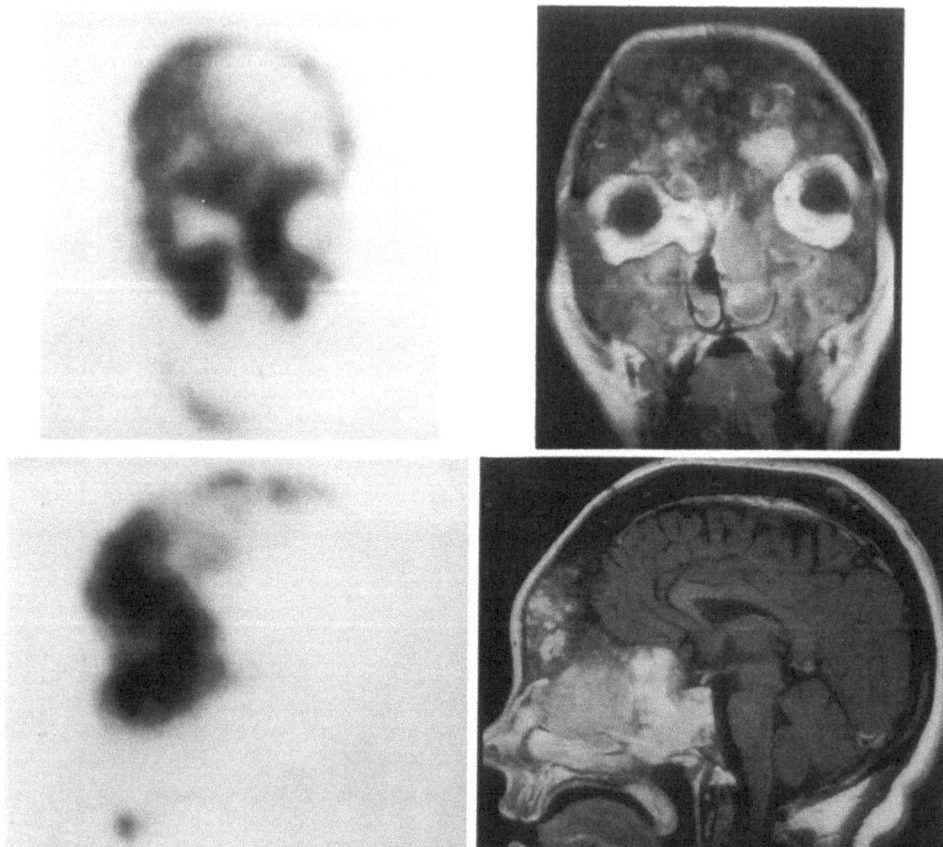

Osteofibrous Dysplasia

Osteofibrous dysplasia (ossifying fibroma, Campanacci disease) is a rare disorder in which fibrous tissue proliferates. It is distinct from fibrous dysplasia in its tendency to involve cortical rather than medullary bone and, histologically, by the presence of osteoblastic rimming and a zonal architecture (woven bone centrally and lamellar bone peripherally). It affects the tibia in the vast majority of cases. Fibular involvement is occasionally reported. Osteofibrous dysplasia is predominantly encountered in the first two decades of life, with two thirds of affected children presenting prior to 5 years of age. Anterior tibial bowing or a pathologic fracture are the typical modes of presentation. The lesion appears radiographically as an expansile, lytic, eccentrically located, multiloculated diaphyseal lesion that characteristically bows the tibial diaphysis anteriorly.[59,116]

Osteofibrous dysplasia may be a precursor to adamantinoma of long bones. The relationship between these two lesions, however, is uncertain.[13,44,74] Adamantinoma of long bones is an unusual malignant neoplasm that predominantly affects adolescents and young adults. It resembles osteofibrous dysplasia radiographically and in its tendency to involve the tibia. Due to the radiographic similarity, skeletal scintigraphy is occasionally requested to exclude the possibility of bone metastases, which are rare, prior to biopsy. Both osteofibrous dysplasia and adamantinoma demonstrate increased skeletal tracer localization and cannot be differentiated scintigraphically (Fig. 4.31).

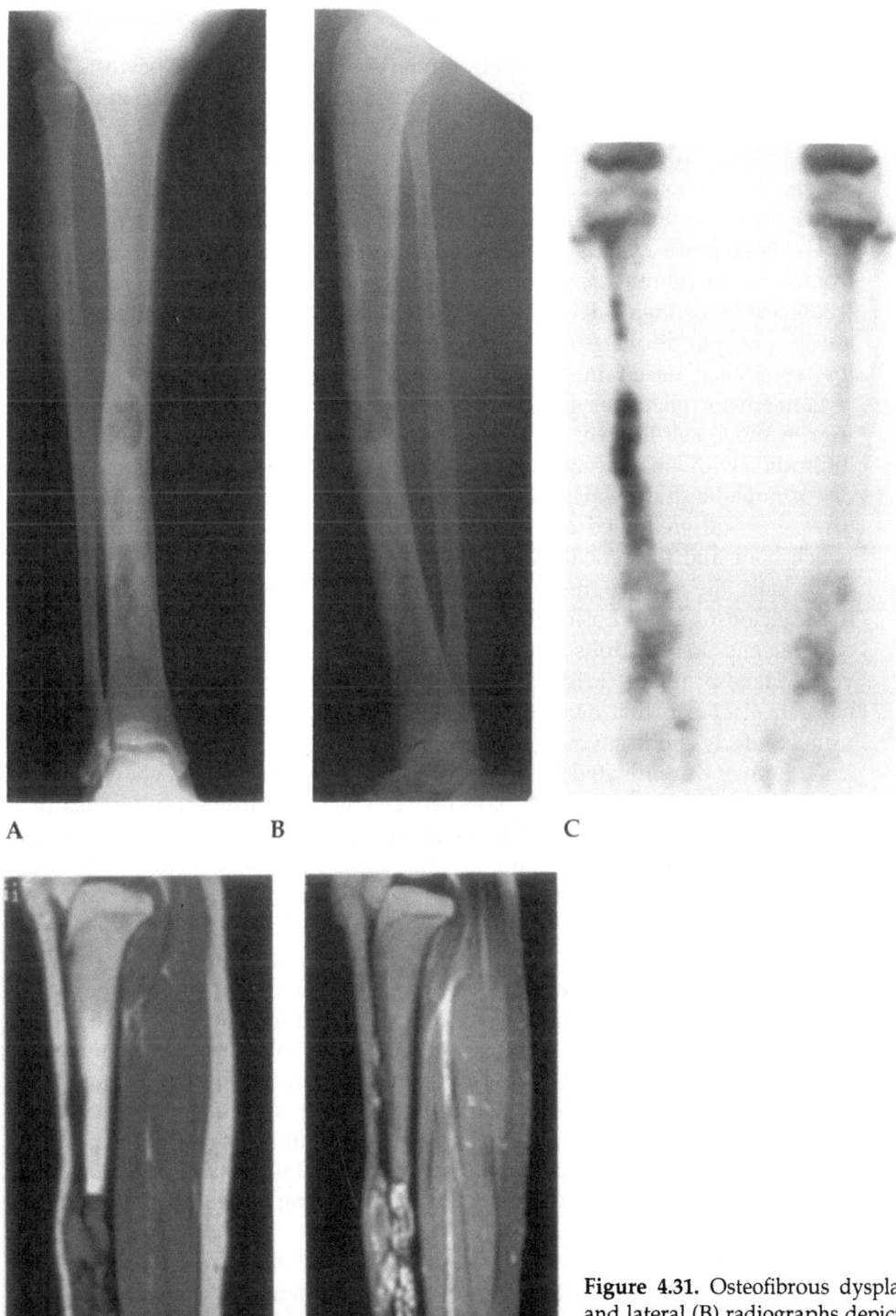

A

B

C

D

E

Figure 4.31. Osteofibrous dysplasia. Anteroposterior (A) and lateral (B) radiographs depict a right tibial diaphyseal lesion with mixed areas of sclerosis and radiolucency. The tibia is bowed anteriorly. Skeletal scintigraphy (C) shows increased tracer localization within the lesion. Magnetic resonance imaging shows a lesion of low signal intensity on T1-weighted imaging (D) with prominent enhancement following gadolinium (E).

Langerhans Cell Histiocytosis

Langerhans cell histiocytosis (LCH), formerly referred to as histiocytosis X, is a disease or group of diseases characterized by proliferation of Langerhans cells and granuloma formation.[107] Langerhans cells arise in the bone marrow (or from cells that originate in the bone marrow) and mature in the epidermis, dermal lymphatics, and lymph nodes. They present antigens to T lymphocytes. Birbeck granules, which are centrally striated rod-shaped organelles, are their distinctive feature.[17]

The etiology of LCH is unknown. The disease has been postulated to result from abnormal immune regulation.[107] Recent work suggests that LCH is a neoplastic process involving clonal cellular proliferation.[123] Whether the proliferating cells are truly neoplastic or are proliferating in response to an undetermined inflammatory stimulus is uncertain, however.

Langerhans cell histiocytosis encompasses a wide pathologic spectrum ranging from a single self-limited skeletal lesion to disseminated visceral and marrow infiltration without associated osseous involvement. The classic clinical groupings of eosinophilic granuloma, Hand-Schüller-Christian disease, and Letterer-Siwe disease are differentiated on the basis of their clinical course and the extent to which bone and the reticuloendothelial system are involved. With eosinophilic granuloma, the most common clinical variant of LCH, involvement is limited to the skeleton or lung. Eosinophilic granuloma is seen most frequently in older children and young adults, with an average age of diagnosis between 10 and 14 years. Hand-Schüller-Christian disease is a chronic, recurrent form of disseminated histiocytosis that involves bone and extraosseous sites. This form of LCH usually affects children younger than 5 years of age. Letterer-Siwe disease is an acute form of disseminated histiocytosis typically seen in children younger than 2 years of age. Significant overlap exists between these syndromes, and transformation from one form of the disease to another occurs.[107] Cases of LCH, therefore, are more accurately classified on an individual basis without reference to these eponyms. Nevertheless, they remain in common usage.

Children with osseous LCH, often present with localized pain, soft tissue swelling, and tenderness. Skeletal involvement, especially when monostotic, may not produce symptoms and may be detected as an incidental radiographic finding. An occasional clinical presentation of osseous LCH with fever, elevated erythrocyte sedimentation rate, mild leukocytosis, and anemia mimics that of osteomyelitis.[107] Children with disseminated disease may present with nonspecific systemic signs or with complaints referable to sites of involvement, such as the liver or lungs. Diabetes insipidus can result from extension of skull or orbital lesions or from neurohypophyseal infiltration of Langerhans cells.[8] Otologic manifestations, such as aural discharge, postauricular swelling, and hearing loss may occur with temporal bone involvement.[21]

Extent of disease and age at presentation are the most important prognostic indicators.[59] Clinicians must perform a thorough diagnostic evaluation to accurately determine the extent of disease.[23] Children who present prior to 2 years of age with disseminated disease have a high likelihood of disease progression and the poorest prognosis. Children who present with disease limited to bone are unlikely to develop systemic disease and have an excellent prognosis.[23,107]

Treatments of osseous LCH include observation without intervention, surgical excision, radiation therapy, and intralesional steroid administration. Multiagent chemotherapy is used in cases with systemic involvement.[107] Bone marrow transplantation is used in some children with disseminated involvement whose initial treatment proved unsuccessful and whose prognosis is poor.[106]

Osseous involvement is the most common manifestation of LCH. Lesions in the skull, ribs, mandible, spine, and pelvis account for approximately 65% of osseous LCH (Figs. 4.32 to 4.35).[52] Long bones, where the lesions are usually diaphyseal (Fig. 4.36), occasionally metaphyseal, and rarely epiphyseal,[107] are involved in about 30% of cases.[52]

Imaging is used primarily in determining disease extent and in localizing lesions for biopsy. A complete radiographic skeletal survey and whole-body skeletal scintigraphy are useful for these purposes.

The radiographic appearance of osseous LCH varies. The typical appearance is a lytic lesion, the margins of which may show sclerosis. There may be associated bone expansion and pathologic fracture. Periosteal new bone is common with lesions of the long bones but rare with those of flat bones. A soft tissue mass is frequently present.[59] Diffuse osteopenia is the only skeletal manifestation in some cases with disseminated involvement.

Certain patterns of involvement and radiographic appearances are characteristic of osseous LCH. A radiolucent skull lesion with beveled edges due to uneven destruction of the inner and outer tables is a classic radiographic manifestation (Fig. 4.33). Destruction of alveolar bone due to mandibular or maxillary involvement causes multiple "floating teeth." A button sequestrum, a central fragment of intact bone, may be demonstrated in calvarial or pelvic lesions. Rib lesions, which are frequently multiple, appear as expansile or permeative osteolysis. In the spine, the vertebral body is primarily involved. Vertebra plana, complete collapse of a vertebral body, occurs in some cases.[59,107,109] Sclerosis, prominent trabeculae, and cortical thickening become evident with healing. An involved bone may eventually return to a normal appearance and a collapsed vertebra may show considerable reconstitution of vertebral height over years of follow-up.[59]

With skeletal scintigraphy, LCH lesions often appear as foci of low tracer localization. Adjacent high tracer localization, reflecting bone repair, may be present. In the skull, a typical appearance is one of high localization circumferentially outlining a zone of decreased localization. Only increased tracer localization, which may be intense, is apparent in some cases. Lesions that do not incite an adjacent osteoblastic response are quite subtle and difficult to identify. New aggressive lesions are likely to be detected with skeletal scintigraphy. Older, quiescent, or treated lesions are less likely to exhibit a scintigraphic abnormality.

The sensitivity of radiography relative to that of skeletal scintigraphy for detecting osseous LCH has been widely debated. A review of multiple published series that have led to radiography being accepted as a more sensitive approach showed significant biases favoring radiography. Biases included the use of early generation relatively low-resolution gamma cameras, scintigrams performed following therapy being compared with radiographs obtained prior to therapy, and the direction of radiographic examinations by scintigraphic findings.[98] A recent report showed a higher overall sensitivity for skeletal scintigraphy than radiography in detecting osseous LCH and supported prior studies in showing that some lesions are demonstrated only with scintigraphy, some lesions only with radiography, and the majority of lesions with both.[24] Lesions of the spine, pelvis, and ribs may be difficult to detect radiographically due to the complex radiographic anatomy of these regions. Calvarial lesions can be missed by either technique, but tend to go undetected somewhat more frequently with scintigraphy. The extent of osseous involvement in children with LCH is optimally determined by a combined scintigraphic and radiographic approach. Additionally, it has been suggested that lesions detected with skeletal scintigraphy are clinically active while those detected radiographically, but not scintigraphically, are more likely to have healed.[42a]

Attempts have been made at using other radiopharmaceuticals in LCH patients. Gallium-67 imaging and ^{99m}Tc sulfur colloid bone marrow scintigraphy have proven to be significantly less effective at demonstrating osseous LCH than either skeletal scintigraphy or radiography.[101] Localization of thallium-201 (^{201}Tl) in the highly cellular sheets of Langerhans cells that characterize the early phase of LCH has been reported (Fig. 4.36).[3,28] Since ^{201}Tl localization reflects cellularity, a paucity of Langerhans cells in older active LCH lesions limits the potential utility of this agent for long-term follow-up of children with LCH.

Imaging with CT or MRI is valuable in defining the soft tissue component of an osseous lesion. This is particularly important when extension into the epidural space is suspected. The excellent anatomic delineation provided by CT or MRI is also useful in assessing local osseous involvement, especially with calvarial, facial, spinal, and pelvic lesions. With MRI, osseous LCH typically appears hypointense on T1-weighted images, hyperintense on T2-weighted images, and hyperintense on gadolinium-enhanced T1-weighted images. Abnormal bone marrow and soft tissue signal are prominent features. Accurate differentiation between LCH involvement and edema has not been achieved with MRI. A decrease in T2 and postgadolinium T1 signal intensity occur with therapeutic response.[33]

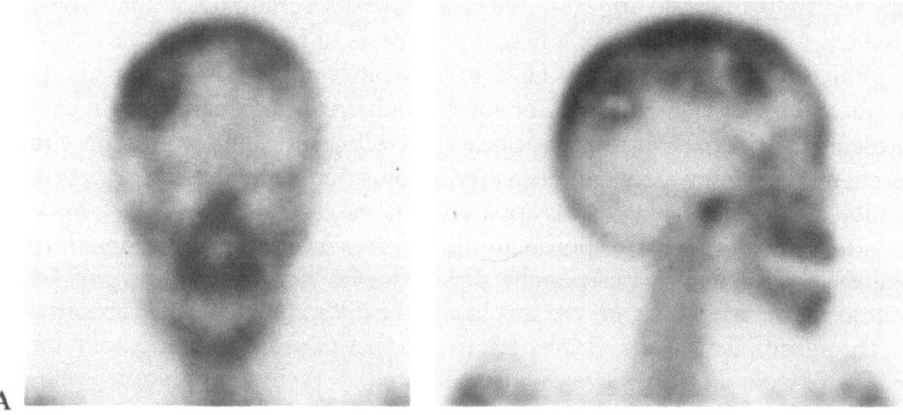

A

Figure 4.32. Langerhans cell histiocytosis. Anterior and lateral images depict extensive areas of increased and decreased tracer localization within the skull (A). Correlative radiographs show multiple radiolucencies (B,C).

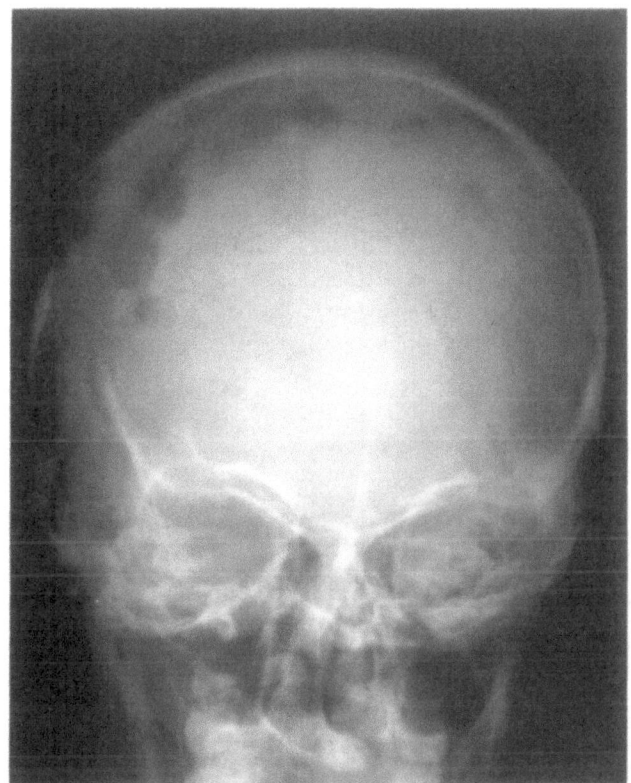

B

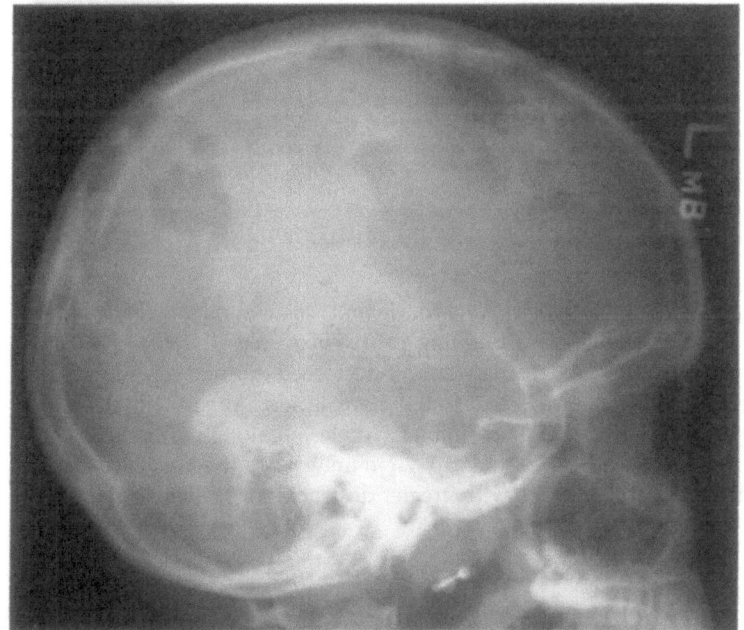

C

Figure 4.32 (*cont'd.*).

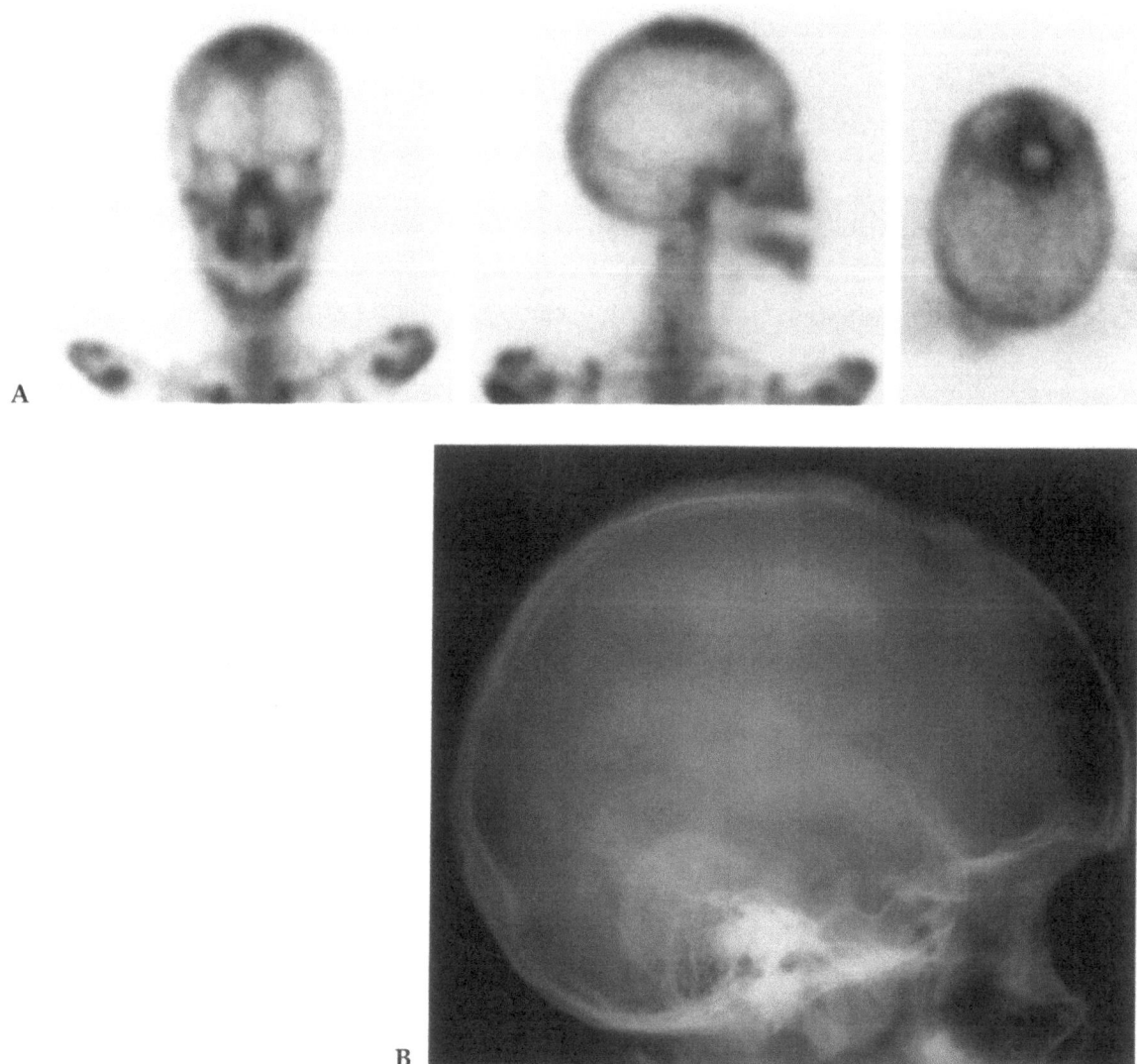

Figure 4.33. Langerhans cell histiocytosis. Anterior, lateral, and vertex projections reveal markedly increased tracer localization surrounding an area of decreased tracer localization in the region of the sagittal suture (A). A subtle area of decreased tracer localization is seen on the anterior projection, inferior and lateral to the more striking abnormality. A lateral radiograph (B) of the skull depicts a 2.5-cm circular lytic lesion along the sagittal suture with a second smaller area of cortical irregularity 2 cm anterior to the larger lesion. The larger lesion demonstrates beveled edges with greater destruction of the inner than outer table.

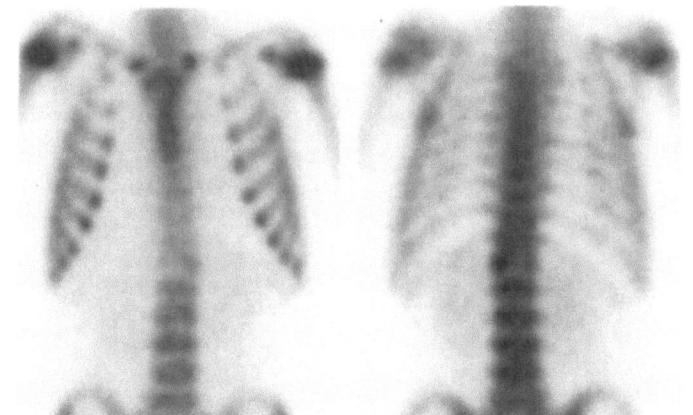

A

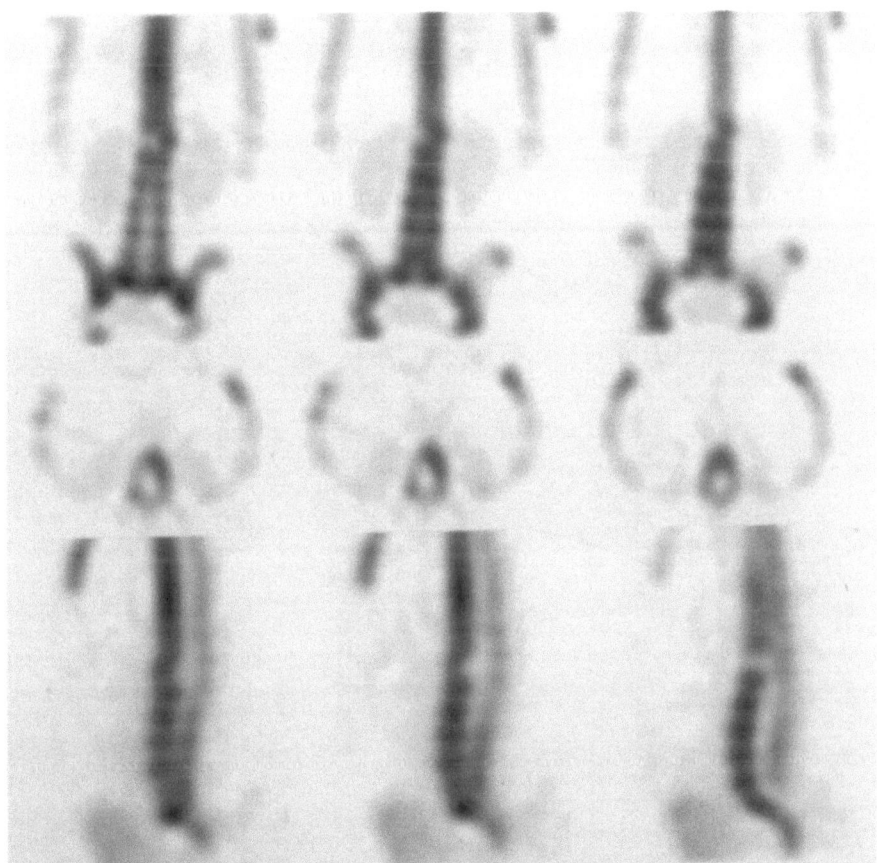

B

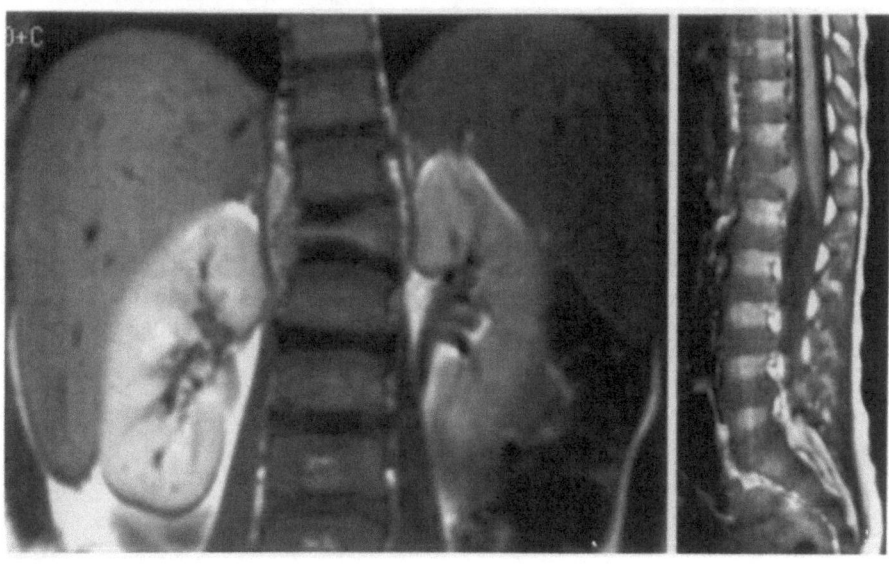

C

Figure 4.34. Langerhans cell histiocytosis. An anterior planar image reveals decreased tracer localization in the right aspect of T12 with increased tracer localization seen in the left aspect of that vertebrae on anterior and posterior images (A). The distribution of ^{99m}Tc-MDP is better depicted with SPECT (B). Complete collapse of the central and right sided portions of the T12 vertebral body are shown with coronal MRI. Posterior displacement of the conus is depicted on the sagittal MR image. The disk spaces are preserved at all levels including T11–T12 and T12–L1 (C).

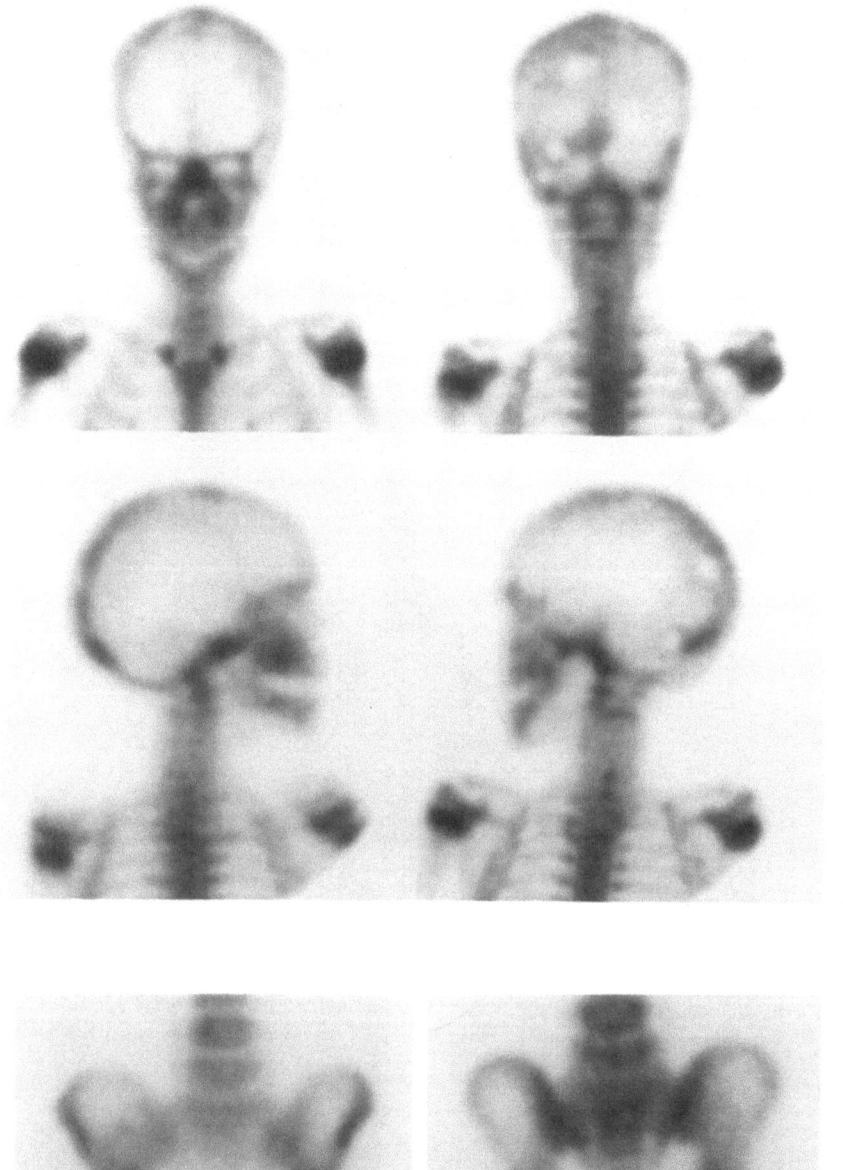

A

B

Figure 4.35. Langerhans cell histiocytosis. Anterior, posterior, right lateral, and left lateral images of the skull reveal rounded areas of decreased tracer localization in the region of the lambdoid suture on the left and inferiorly in the left occipital bone (A). The perilambdoid lesion has minimal surrounding increased tracer localization while the occipital lesion has more prominently increased adjacent tracer localization. Anterior and posterior images of the pelvis show slightly increased tracer localization relative to adjacent bone in the right ilium (B).

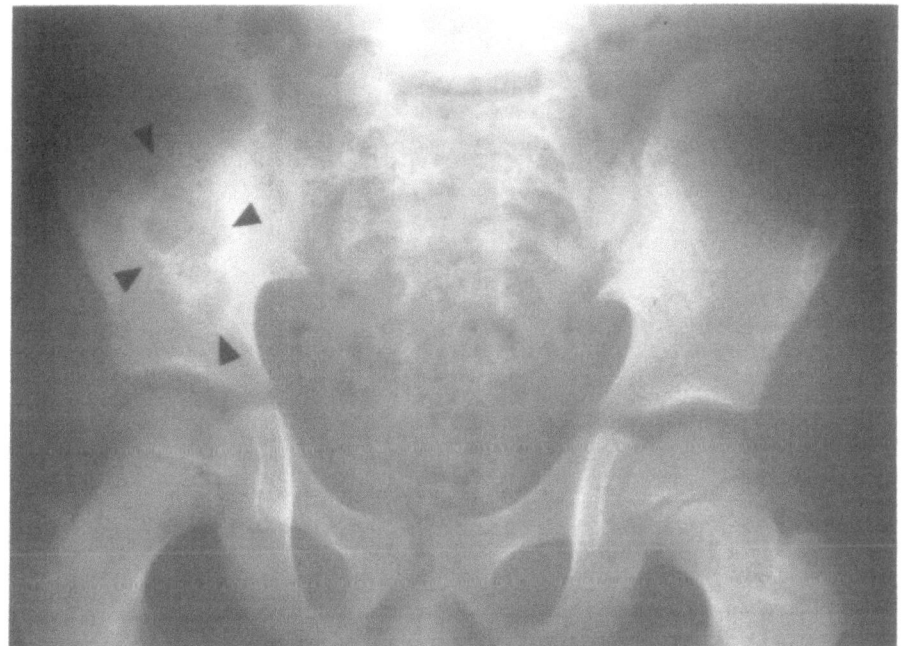

C

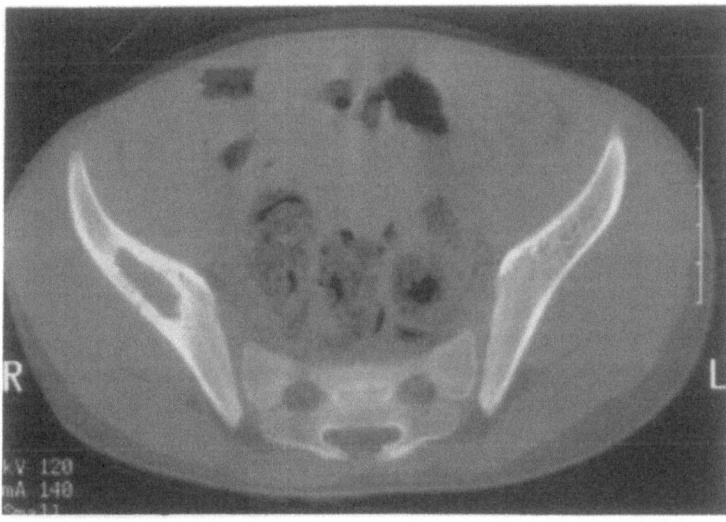

D

Figure 4.35 (*cont'd.*). A pelvic radiograph (C) shows a lytic lesion with sclerotic margins corresponding to the scintigraphic abnormality (arrows). The lesion is well delineated by CT (D).

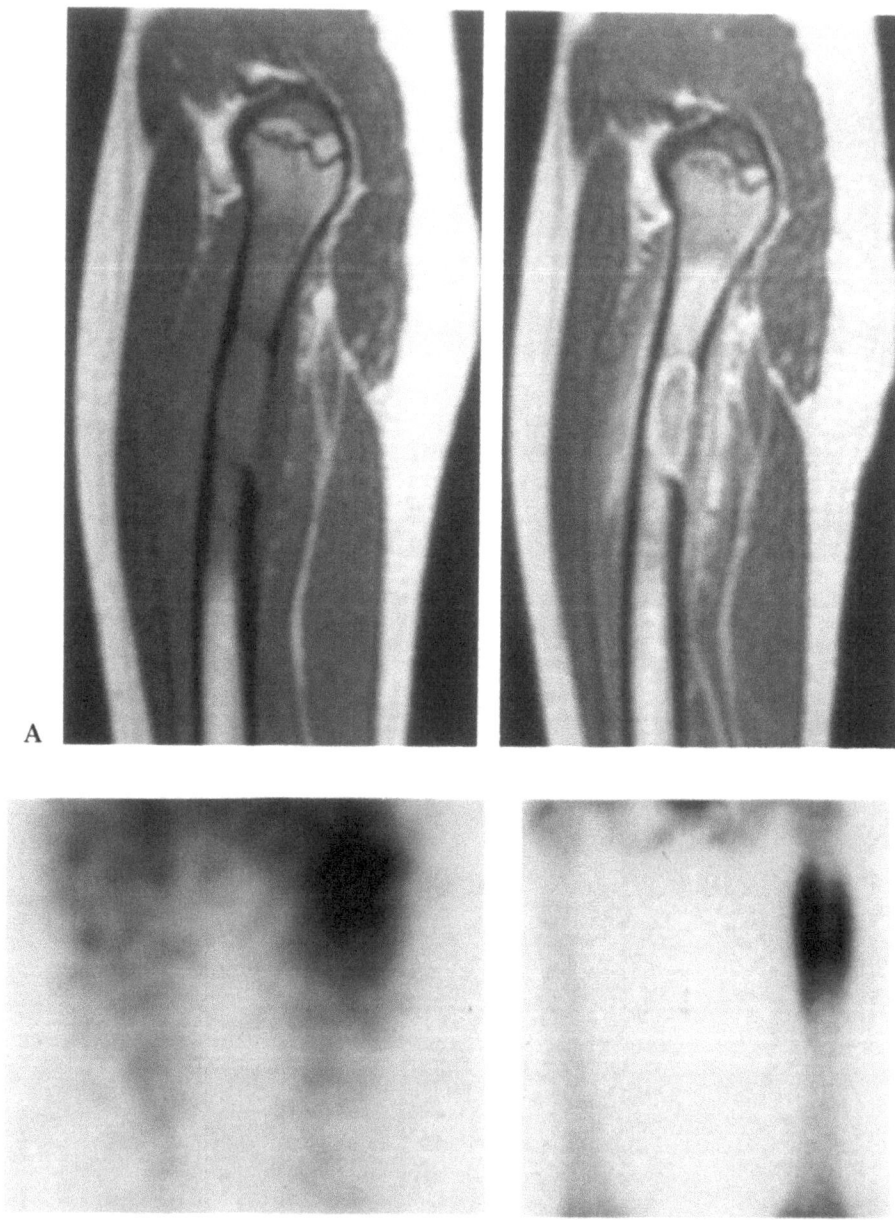

Figure 4.36. Langerhans cell histiocytosis. Sagittal T1-weighted images of the left femur demonstrates an intramedullary mass that violates the posterior cortex and enhances following gadolinium(A). Thallium-201 localizes in the lesion (B, left panel), which is associated with increased ^{99m}Tc-MDP localization in the medial and lateral cortices of the proximal left femur (B, right panel).

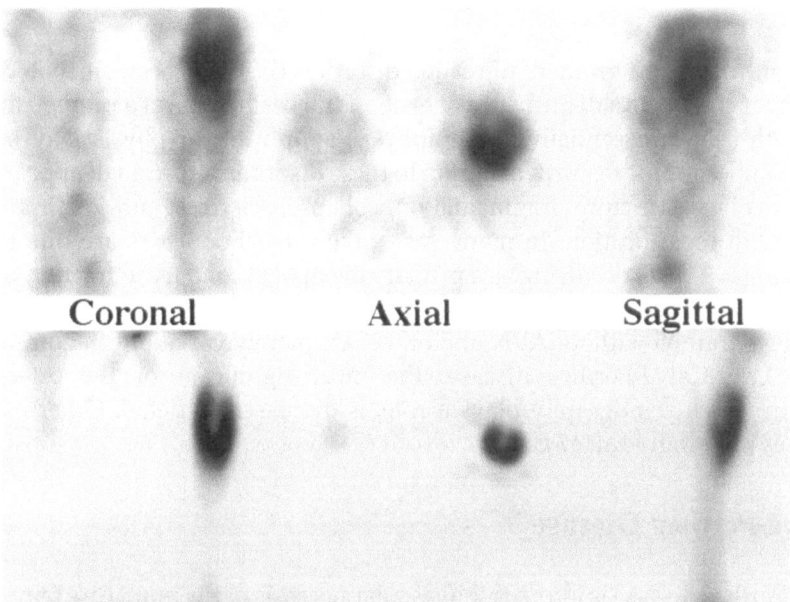

Coronal   Axial   Sagittal

C

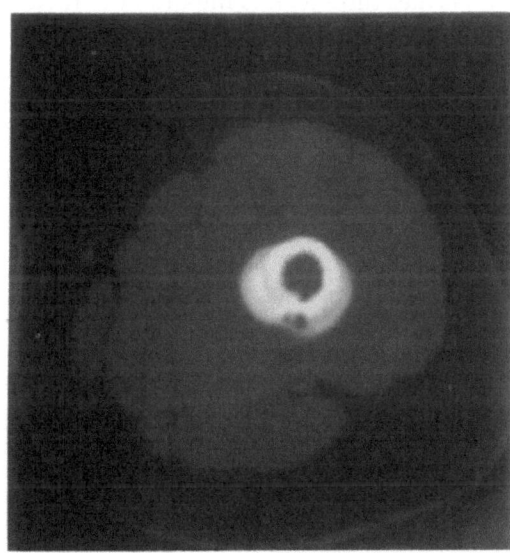

D

Figure 4.36 (*cont'd.*). The difference between the distribution of ^{99m}Tc-MDP and [201]T1 in the lesion is shown with SPECT (C). Transaxial CT scan through the superior aspect of the lesion demonstrates cortical expansion, endosteal scalloping, and solid periosteal reaction. Correlating scintigraphy with CT (D), it is likely that the high ^{99m}Tc-MDP localization relates to extensive reparative bone formation, while [201]T1 uptake reflects cellular deposits. (Reprinted from Bar-Sever et al,[3] with permission.)

The Osteochondroses

The osteochondroses are a group of unrelated disorders that have been attributed, sometimes erroneously, to a disturbance of enchondral ossification at a previously normal growth center. Essentially any epiphysis, apophysis, or physis may be affected. The radiographic features common to these disorders are a small appearance to the involved structure, fragmentation, collapse, sclerosis, and, often, reconstitution with reossification. In many cases, the osteochondroses are due to avascular necrosis (AVN) occurring as a primary event or secondary to fracture or other trauma. Some conditions that are traditionally considered osteochondroses are likely due to trauma without AVN and others are merely variations in normal ossification. Legg-Calvé-Perthes disease, the most significant of the osteochondroses in which scintigraphy plays a role, is discussed in detail. Other osteochondroses are briefly reviewed.

Legg-Calvé-Perthes Disease

Legg-Calvé-Perthes disease is idiopathic avascular necrosis of the immature femoral capital epiphysis.

For an understanding of Legg-Calvé-Perthes disease, it is important to review the vascular supply of the femoral capital epiphysis in young children (Fig. 4.37).[16] The proximal femur receives its blood supply via an extracapsular vascular ring

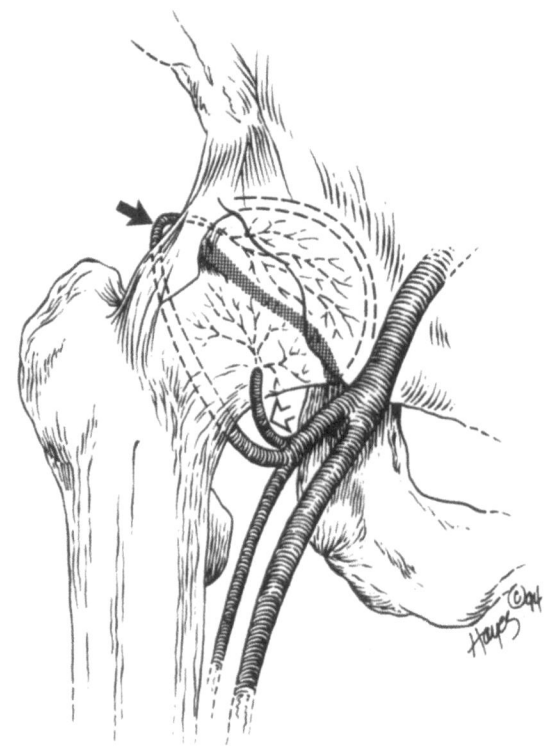

Figure 4.37. Arterial supply to the femoral capital epiphysis. The medial circumflex artery (solid arrow) arises from the deep femoral artery, passes posterior to the femoral neck, and enters the lateral aspect of the joint. Branches of this vessel supply the epiphysis. The lateral circumflex artery (open arrow) primarily supplies the femoral neck. (Diagram courtesy of James J. Conway, M.D., Children's Memorial Hospital, Chicago. Reprinted from Conway,[19] with permission.)

formed by two primary branches of the deep femoral artery, the medial circumflex and lateral circumflex arteries, and the artery of the ligamentum teres. Ascending cervical vessels that arise from the vascular ring are the most important source of blood to the epiphysis. The posterior and lateral aspects of the ring are formed by the medial circumflex artery. The terminal branch of the medial circumflex artery, the lateral ascending cervical artery, provides the largest volume of blood to the epiphysis. This vessel enters the capsule posterolaterally and gives off a rete of branching arterioles that extend medially and anteriorly to supply the entire epiphysis. The anastomotic network of the anterior portion of the ring, which is formed by the lateral circumflex artery, is much less extensive than that of the posterior portion of the ring. This is particularly true in males between the ages of 3 and 10 years. The importance of a single branch, the lateral ascending cervical artery, of one vessel, the medial circumflex artery, places the femoral capital epiphysis at risk of AVN.[18]

Despite extensive study, the etiology of Legg-Calvé-Perthes disease remains an enigma. Proposed mechanisms include vascular tamponade due to processes within the hip joint that produce effusions (e.g., septic arthritis, transient synovitis, trauma with or without fracture), compression of intraepiphyseal vessels as a direct result of trauma, and increased blood viscosity. These conditions produce varying degrees of ischemia with repeated or prolonged ischemia leading to AVN.[47,97] It has been suggested that Legg-Calvé-Perthes disease is the result not of AVN alone, but rather of a resorptive process initiated by a subchondral fracture complicating AVN.[96]

Legg-Calvé-Perthes disease most often occurs in children between the ages of 5 and 8 years. It is rare in children younger than 4 years or older than 12 years of age and in nonwhites of any age. In a child of African descent, hemoglobin analysis to assess for sickle cell anemia should be performed prior to attributing the imaging findings of femoral head AVN to Legg-Calvé-Perthes disease. A marked male predilection of approximately 4:1 is consistently reported. Legg-Calvé-Perthes disease is typically unilateral; only approximately 13% of cases are bilateral.[26,78] Skeletal maturation is typically delayed; bone age is more than 2 standard deviations below the mean in almost 75% of Legg-Calvé-Perthes disease patients.[36] Clinically, children with Legg-Calvé-Perthes disease typically present with limping. Hip, thigh, or knee pain may be present. Physical examination may reveal muscular spasm and limited internal rotation at the hip.

Four identifiable radiographic stages are described. Early in the initial stage (devascularization stage), the affected femoral capital epiphysis appears normal, as dead avascular bone has a normal radiographic appearance.[18,20] Small size of the affected epiphysis, due to a growth failure induced by the absence of its blood supply, is the earliest radiographic finding. Synovial overgrowth and femoral and acetabular cartilage hypertrophy result in widening of the joint space medially.[95] A subchondral radiolucency, representing a stress fracture, is a characteristic finding. The extent of this fracture corresponds to the extent of the necrotic zone and is useful prognostically.[122] Later in this stage the physis appears irregular and the metaphysis relatively osteopenic, while the femoral head appears relatively dense. In the second stage (revascularization stage), changes due to repair become evident. The epiphysis is fragmented with variable areas of radiolucency and increased radiodensity. These findings reflect bone resorption and reparative bone formation. Cyst-like metaphyseal radiolucencies, representing extensions of physeal cartilage,[83] are demonstrated in approximately one third of patients.[78] The presence of these metaphyseal lesions is an unfavorable prognostic sign, predictive of growth arrest.[50] During the third stage (the reparative or reossification stage), the epiphysis returns to normal radiodensity. Changes in the shape of the proximal femur, including coxa magna, a shortened femoral neck, and an irregular epiphyseal contour are often evident. In the final stage (healed stage) the epiphysis has ossified into a shape determined by the extent of AVN, the effects of cartilaginous overgrowth, the impact of abnormal vector forces on the reossifying epiphysis, and the results of surgical or orthotic treatment. There may be complete restoration to a normal femoral head or a flattened, misshapen femoral head with a short femoral neck, producing a coxa magna deformity. The degree to which the epiphysis reconstitutes and attains a normal morphology determines the degree of long-term symptoms and arthritic changes.

The insidious nature of the clinical syndrome results in radiographs being positive in the majority of children at presentation. Scintigraphic changes are present 4 to 6 weeks earlier than radiographic changes, however.[5] The sensitivity of skeletal scintigraphy for early detection of Legg-Calvé-Perthes disease is between 90% and 98%.[12,15,110] Scintigraphy, therefore, is extremely valuable whenever radiographs do not confirm a suspected diagnosis of Legg-Calvé-Perthes disease. Absence of radionuclide localization in the femoral capital epiphysis, best demonstrated with pinhole magnification, is the earliest scintigraphic finding (Fig. 4.38).

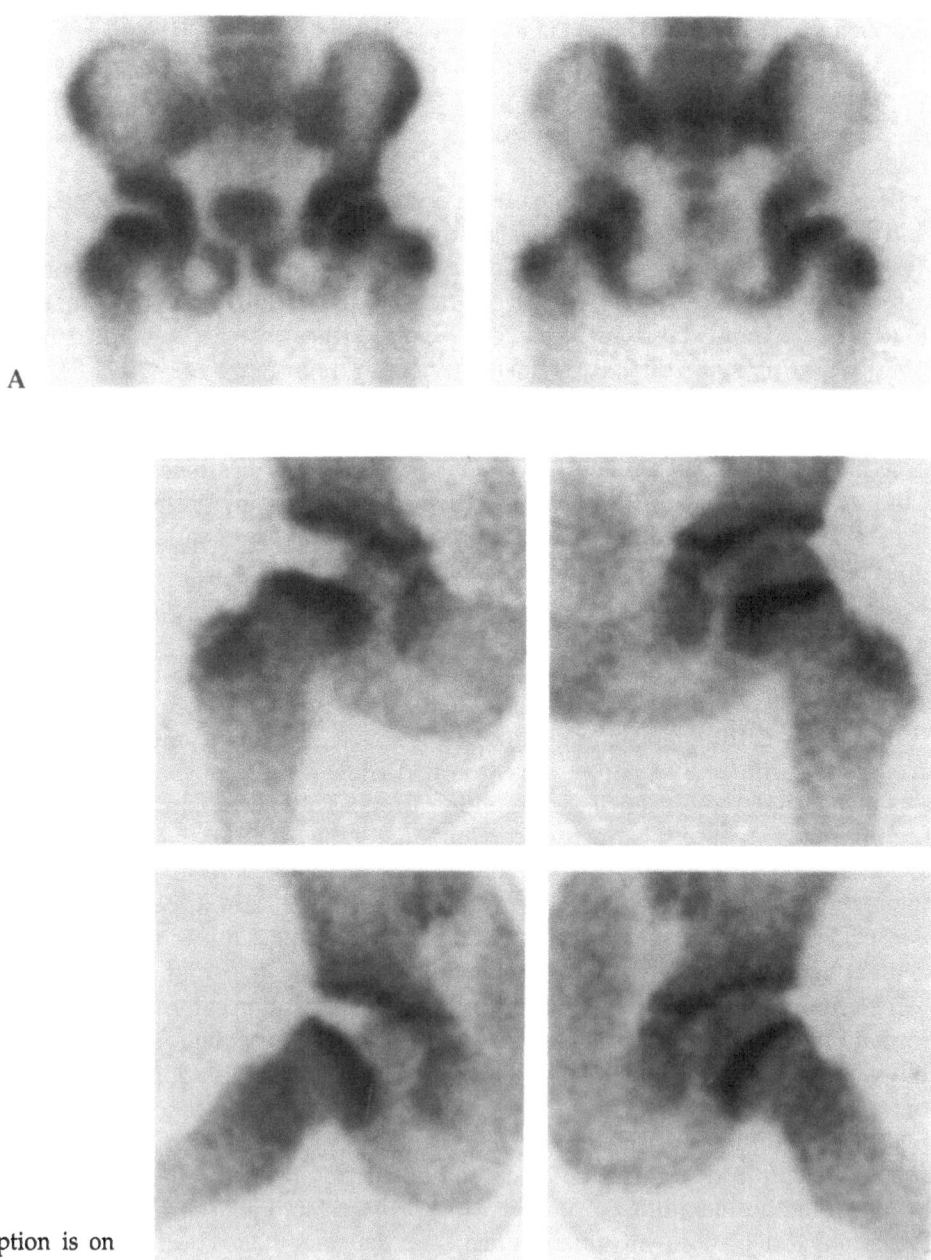

A

B

Figure 4.38 (A) and (B). Caption is on p. 197.

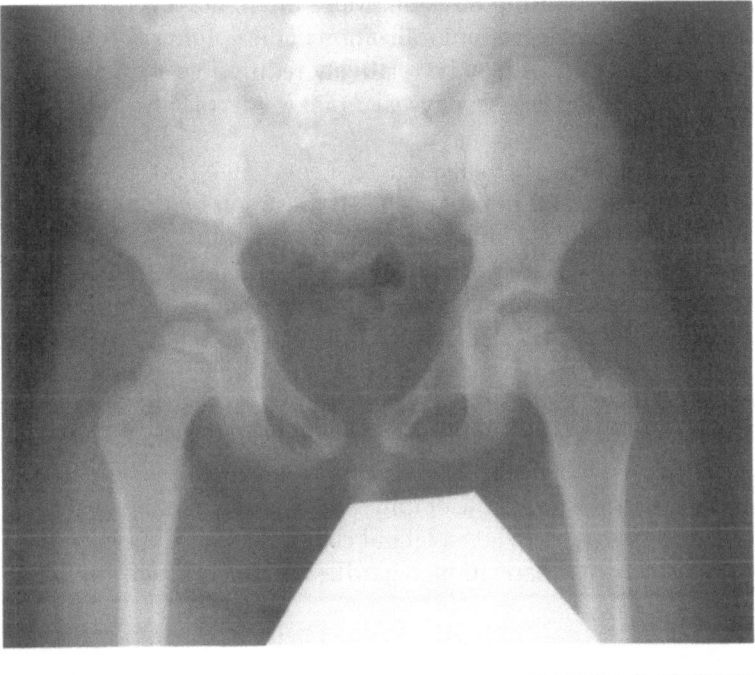

C

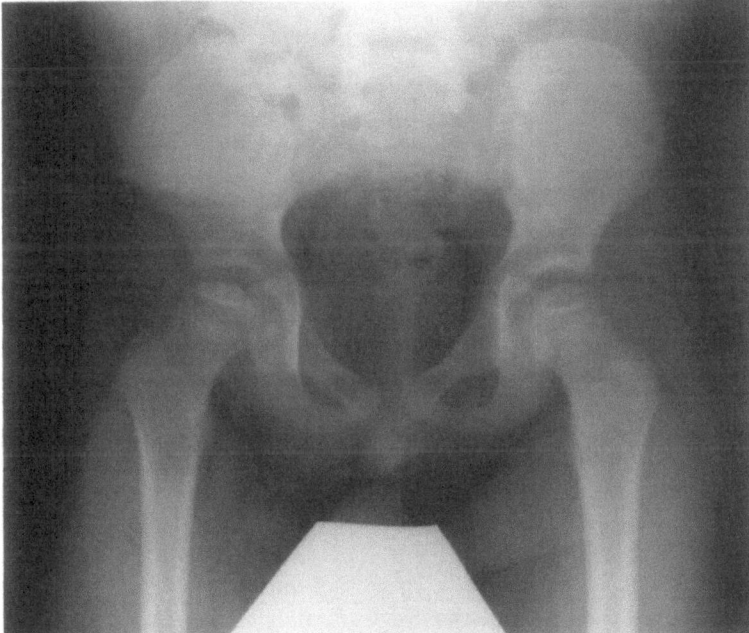

D

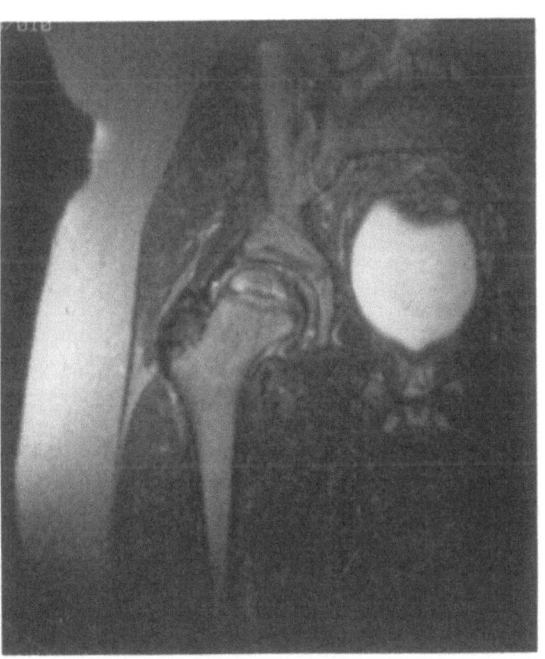

E

Figure 4.38. Legg-Calvé-Perthes disease. Absence of tracer localization in the right femoral capital epiphysis is demonstrated with high-resolution (A, anterior projection and posterior projection) and pinhole (B, anterior and frog-leg lateral projections) scintigraphy. Note that tracer localization in the acetabulum should not be misinterpreted as being within the medial portions of the epiphysis. The affected epiphysis appeared normal radiographically (C) at the time of diagnostic scintigraphy. Six months later (D), the epiphysis appeared small, sclerotic, and fragmented, and radiolucencies extended from the physis into the metaphysis. Magnetic resonance imaging, performed one week after scintigraphy (E), shows increased T2 signal, consistent with edema, in the epiphyseal marrow. The physis is slightly widened. An effusion is not identified.

This finding is not entirely specific as it is also seen when ischemia results from vascular tamponade induced by a hip effusion. More often, however, hip effusions decrease, but do not eliminate, tracer localization in the epiphysis. Additionally, tracer localization in the physis may be relatively reduced with an effusion, whereas in Legg-Calvé-Perthes disease physeal uptake is typically normal or increased.[109]

In addition to its value in early detection of Legg-Calvé-Perthes disease, skeletal scintigraphy may be useful in prognostic stratification by depicting two different patterns during the revascularization and reparative stages.[18] The first scintigraphic pattern (the lateral column sign) is postulated to result from recanalization of existing vessels. Pinhole imaging of an epiphysis that is healing through recanalization demonstrates a posterolateral epiphyseal column of tracer localization (Fig. 4.39). This is best depicted with anterior imaging. In the frog position, the lateral column may not be visualized due to its being rotated posteriorly. With recanalization, radiographic findings of sclerosis and resorption first appear during the period in which the lateral column becomes visible. Tracer localization returns in the remainder of the epiphysis as revascularization extends to its medial and anterior portions. When a lateral column sign is demonstrated, healing is inferred to be by revascularization, regardless of radiographic findings.

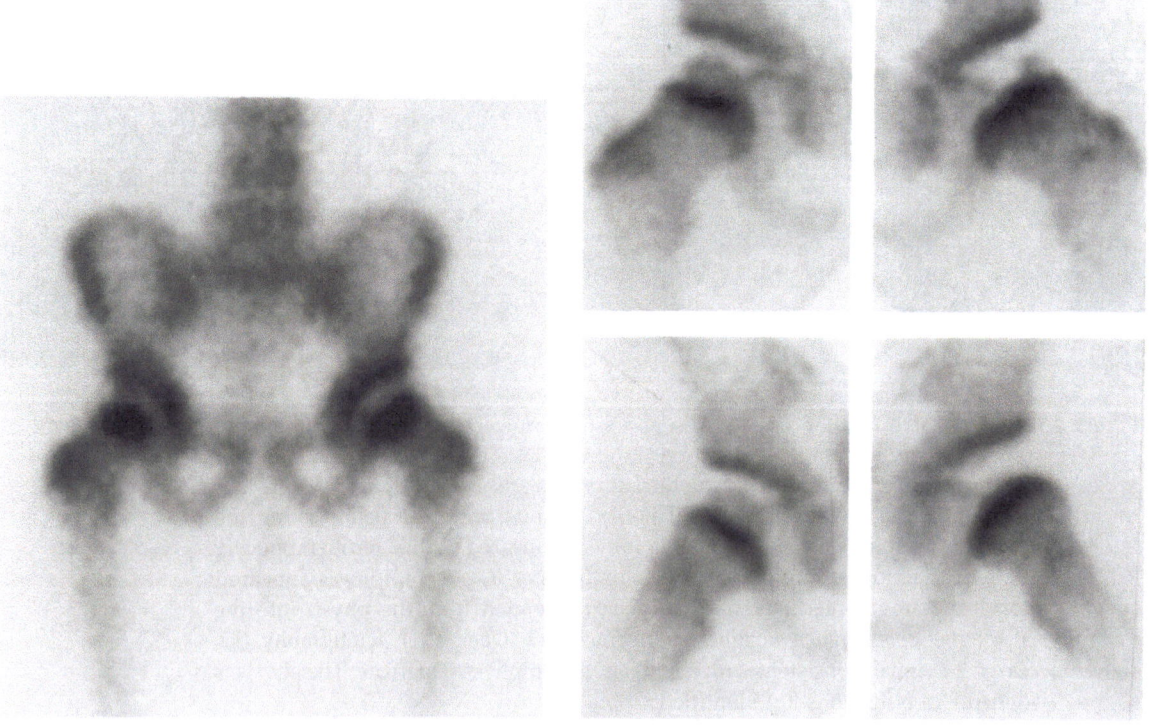

A   B

Figure 4.39. Legg-Calvé-Perthes disease. Skeletal scintigraphy shows asymmetrically decreased tracer localization in the left femoral capital epiphysis (A). Pinhole imaging in the anterior projection shows a prominent lateral column (B, upper row). This is not visualized in the frog lateral position (B, lower row).

The second pattern is proposed to reflect neovascularization, the development of new vessels that supply the epiphysis. The earliest clue that this is the operative healing mechanism is that radiographic findings of sclerosis and, sometimes, resorption are present while the epiphysis continues to be void of tracer localization. With neovascularization, tracer localization first returns to the epiphysis as apparent physeal widening due to tracer delivery across the base of the epiphysis by new vessels arising from the lateral circumflex artery (Fig. 4.40). Gradually tracer localization extends to the dome of the epiphysis (mushrooming). Neovascularization is implied when skeletal scintigraphy reveals this pattern or the complete absence of tracer localization in the epiphysis, while radiographs demonstrate sclerosis and/or resorption. When radiographs are normal and scintigraphy demonstrates absent tracer localization in the entire femoral capital epiphysis, the revascularization mechanism cannot be established. The progosis is reported to be markedly better for those who revascularize by recanalization than for those who revascularize by neovascularization.[18,19] Healing by recanalization may be complicated by epiphyseal fracture or collapse and subsequent conversion to the neovascularization process. The significance of early reports estimating prognosis scintigraphically by the extent of epiphyseal abnormality is limited by a failure to adequately account for the contribution of tracer localization in the acetabulum (shine through).[27,58]

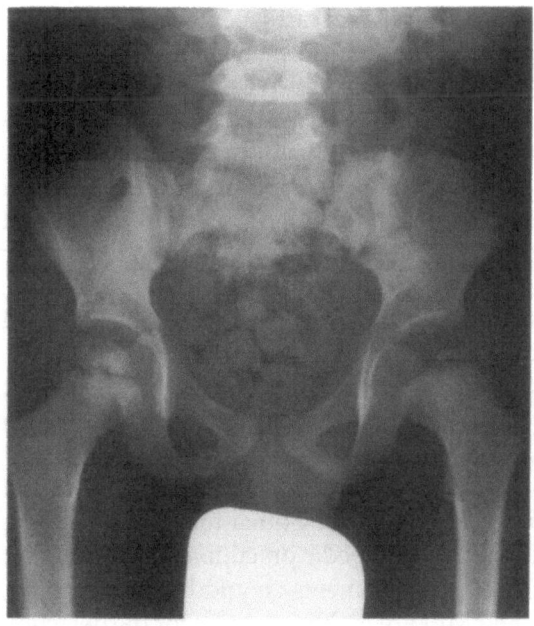
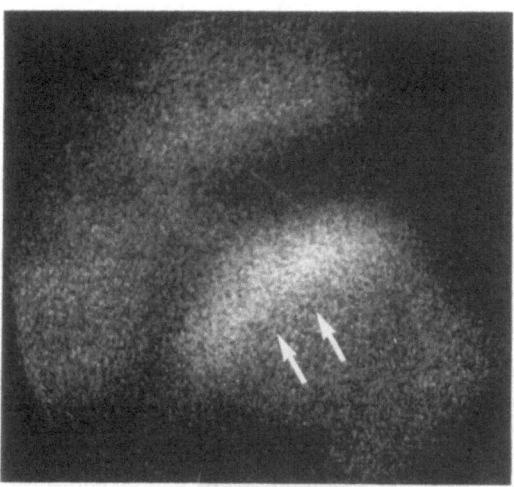

A   B

Figure 4.40. Legg-Calvé-Perthes disease. Extensive fragmentation of the left femoral capital epiphysis is shown radiographically (A). Pinhole imaging in the anterior projection (B) depicts tracer localization across the base of the epiphysis without evidence of a lateral column. (Case courtesy of James J. Conway, M.D. Children's Memorial Hospital, Chicago. Reprinted from Conway,[19] with permission.)

Because MRI is highly sensitive for the early detection of ischemia, it is also useful in cases of clinically suspected Legg-Calvé-Perthes disease when radiographs are unrevealing (Fig. 4.38). A nonuniform appearance to the femoral head with areas of low signal on T1-weighted images and high signal on T2-weighted images indicates marrow edema, an early and possibly reversible sign of Legg-Calvé-Perthes disease.[6,80] Absence of marrow enhancement following gadolinium helps to confirm the diagnosis of AVN.[25,118] Magnetic resonance imaging is also valuable in revealing anatomic abnormalities such as synovial proliferation and epiphyseal cartilage overgrowth that lead to loss of containment of the femoral head within the acetabulum and increase the need for surgery. These findings result from unimpeded nourishment of the synovium and epiphyseal cartilage by synovial fluid.[6,50,95] Impaired delivery of oxygen and nutrients to the physis may lead to abnormalities, including osseous bridging, that are also well demonstrated with MRI. Demonstration of bridging is particularly important in identifying children who are at increased risk for growth arrest. Tongues of physeal cartilage extending into the metaphysis, similar to that seen after experimental damage to the metaphyseal vasculature, are frequently present. These metaphyseal abnormalities reflect the same process responsible for the metaphyseal radiolucencies seen radiographically. When detected only with MRI, they carry less prognostic significance than when demonstrated radiographically, however.[50]

Through 40 years of follow-up, the vast majority of patients with Legg-Calvé-Perthes disease are pain-free and active. Beyond this point, osteoarthritis is significantly more prevalent than in the general population.[122] Treatment is aimed at children with Legg-Calvé-Perthes disease who are at increased risk of early disability. Preventing, or at least limiting, the late onset of degenerative joint disease is also a desirable, but perhaps more elusive, goal. Identifying children who will benefit from treatment for Legg-Calvé-Perthes disease and the determination of the optimum therapeutic approach are significant clinical challenges that have produced much debate and controversy. It is estimated that 60% of children with Legg-Calvé-Perthes disease do not require therapy. The foundation of treatment is containment, the maintenance of the developing femoral head in the acetabulum to reduce stress on the femoral head, allow normal epiphyseal molding, and prevent extrusion of the lateral segment of epiphyseal cartilage. Treatment options include the use of an abduction orthosis and surgical management with varus and/or innominate osteotomy or a shelf arthroplasty.[122]

Clinically, age at diagnosis is the most significant prognostic indicator. Children who are older than 8 years of age[70] are more likely to develop disability. Various radiographic grading systems, including those based on the work of Catterall[14] and Salter and Thompson,[96] are used for prognostic stratification and determining the need for early therapy. Prognostically unfavorable radiographic signs include extensive femoral head involvement, persistent lateral subluxation, and metaphyseal radiolucencies. As noted above, skeletal scintigraphy and MRI may also be of value in assessing prognosis.

Questions regarding when to perform imaging other than radiographs and which modality to use in children with Legg-Calvé-Perthes disease have been raised but not settled. Uncertainty over the value of information provided by different imaging studies reflects a lack of consensus regarding the merits of various therapeutic options. The optimal use of imaging other than radiographs is determined by the philosophy of individual orthopedic practitioners in managing Legg-Calvé-Perthes disease. Certain general statements should be kept in mind, however. Both skeletal scintigraphy and MRI are highly sensitive for the detection of AVN. In children with nonspecific symptoms, the whole-body evaluation afforded by scintigraphy is advantageous. After a diagnosis of Legg-Calvé-Perthes disease is established, skeletal scintigraphy may provide information regarding the revascularization mechanism. Magnetic resonance imaging provides information regarding the congruity of the articular surfaces, the degree of cartilaginous coverage of the femoral head, and the presence of physeal bridging. Scintigraphy and MRI are, therefore, complementary modalities for the evaluation of Legg-Calvé-Perthes disease.

Conditions that cause AVN must be considered in the differential diagnosis of children with the imaging findings of Legg-Calvé-Perthes disease. The femoral capital epiphysis may develop AVN as a sequela of synovitis, septic arthritis, trauma, developmental dysplasia of the hip, radiation, and secondary to systemic disorders including hypothyroidism, sickle cell anemia, and Gaucher's disease. Radiographically symmetric bilateral involvement suggests a generalized disorder.

Femoral head deformity, resembling that of Legg-Calvé-Perthes disease, is also seen in epiphyseal dysplasias. Meyer's dysplasia, in particular, should be considered in children under 5 years of age. Meyer's dysplasia is most likely a variant of multiple epiphyseal dysplasia that is limited to the femoral head. It is seen almost exclusively in males. With Meyer's dysplasia, the femoral head ossification centers show delayed ossification at approximately 2 years rather than at 6 months of age. The femoral head ossifies in an abnormal pattern of multiple granular-appearing flattened centers.[71] Meyer's dysplasia may be detected incidentally on radiographs that include the pelvis or in children who experience joint pain and stiffness. Radiographically, there is neither epiphyseal sclerosis nor subchondral fracture with Meyer's dysplasia. The hips are involved bilaterally, often symmetrically, in close to 50% of cases.[71] Serial radiographs typically show the femoral head assuming a normal appearance over 3 years.[59] Skeletal scintigraphy demonstrates tracer localization in the ossification centers that are seen radiographically in contrast to the appearance of Legg-Calvé-Perthes disease described above.[66]

Other Osteochondroses

Blount Disease (Tibia Vara)

Physiologic bowing of the tibiae is present in the first 2 years of life. When bowing is identified after 2 years of age, Blount disease should be considered. Blount disease occurs in infantile and late-onset forms. Infantile Blount disease is believed to reflect disturbed enchondral ossification resulting from mechanical forces acting on the proximal medial tibial physis. The cause of the adolescent type, which is typically seen between 6 and 15 years of age, is uncertain. Segmental physeal arrest secondary to trauma or infection has been implicated. Radiographically, there is beaking of the medial tibial metaphysis, which appears depressed, irregular, and fragmented.[59] Skeletal scintigraphy is not useful in diagnosis but may reveal increased tracer localization in the proximal tibial growth plate and metaphysis.

Scheuermann Disease (Juvenile Kyphosis)

Scheuermann disease is a structural kyphosis of the spine detected in children after ossification of the vertebral apophysis around 10 years of age. The etiology is uncertain. End-plate fractures during growth may be contributory. Typically, Scheuermann's disease affects the thoracic spine with the apex of the kyphosis at the T7 to T9 levels. Less commonly, the lumbar spine is affected. Radiographic demonstration of anterior wedging of three adjacent vertebrae by 5° or greater is required for the diagnosis. The end plates appear irregular and the disk spaces are narrowed.[59] Skeletal scintigraphy is occasionally requested to exclude pars interarticularis stress, diskitis, or other etiologies of the back pain, which children with Scheuermann disease may experience. The distribution of tracer in the spine of children with thoracic Scheuermann disease is usually normal on planar imaging.[124] With lumbar involvement, mild increased tracer localization has been described.[67]

Osgood-Schlatter Disease

Osgood-Schlatter disease is either a traction apophysitis of the tibial tubercle resulting from forces applied by the quadriceps femoris on the tubercle via the patellar tendon or primarily a patellar tendinitis. This disorder, characterized by localized pain, swelling, and tenderness occurs most frequently in boys between 10 and 15 years of age.[77,78] The diagnosis of Osgood-Schlatter disease is almost always established clinically. Imaging is most useful in excluding other pathology. Radiographs may reveal soft tissue swelling anterior to the tibial tubercle, thickening of the patellar tendon, and inhomogeneity of the infrapatellar fat pad. The tibial tubercle may appear irregularly ossified and fragmented, although in the absence of symptoms this may represent a normal variant. Skeletal scintigraphy and MRI are requested to address a diagnostic uncertainty but are not used routinely in the diagnosis of this entity. Increased tracer localization may occur in or about the patellar tendon. Skeletal tracer localization in the tibial tubercle of an asymptomatic individual should not be taken as evidence of Osgood-Schlatter disease as this is part of the normal distribution of tracer in the growing skeleton. High T2-weighted signal in the patellar tendon at its insertion into the tibial tuberosity and in the surrounding soft tissues may be demonstrated with MRI. Adjacent bone marrow edema may be present.[93]

Sinding-Larsen-Johansson Disease

Originally thought to be a traction apophysitis of the patella, Sinding-Larsen-Johansson disease is now believed to result from injury to the proximal patellar tendon. Calcification or irregular ossification in the injured tendon may follow. This condition is most frequently encountered in boys between 10 and 12 years of age who present with knee pain. As with Osgood-Schlatter disease, the diagnosis is a clinical one with imaging used to exclude other pathologic conditions in difficult cases.

Sever Disease and Van Neck Disease

A sclerotic irregular appearance to the calcaneal apophysis and an irregular bubbly appearance to the ischiopubic synchondrosis have previously been labeled Sever disease and Van Neck disease, respectively. Both of these radiographic appearances, however, reflect normal patterns of ossification and carry no clinical significance.

Köhler Disease

Midtarsal pain in association with radiographic evidence of resorption, fragmentation, and eventual reossification of the tarsal navicular constitutes Köhler disease. Clinically, this is most commonly seen in boys who are younger than 6 years of age. It is uncertain whether this represents a normal pattern of ossification or is a form of AVN. Support for the latter hypothesis is indirectly derived from anatomic studies showing that the tarsal navicular derives its blood supply from a single vessel and is therefore presumably at risk for AVN from repetitive mechanical stress.[121] A role for scintigraphy in evaluating this controversial entity has not been established.

Trauma-Related Osteochondroses

Repetitive trauma and microtrabecular fracturing without sufficient healing, can cause complete interruption of the blood supply to the capitellum (Panner disease, "Little Leaguer's elbow"), lunate (Kienböck disease), phalangeal epiphyses of the hand (Thiemann disease), or a metatarsal head (Freiberg's infraction). Unlike processes in which AVN occurs as a primary event, these entities are often associated with increased tracer localization early in their course. Decreased or absent tracer localization in necrotic bone may also be demonstrated.[65]

Miscellaneous Conditions

Metabolic Bone Disease

Manifestations of metabolic bone disease, particularly rickets and secondary hyperparathyroidism, are demonstrated with skeletal scintigraphy (Fig. 4.41).

Rickets is a condition in which the growing skeleton fails to mineralize properly due to a relative or absolute insufficiency of vitamin D or its hormonal derivative 1,25-dihydroxycholecalciferol. Etiologies include dietary deficiency and malabsorption of vitamin D, liver disease, renal disease, and metabolic effects of various medications, most notably phenobarbital and phenytoin. Osteomalacia, a state of defective mineralization of osteoid in mature bone, coexists with rickets in the growing skeleton.[81,82] Children with rickets of renal etiology often have associated evidence of secondary hyperparathyroidism (renal osteodystrophy).

The radiographic features of rickets are best seen in areas of rapid bone growth. In the long bones, failure of physeal cartilage ossification results in irregularity of the physis, decreased density or absence of the thin sclerotic line normally associated with the zone of provisional calcification, and metaphyseal cupping and fraying. The anterior rib ends appear frayed and widened. Coexistent osteomalacia results in indistinct cortical margins and thin coarse bony trabeculae. Linear radiolucencies due to focal osteoid accumulation (Milkman pseudofractures, Looser lines) may be demonstrated at multiple sites, especially the medial femoral neck, ischium, pubis, ribs, clavicles, and scapulae. Bowing of the long bones and insufficiency fractures develop. When associated with secondary hyperparathyroidism there may be periostitis due to bone resorption, osteosclerosis due to stimulation of osteoblastic activity, and soft tissue calcification as a result of an increased calcium-phosphate product in extracellular fluid.[59,76,109] Epiphyseal separations, particularly a slipped capital femoral epiphysis, can result from rickets and hyperparathyroidism.

The scintigraphic manifestations of rickets have received little note in the literature. Two reported cases of neonatal rickets demonstrated diminished overall tracer localization within the skeleton of both neonates and focally increased tracer localization at sites of insufficiency fractures in one neonate. Following therapy with vitamin D, tracer localization in the skeleton improved and additional focal abnormalities, possibly representing healing insufficiency fractures, were seen in that neonate.[81,82] Prominent tracer localization in the axial and appendicular skeleton are scintigraphic findings in both osteomalacia and secondary hyperparathyroidism. Tracer localization in the bones of the skull, mandible, and sternum are often particularly prominent. Relative increased tracer localization in the anterior rib ends, a feature of osteomalacia and hyperparathyroidism in adults, is difficult to appreciate in children due to the normal high intensity of tracer localization at these sites in the immature skeleton. Focally increased tracer localization corresponding to Milkman pseudofractures or true fractures may be

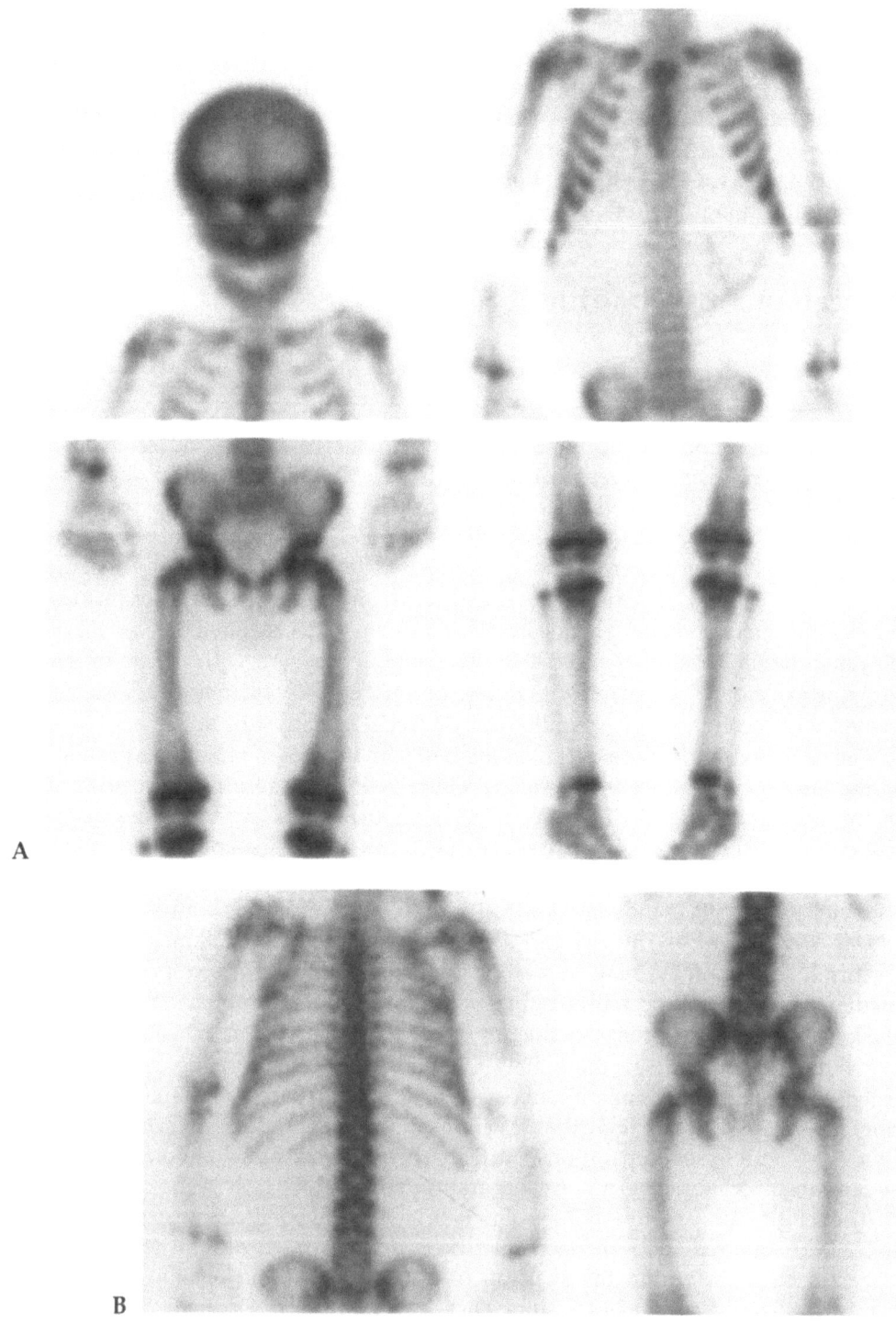

Figure 4.41. Renal osteodystrophy. Anterior images (A) demonstrate prominent tracer localization in the skull, sternum, and the lower extremities. The femoral diaphyses are bowed and the proximal femoral metaphyses appear deformed. Extraosseous tracer localization in the left upper quadrant is likely within the stomach walls. The kidneys are not visualized on the posterior images (B).

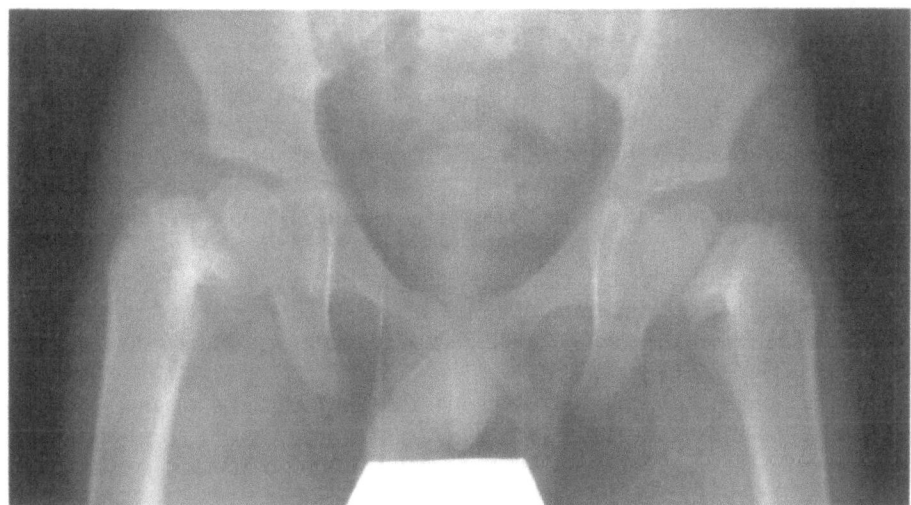

C

Figure 4.41 (*cont'd.*). Bilateral coxa vara deformities secondary to slipped capital femoral epiphyses and coarsened trabeculae are demonstrated radiographically (C).

visualized. The kidneys are often seen faintly due to relatively decreased renal tracer excretion.[29] Extraosseous tracer localization may occur at sites of soft tissue calcification in secondary hyperparathyroidism.

Infantile Cortical Hyperostosis

Infantile cortical hyperostosis, also known as Caffey's disease, is a self-limited disease of unknown etiology characterized by hyperplasia of subperiosteal bone over which there is soft tissue swelling and sometimes a brawny discoloration. Lesions of Caffey's disease have been observed in the skull, mandible, clavicles, ribs, scapulae, long bones of the extremities, and metatarsals. Recovery is the rule and usually occurs within weeks to a year. Radiologically, there is periosteal new bone formation and cortical thickening of underlying bone. During healing, radiographs may show laminated periosteal reaction and, in the more chronic forms, show cortical thinning and shaft expansion.[11,79] Scintigraphy is not indicated in this condition. During the active phase of the disease scintigraphy reveals intense accumulation of radiopharmaceutical in the involved bones.

References

1. Aoki J, Sone A, Fujioka F, et al. MR of enchondroma and chondrosarcoma: rings and arcs of Gd-DTPA enhancement. *J Comput Assist Tomogr* 1991;15:1011–1016.
2. Assoun J, Richardi G, Railhac JJ, et al. Osteoid osteoma: MR imaging versus CT. *Radiology* 1994;191:217–223.
3. Bar-Sever Z, Connolly LP, Jaramillo D, et al. Thallium-201 uptake in Langerhans cell histiocytosis of bone. *Pediatr Radiol* 1996;26:739–741.
4. Baunin C, Puget C, Assoun J, et al. Percutaneous resection of osteoid osteoma under CT guidance in 8 children. *Pediatr Radiol* 1994;24:185–188.
5. Bensahel H, Bok B, Cavailloles F, et al. Bone scintigraphy in Perthes disease. *J Pediatr Orthop* 1985;3:302–305.
6. Bos CFA, Bloem JL, Bloem RM. Sequential magnetic resonance imaging in Perthes disease. *J Bone Joint Surg [B]* 1991;73:219–224.
7. Brenner RJ, Hattner RS, Lilien DL. Scintigraphic features of nonosteogenic fibroma. *Radiology* 1979;131:727–730.
8. Broadbent V, Dunger DB, Yeomans E, et al. Anterior pituitary function and computed tomography/magnetic resonance imaging in patients with Langerhans cell histiocytosis and diabetes insipidus. *Med Pediatr Oncol* 1993;21:649–654.
9. Burr BA, Resnick D, Syklawer R, et al. Fluid-fluid levels in a unicameral bone cyst: CT and MR findings. *J Comput Assist Tomogr* 1993;17:134–136.
10. Burrows PE, Greenbert ID, Reed MH. The distal femoral defect: technetium-99m pyrophosphate bone scan results. *J Can Assoc Radiol* 1982;33:91–93.
11. Caffey J, Silverman FA. Infantile cortical hyperostoses: preliminary report on a new syndrome. *AJR* 1945;54:1–3.
12. Calver R, Venugopal V, Dorgan J, et al. Radionuclide scanning in the early diagnosis of Perthes' disease. *J Bone Joint Surg [B]* 1981;63:379–382.
13. Campanacci M. Osteofibrous dysplasia of long bones. A new clinical entity. *Ital J Orthop Traumatol* 1976;2:221–225.
14. Catterall A. The natural history of Perthes' disease. *J Bone Joint Surg [B]* 1971;53:37–53.
15. Cavaillos F, Bok B, Bensahel H. Bone scintigraphy in the diagnosis and follow-up of Perthes disease. *Eur J Nucl Med* 1982;7:327–330.
16. Chung SMK. The arterial supply of the developing proximal end of the human femur. *J Bone Joint Surg [A]* 1976;58:961–970.
17. Cline MJ. Histiocytes and histiocytosis. *Blood* 1994;84:2840–2853.
18. Conway JJ. Scintigraphic classification of Legg-Calvé-Perthes disease. *Semin Nucl Med* 1993;23:274–295.
19. Conway JJ. Radionuclide evaluation of Legg-Calvé-Perthes disease. In: Treves ST, ed. *Pediatric Nuclear Medicine.* 2nd ed. New York: Springer-Verlag; 1995:302–315.
20. Conway JJ, Weiss SC, Maldonado V. Scintigraphic patterns in Legg-Calvé-Perthes disease [abstract]. *Radiology* 1983;149(suppl):102.
21. Cunningham MJ, Curtin HD, Jaffe R, et al. Otologic manifestations of Langerhans cell histiocytosis. *Arch Otolaryngol* 1989;115:807–813.
22. DeCristofaro R, Biagini R, Boriani S, et al. Selective arterial embolization in the treatment of aneurysmal bone cyst and angioma of bone. *Skeletal Radiol* 1992;21:523–527.
23. Dimentberg RA, Brown KLB. Diagnostic evaluation of patients with histiocytosis X. *J Pediatr Orthop* 1990;10:733–741.
24. Dogan AS, Conway JJ, Miller JH, et al. Detection of bone lesions in Langerhans cell histiocytosis: complementary roles of scintigraphy and conventional radiography. *J Pediatr Hematol* 1996;18:51–58.
25. Ducou le Pointe H, Haddad S, Silberman B, et al. Legg-Perthes-Calvé disease: staging by MRI using gadolinium. *Pediatr Radiol* 1994;24:88–91.
26. Fisher RL. An epidemiological study of Legg-Perthes disease. *J Bone Joint Surg [A]* 1972;54:769–774.
27. Fisher RL, Roderique JW, Brown DC, et al. The relationship of isotopic bone imaging findings to prognosis in Legg-Perthes disease. *Clin Orthop* 1980;150:23–29.

28. Flores LG, Hoshi H, Nagamachi S, et al. Thallium-201 uptake in eosinophilic granuloma of the frontal bone: comparison with technetium-99m-MDP imaging. *J Nucl Med* 1995;36:107–110.

29. Fogelman I, McKillop JH, Bessent RG, et al. The role of bone scanning in osteomalacia. *J Nucl Med* 1978;19:245–248.

30. Freiberger RH, Loitman BS, Helpern M, et al. Osteoid osteoma: a report of 80 cases. *AJR* 1959;82:194–205.

31. Garrison RC, Unni KK, McLeod RA, et al. Chondrosarcoma arising in osteochondroma. *Cancer* 1982;49:1890–1897.

32. Geirnaerdt MJ, Bloem JL, Eulderink F, et al. Cartilaginous tumors: correlation of gadolinium-enhanced MR imaging and histopathologic findings. *Radiology* 1993; 186:813–817.

33. George JC, Buckwalter KA, Cohen MD, et al. Langerhans cell histiocytosis of bone: MR imaging. *Pediatr Radiol* 1994;24:29–32.

34. Ghelman B, Vigorita V. Postoperative radionuclide evaluation of osteoid osteomas. *Radiology* 1983;146:509–512.

35. Gilday DL, Ash JM. Benign bone tumors. *Semin Nucl Med* 1976;6:33–46.

36. Girdany BR, Osman MZ. Longitudinal growth and skeletal maturation in Perthes' disease. *Radiol Clin North Am* 1968;6:245–251.

37. Giudici MA, Moser RP, Kransdorf MJ. Cartilaginous bone tumors. *Radiol Clin North Am* 1993;31:237–259.

38. Golding JSR. The natural history of osteoid osteoma. With a report of 20 cases. *J Bone Joint Surg [B]* 1954;36:218–229.

39. Harris WH, Dudley HR, Barry RV. The natural history of fibrous dysplasia. *J Bone Joint Surg [A]* 1962;44:207–233.

40. Hayes CW, Conway WF, Sundaram M. Misleading aggressive MR imaging appearance of some benign musculoskeletal lesions. *Radiographics* 1992;12:1119–1134.

41. Helms CA. Osteoid osteoma: the double density sign. *Clin Orthop* 1987;222:167–173.

42. Helms CA, Hattner RS, Vogler JB III. Osteoid osteoma: radionuclide diagnosis. *Radiology* 1984;151:779–784.

42a. Howarth DM, Mullan BP, Wiseman GA, et al. Bone scintigraphy evaluated in diagnosing and staging Langerhans cell histiocytosis and related disorders. *J Nucl Med* 1996;37:1456–1460.

43. Hudson TM. Scintigraphy of aneurysmal bone cysts. *AJR* 1984;142:761–765.

44. Hudson TM. *Radiologic-Pathologic Correlation of Musculoskeletal Lesions.* Baltimore: Williams & Wilkins; 1987.

45. Hudson TM, Hamlin DJ, Fitzsimmons JR. Magnetic resonance imaging of fluid levels in an aneurysmal bone cyst and in anticoagulated human blood. *Skeletal Radiol* 1985;13:267–270.

46. Hudson TM, Springfield DS, Spanierr SS, et al. Benign exostoses and exostotic chondrosarcomas: evaluation of cartilage thickness by CT. *Radiology* 1984;152:595–599.

47. Inoue A, Freeman MAR, Vernon-Roberts B, et al. The pathogenesis of Perthes' disease. *J Bone Joint Surg [B]* 1976; 58:453–461.

48. Israeli A, Zwas ST, Horoszowski H, et al. Use of radionuclide method in preoperative and intraoperative diagnosis of osteoid osteoma of the spine. Case report. *Clin Orthop* 1983;175:194–196.

49. Jaffe HL. *Tumor and Tumorous Conditions of the Bones and Joints.* Philadelphia: Lee & Febiger; 1958.

50. Jaramillo D, Kasser JR, Villegas-Medina OL, et al. Cartilaginous abnormalities and growth disturbances in Legg-Calvé-Perthes disease: evaluation with MR imaging. *Radiology* 1995;197:767–773.

51. Keats TE, Joyce JM. Metaphyseal, cortical irregularities in children. *Skeletal Radiol* 1985;12:112–118.

52. Kirks DR, Taybi H. Histiocytosis X. In: Parker BD, Castellino RA, eds. *Pediatric Oncologic Radiology.* St. Louis: Mosby; 1977:209–234.

53. Kneisl JS, Simon MA. Medical management compared with operative treatment for osteoid osteoma. *J Bone Joint Surg [A]* 1992;74:179–185.

54. Kransdorf MJ, Moser RP, Gilkey FW. Fibrous dysplasia. *Radiographics* 1990;10:519–537.

55. Kransdorf MJ, Stull MA, Gilkey FW, et al. Osteoid osteoma. *Radiographics* 1991;11:671–696.

56. Kransdorf MJ, Sweet DE. Aneurysmal bone cyst: concept, controversy, clinical presentation and imaging. *AJR* 1995;164:573–580.

57. Kumas R, Madewell JE, Lindell MM, et al. Fibrous lesions of bones. *Radiographics* 1990;10:237–250.

58. LaMont RL, Muz J, Heilbronner D, et al. Quantitative assessment of femoral head involvement in Legg-Calvé-Perthes disease. *J Bone Joint Surg [A]* 1981;63:746–752.

59. Laor T, Jaramillo D, Oestrich A. Skeletal system. In: Kirks DR, ed. *Practical Pediatric Imaging. Diagnostic Radiology of Infants and Children.* 3rd ed. Philadelphia: Lippincott-Raven; 1997:327–510.

60. Lee JK, Yao L, Wirth CR. MR Imaging of solitary osteochondromas: report of eight cases. *AJR* 1987;149:557–560.

61. Libshitz HI, Cohen MA. Radiation-induced osteochondromas. *Radiology* 1982;142:643–647.

62. Lisbona R, Rosenthall L. Role of radionuclide imaging in osteoid osteoma. *AJR* 1979;132:77–80.

63. Makley JT. Prostaglandins—a mechanism for pain mediation in osteoid osteoma. *Orthop Trans* 1982;6:72.

64. Mandell GA, Dalinka MK, Coleman BG. Fibrous lesions in the lower extremities in neurofibromatosis. *AJR* 1979;133:1135–1138.

65. Mandell GA, Harcke HT. Scintigraphic manifestations of infraction of the second metatarsal (Freiberg's disease). *J Nucl Med* 1987;28:249–251.

66. Mandell GA, MacKenzie WG, Scott CI, et al. Identification of avascular necrosis in the dysplastic proximal femoral epiphysis. *Skeletal Radiol* 1989;18:273–281.

67. Mandell GA, Morales RW, Harcke HT, et al. Bone scintigraphy in patients with atypical lumbar Scheuermann's disease. *J Pediatr Orthop* 1993;13:622–627.

68. Marcove RC, Sheth DS, Takemoto S, et al. The treatment of aneurysmal bone cyst. *Clin Orthop* 1995;311:157–163.

69. Mazoyer JF, Kohler R, Bossard D. Osteoid osteoma. CT-guided percutaneous treatment. *Radiology* 1991;181:269–271.

70. McAndrew MP, Weinstein SL. A long term follow-up of Legg-Calvé-Perthes disease. *J Bone Joint Surg [A]* 1984;66:860–869.

71. Meyer J. Dysplasia epiphysealis capitis femoris. *Acta Orthop Scand* 1964;34:183–197.

72. Milgram JW. The origins of osteochondromas and echondromas. *Clin Orthop* 1983;174:264–284.

73. Mirra JM, Gold RH. Fibrous dysplasia. In: Mirra JM, Picci P, Gold RH, eds. *Bone Tumors.* Philadelphia: Lea & Febiger; 1989:191–226.

74. Mirra JM, Picci P. Adamantinoma and osteofibrous dysplasia. In: Mirra JM, Picci P, Gold RH, eds. *Bone Tumors.* Philadelphia: Lea & Febiger; 1989:1203–1239.

75. Moberg E. The natural course of osteoid osteoma. *J Bone Joint Surg [A]* 1951;33:166–170.

76. Murphey MD, Sartoris DJ, Quale JL, et al. Musculoskeletal manifestations of chronic renal insufficiency. *Radiographics* 1993;13:357–379.

77. Ogden JA. Radiology of postnatal skeletal development: X. Patella and tibial tuberosity. *Skeletal Radiol* 1984;11:246–247.

78. Ozonoff MB. *Pediatric Orthopedic Radiology.* 2nd ed. Philadelphia: W.B. Saunders; 1992.

79. Padfield E, Hicken P. Cortical hyperostosis in infants: a radiological study of 16 patients. *Br J Radiol* 1970;143:231–237.

80. Pinto MR, Peterson HA, Berquist TH. Magnetic resonance imaging in early diagnosis of Legg-Calvé-Perthes disease. *J Pediatr Orthop* 1989;9:19–22.

81. Pitt MJ. Rickets and osteomalacia are still around. *Radiol Clin North Am* 1991;29:97–118.

82. Pitt MJ. Rickets and osteomalacia. In: Resnick D., ed. *Diagnosis of Bone and Joint Disorders.* 3rd ed. Philadelphia: W.B. Saunders; 1995:1885–1922.

83. Ponseti IV, Maynard JA, Weinstein JL, et al. Legg-Calvé-Perthes disease: histochemical and ultrastructural observations of the epiphyseal cartilage and physis. *J Bone Joint Surg [A]* 1983;65:797–807.

84. Resnick D. Tumors and tumor-like lesions of bone: radiographic principles. In: Resnick D, ed. *Diagnosis of Bone and Joint Disorders.* 3rd ed. Philadelphia: W.B. Saunders; 1995:3613–3627.

85. Resnick D, Greenway G. Distal femoral cortical defects, irregularities, and excavations. *Radiology* 1982;143:345–354.

86. Resnick D, Kyriakos K, Greenway GD. Tumors and tumor-like lesions of bone: imaging and pathology of specific tumors. In: Resnick D, ed. *Diagnosis of Bone and Joint Disorders.* 3rd ed. Philadelphia: W.B. Saunders; 1995:3662–3697.

87. Reynolds J. The "fallen fragment sign" in the diagnosis of unicameral bone cysts. *Radiology* 1969;92:949–953.

88. Rinski LA, Goris M, Bleck E, et al. Intraoperative skeletal scintigraphy for localization of osteoid osteoma of the spine. *J Bone Joint Surg [A]* 1980;62:143–144.

89. Ritschl P, Hajek PC, Pechmann U. Fibrous metaphyseal defects, magnetic resonance imaging appearances. *Skeletal Radiol* 1989;18:253–259.

90. Ritschl P, Karnel F, Hajek P. Fibrous metaphyseal defects—determination of their origin and natural history using a radiomorphological study. *Skeletal Radiol* 1988;17:8–15.

91. Roach PJ, Connolly LP, Zurakowski D, et al. Osteoid osteoma: comparative utility of high resolution planar and pinhole magnification scintigraphy. *Pediatr Radiol* 1995;26:222–225.

92. Roger B, Bellin MF, Wioland M, et al. Osteoid osteoma: CT-guided percutaneous excision confirmed with immediate follow-up scintigraphy in 16 outpatients. *Radiology* 1996;201:239–242.

93. Rosenberg ZS, Kawelblum M, Cheung YY, et al. Osgood-Schlatter lesion: scintigraphic, CT and MR imaging features. *Radiology* 1992;185:853–858.

94. Rosenthal DI, Alexander A, Rosenberg AE, et al. Ablation of osteoid osteoma with a percutaneously placed electrode: a new procedure. *Radiology* 1992;183:29–33.

95. Rush BH, Bramson RT, Ogden JA. Legg-Calvé-Perthes disease: detection of cartilaginous and synovial changes with MR imaging. *Radiology* 1988;167:473–476.

96. Salter RB, Thompson GH. Legg-Calvé-Perthes disease. The prognostic significance of the subchondral fracture and a two group classification of the femoral head involvement. *J Bone Joint Surg [A]* 1984;66:479–489.

97. Sachis M, Zahir A, Freeman MA. The experimental simulation of Perthes disease by consecutive interruptions of the blood supply to the capital epiphysis in the puppy. *J Bone Joint Surg [A]* 1973;55:335–342.

98. Schaub T, Ash JM, Gilday DL. Radionuclide imaging in histiocytosis X. *Pediatr Radiol* 1987;17:397–404.

99. Schulman L, Dorfman HD. Nerve fibers in osteoid osteoma. *J Bone Joint Surg [A]* 1970;52:1351–1356.

100. Shore RM, Poznanski AK, Annadappa EC, et al. Arterial and venous compromise by an osteochondroma. *Pediatr Radiol* 1994;24:39–40.

101. Siddiqui AR, Tashjian JH, Lazurua K, et al. Nuclear medicine studies in evaluation of skeletal lesions in children with histiocytosis X. *Radiology* 1981;140:787–789.

102. Silverman FN. The bones. In: Silverman FN, ed. *Caffey's Pediatric X-Ray Diagnosis.* 8th ed. Chicago: Year Book; 1985:389–914.

103. Simons GN, Sty J. Intraoperative bone imaging in the treatment of osteoid-osteoma of the femoral neck. *J Pediatr Orthop* 1983;3:399–402.

104. Springfield DS. Bone and soft tissue tumors. In: Morrisy RT, Weinstein SL, eds. *Lovell and Winter's Pediatric Orthopedics.* 4th ed. Philadelphia: Lippincott-Raven; 1996:423–468.

105. Steinmetz JC, Pilon VA, Lee JK. Jaffe-Campanacci syndrome. *J Pediatr Orthop* 1988;8:602–604.

106. Stoll M, Freund M, Schmid H, et al. Allogeneic bone marrow transplantation for Langerhans cell histiocytosis. *Cancer* 1990;66:284–288.

107. Stull MA, Kransdorf MJ, Devaney KO. Langerhans cell histiocytosis of bone. *Radiographics* 1992;12:801–823.

108. Sty J, Simons G. Intraoperative 99m-technetium bone imaging in the treatment of osteoblastic tumors. *Clin Orthop* 1982;165:223–227.

109. Sty JR, Wells RG, Starshak RJ, Gregg D. The musculoskeletal system. In: Sty J, Wells R, Starshak R, Gregg D, eds. *Diagnostic Imaging of Infants and Children.* Vol. 3. Gaithesburg: Aspen; 1992:233–405.

110. Sutherland AD, Savage JP, Paterson DC, et al. The nuclide bone scan in the diagnosis and management of Perthes disease. *J Bone Joint Surg [B]* 1980;62:300–306.

111. Swee RG, McLeod RA, Beabout JW. Osteoid osteoma: detection, diagnosis and localization. *Radiology* 1979;130:117–123.

112. Taylor GA, Shea N, O'Brien TO, et al. Osteoid osteoma: localization by intraoperative magnification scintigraphy. *Pediatr Radiol* 1986;16:313–316.

113. Towbin R, Kaye R, Meza MP, et al. Osteoid osteoma: percutaneous excision using a CT-guided coaxial technique. *Am J Radiol* 1995;164:945–949.

113a. Treves ST, Connolly LP, Kirkpatrick JA et al Bone. In Treves ST (ed) Pediatric Nuclear Medicine. 2nd ed. 1995 New York: Springer-Verlag; 233–301.

114. Tsai JC, Dalinka MK, Fallon MD, et al. Fluid-fluid level: a nonspecific finding in tumors of bone and soft tissue. *Radiology* 1990;175:779–782.

115. Tupler RH, Turbiner EH. Tc-99m labeled RBC scan in Maffucci's syndrome. *Clin Nucl Med* 1991;16:872–873.

116. Unni KK. *Dahlin's Bone Tumors: General Aspects and Data on 11,087 Cases*. Philadelphia: Lippincott-Raven; 1996.

117. Utz JA, Kransdorf MJ, Jelinek JS, et al. MR appearance of fibrous dysplasia. *J Comput Assist Tomogr* 1989;13:845–851.

118. VandeBerg B, Malghem J, Labaisse MA, et al. Avascular necrosis of the hip: comparison of contrast-enhanced and nonenhanced MR imaging with histologic correlation. Work in progress. *Radiology* 1992;182:445–450.

119. Vickers CW, Pugh DC, Ivins JC. Osteoid osteoma. A fifteen year follow-up in an untreated patient. *J Bone Joint Surg [A]* 1959;41:357–358.

120. Vigorita VJ, Ghelman B. Localization of osteoid osteoma—use of radionuclide scanning and autoimaging in identifying the nidus. *Am J Clin Pathol* 1983;79:223–225.

121. Waugh W. The ossification and vascularization of the tarsal navicular and their relation to Köhler disease. *J Bone Joint Surg [B]* 1958;68:834–839.

122. Weinstein SL. Legg-Calvé-Perthes disease. In: Morrisy RT, Weinstein SL, eds. *Lovell and Winter's Pediatric Orthopedics*. 4th ed. Philadelphia: Lippincott-Raven; 1996:951–992.

123. Willman CL. Detection of conal histiocytes in Langerhans cell histiocytosis: biology and clinical significance. *Br J Cancer* 1994;70:S29–S33.

124. Winter WA, Veraart BE, Vandegaal WP. Bone scintigraphy in patients with juvenile kyphosis (M. Scheuermann). *Diagn Imaging* 1981;50:186–190.

125. Yamazaki T, Maruoka S, Takahashi S, et al. MR findings of avulsive cortical irregularities of the distal femur. *Skeletal Radiol* 1995;24:43–46.

5
Primary and Metastatic Bone Malignancies

The uses of skeletal scintigraphy and other scintigraphic studies in evaluating children with primary bone tumors and children with skeletal metastases are reviewed in this chapter. The chapter emphasizes the relative values of different imaging studies in assessing osteosarcoma and neuroblastoma, which are, respectively, the most common primary and metastatic bone malignancies of childhood.

Primary Bone Malignancies

Osteosarcoma

Clinical Considerations

Osteosarcoma is the most common primary bone malignancy of childhood. This tumor usually originates within the medullary space and occasionally arises from the surface of a bone (periosteal and parosteal forms). Histologically, the diagnosis of osteosarcoma requires demonstration of neoplastic osteoid and osseous tissue.[49,78] Chondroid or fibrous tissue is frequently present. Osteosarcoma is classified as osteoblastic, chondroblastic, fibroblastic, or mixed cellularity, based on the relative distribution of tissue types, or as telangiectatic, when there are large cystic spaces containing blood, scant osteoid, and massive cellular necrosis. In terms of its aggressiveness and degree of cellular differentiation, the tumor is graded as high or low.[78,101] Histologic grading of osteosarcoma is difficult, however, as marked variability is frequently found among tissue samples obtained from different regions of the same tumor.

The highest incidence of osteosarcoma occurs between the ages of 15 and 25 years. The tumor rarely affects children younger than 6 years of age.[78] Patients typically present with localized pain and/or swelling.[48] Pathologic fracture occurs in approximately 5% of patients. This disturbs normal barriers to tumor spread and worsens the prognosis.[1,57]

Osteosarcoma is predominantly a lesion of the long bones, where it is typically metaphyseal in location. The distal femur, proximal tibia, and proximal humerus are most commonly affected.[48,101] Since osteosarcoma is related to production of bone, it is not surprising that it primarily occurs in these, the regions of fastest skeletal growth. Flat bones, particularly the ilium and mandible, are involved in 10% of cases.[57]

The etiology of osteosarcoma is unknown. In a minority of cases, osteosarcoma develops as a late complication of radiation therapy or chemotherapy. A predisposition to osteosarcoma is present in children with the genetic or hereditary type of retinoblastoma. This risk is increased by exposure to radiation or chemotherapy.[62,74,81] Very rarely, osteosarcoma develops in benign lesions. These lesions include fibrous dysplasia, infarction, chronic osteomyelitis, osteoblastoma, and aneurysmal bone cyst.[74,78,81,101]

The most common locations of osteosarcoma metastases are lung and bone. Pulmonary metastases typically, but not invariably, precede skeletal metastases. They are more commonly present at diagnosis than are skeletal metastases. Skeletal metastases involve sites distant from the primary tumor or the same bone in which the primary tumor is located (skip metastasis). A small percentage of patients have multiple skeletal lesions detected at the time of diagnosis (osteosarcomatosis). These lesions most commonly involve metaphyses of the long bones, pelvis, vertebrae, and ribs. Some authors have proposed that osteosarcomatosis represents multiple primary osteosarcomas. It is more likely that osteosarcomatosis is due to skeletal metastases of a single primary lesion as a single radiographically dominant lesion is identified in over 90% of cases.[45]

The treatment of choice for osteosarcoma is wide resection and limb-sparing surgery. Limb-sparing procedures entail the resection of tumor with a cuff of surrounding normal tissue at all margins, skeletal reconstruction, and muscle and soft tissue transfers. Skeletal reconstruction is accomplished with a cadaveric allograft, bone prosthesis, or both.[1] Employing current chemotherapeutic regimens pre- and postoperatively and imaging to define tumor extent and tumor viability preoperatively, limb-sparing procedures can be appropriately performed in 80% of patients with osteosarcoma.[72] An alternative procedure aimed at restoring function, tibiofemoral rotationplasty, is used in some cases of distal femoral osteosarcoma following tumor resection. With tibiofemoral rotationplasty, the tibia is rotated 180° on its axis and fixed to the femur with plate and screws. The ankle, which is positioned so that it should be at the same level as the contralateral knee at the time of growth cessation, acts as a knee joint for a custom-fitted prosthesis that serves as the lower leg. The choice of procedure depends on multiple factors that include the overall prospects for survival, psychologic effects, estimated likelihood of recurrence, and probability of restoring function with a limb-sparing procedure in a given individual.[1]

The 10-year survival rate of osteosarcoma patients treated with current methods exceeds 70%.[33] Death is frequently due to pulmonary metastatic disease and rarely to local recurrence. The highest survival rates are realized in patients without metastatic disease at presentation, whose tumor shows greater than 90% to 95% necrosis prior to resection.[5,76]

Imaging is required to define the extent of the primary tumor at diagnosis, to evaluate the response to preoperative chemotherapy when a limb-sparing procedure is planned, and to detect metastatic disease at diagnosis and during follow-up. Different cross-sectional anatomic imaging studies and scintigraphic techniques are useful in variable degrees for each of these purposes (Figs. 5.1–5.6).

Imaging at Diagnosis

The radiographic appearance of osteosarcoma is related to bone production and bone destruction. Radiographs typically reveal a large bone-forming lesion at the time of initial presentation (Figs. 5.1 and 5.2). Most often, the tumor is eccentrically situated in the metaphysis of a long bone. It is diaphyseal in approximately 10% of cases.[113] Neoplastic bone, the distinguishing feature of osteosarcoma, is visible in 90% of cases. Radiolucent areas of lysis are frequently intermixed with radiodense areas of sclerosis (Figs. 5.3 and 5.4). In some tumors, particularly aggressive and telangiectatic lesions, the lytic component predominates (Figs. 5.5 and 5.6). The cortex is destroyed and an aggressive-appearing periosteal reaction, such as a Codman's triangle or a spiculated "sunburst" pattern, is often present. There is usually an associated soft tissue mass, which may contain areas of malignant bone.[57,78,101] Very rarely, the radiographic appearance is misleading and suggestive of a benign process. This can occur early in the development of an osteosarcoma, with low-grade tumors, and in osteosarcomas arising in benign lesions.[104,113]

Text continued on p. 223

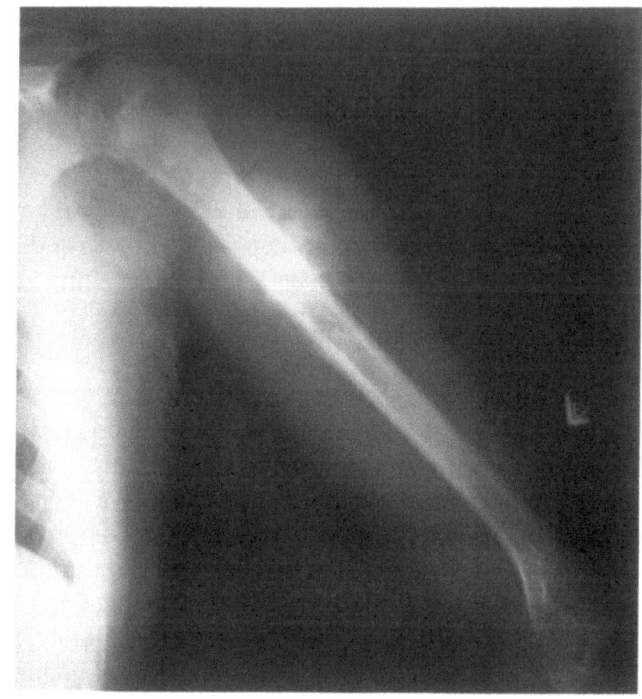

A

Figure 5.1. Metastatic osteosarcoma. A radiograph (A) shows a large osteosarcoma involving the proximal metaphysis and much of the diaphysis of the left humerus. Extensive ossification extends into the adjacent soft tissues.

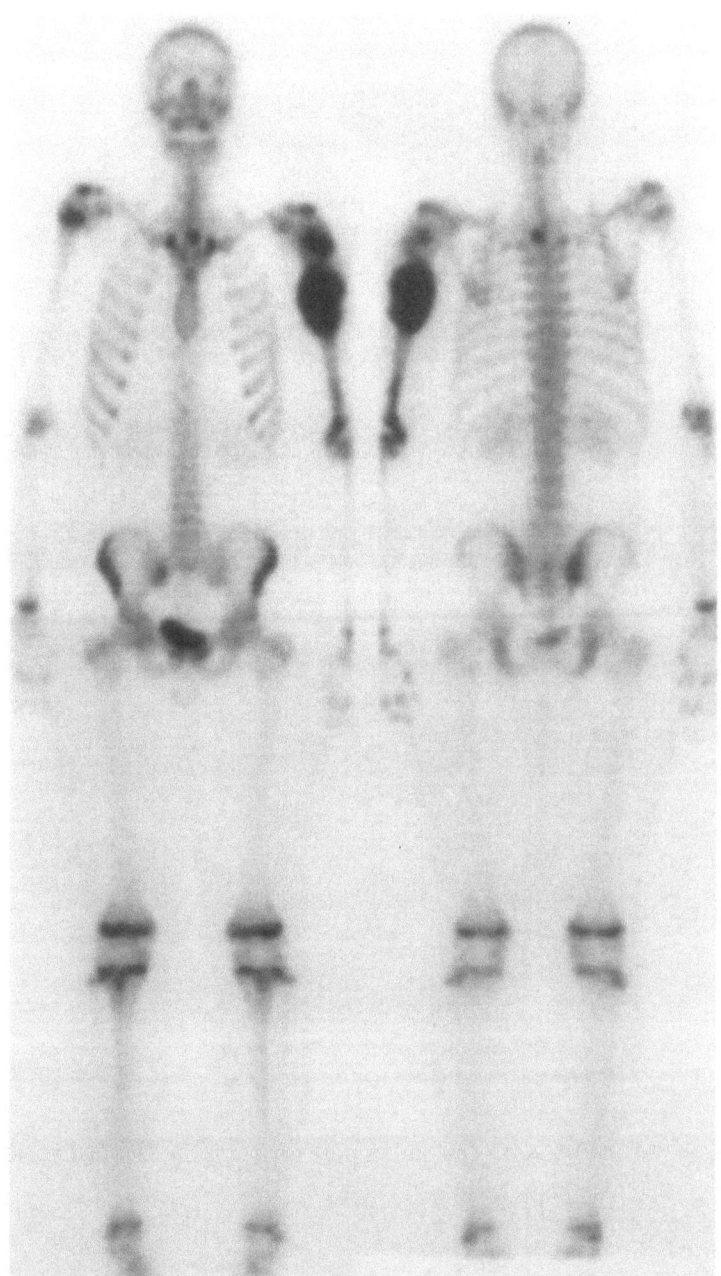

B

Figure 5.1 (*cont'd*). Skeletal scintigraphy (B) demonstrates increased ^{99m}Tc-MDP localization extending to the distal left humeral metaphysis. Focal increased tracer localization in the right aspect of the sacrum and in T2 indicate that this tumor has metastasized to bone. Radiographs of these two areas were normal.

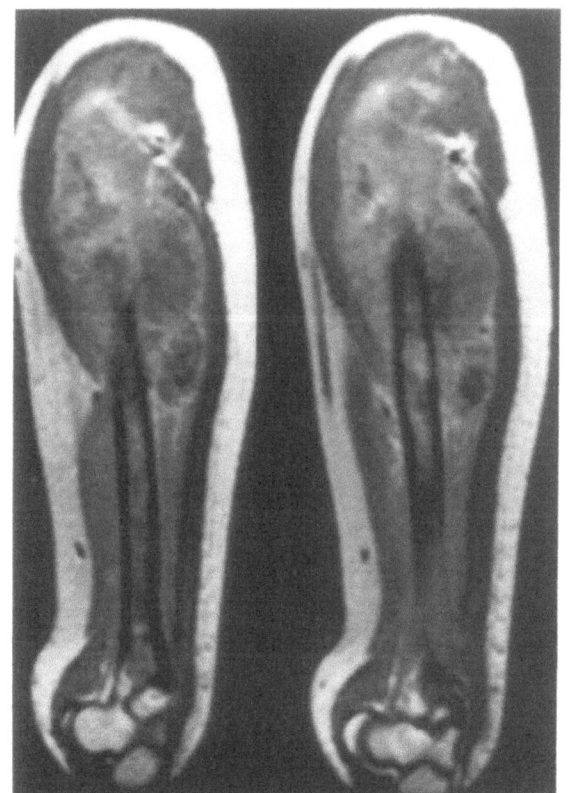

C

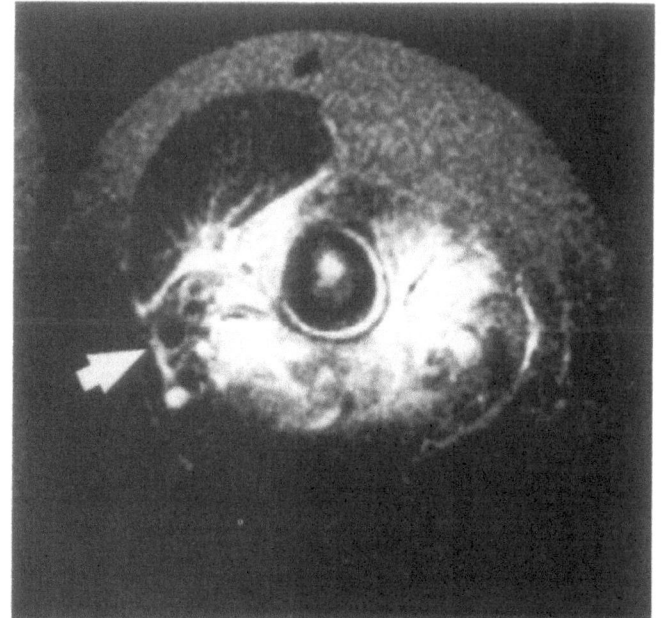

D

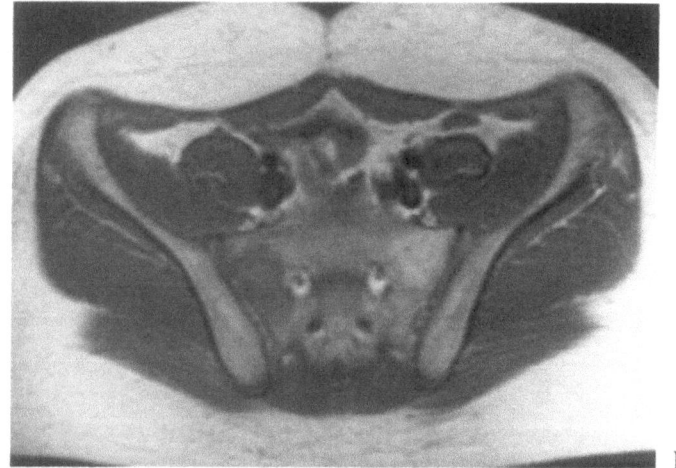

E

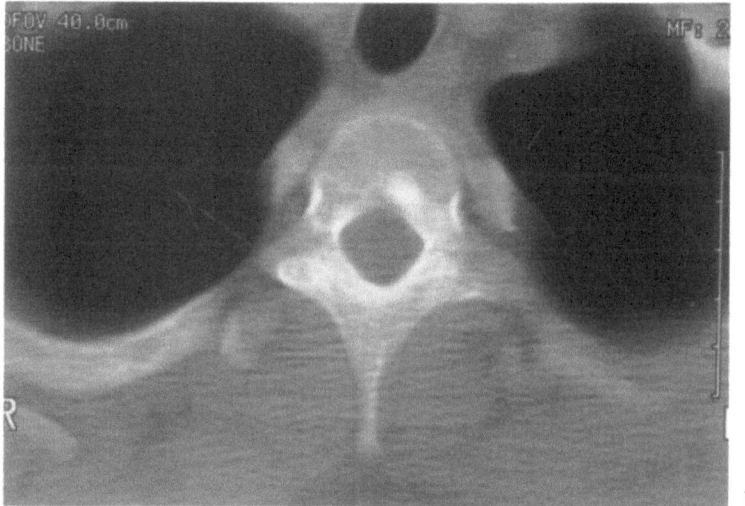

F

Figure 5.1 (cont'd). Sagittal T1-weighted images following gadolinium administration (C) reveal a heterogeneously enhancing tumor arising from the proximal humeral metaphysis extending along the entire diaphysis with a large subperiosteal soft tissue mass. A transaxial T2-weighted image (D) demonstrates the tumor's relationship to the neurovascular bundle (arrow). An MRI (E), obtained to confirm that the sacral abnormality was metastatic rather than stress related in this athletic 15-year-old boy, demonstrates abnormal T1 signal in the right sacrum. A sclerotic metastasis in the T2 vertebral body (F) is identified on a chest CT (displayed with a bone algorithm).

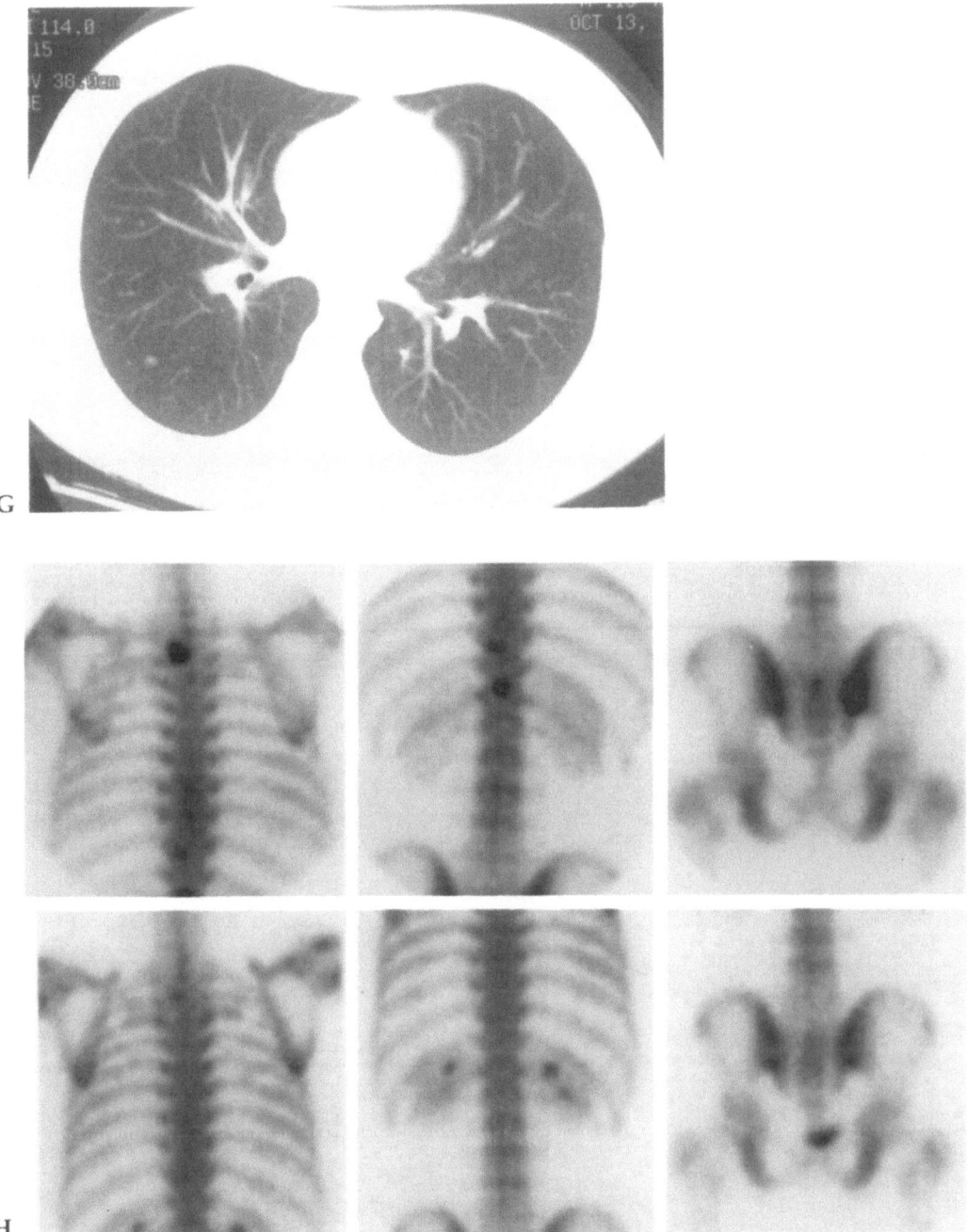

Figure 5.1 (*cont'd*). Chest CT also revealed multiple 2 to 3 mm in diameter pulmonary nodules, such as the one shown in the right lower lobe (G). Small size of pulmonary metastases, which is common with osteosarcoma, can lead to their escaping detection with radiographs. During chemotherapy, the metastatic sites at T2 and in the sacrum showed a greater degree of tracer localization (H, upper row) than at diagnosis. Additional sites of increased tracer localization were detected at T10 and T12. Three months following chemotherapy, tracer localization is minimally increased at T2 and T10 (H, lower row). The serial appearance is consistent with a flare response.

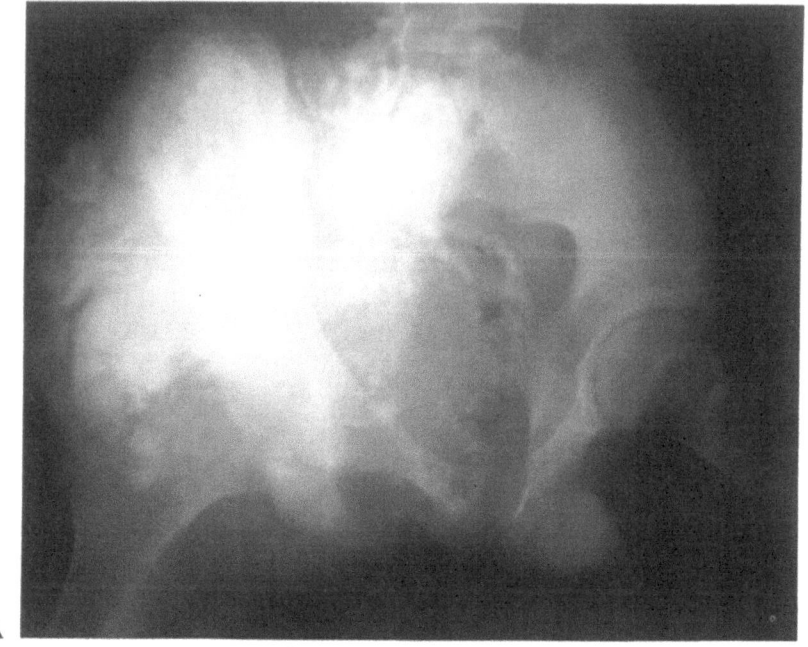

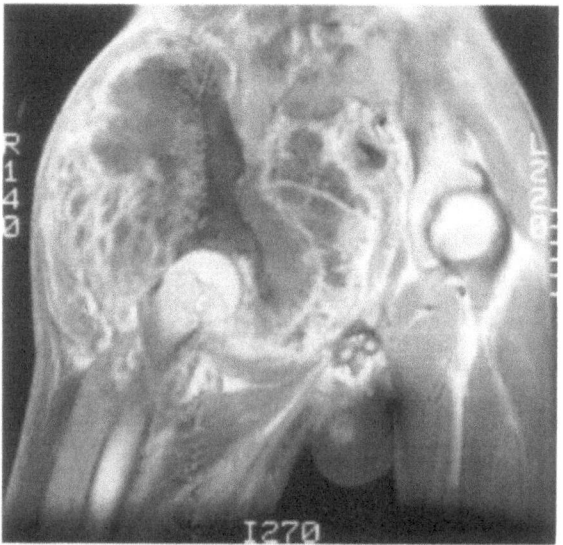

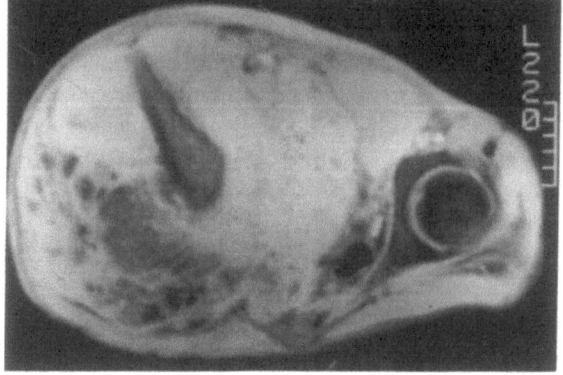

Figure 5.2. Osteosarcoma. A pelvic radiograph (A) demonstrates a large ossified mass projecting over, and likely arising from, the right ilium. A coronal T1-weighted postgadolinium image (B) and a transaxial T2-weighted image (C) show a large heavily calcified, peripherally enhancing, soft tissue mass that envelopes the entire abnormal right iliac bone. The mass crosses the midline and deviates both the rectum and bladder toward the left.

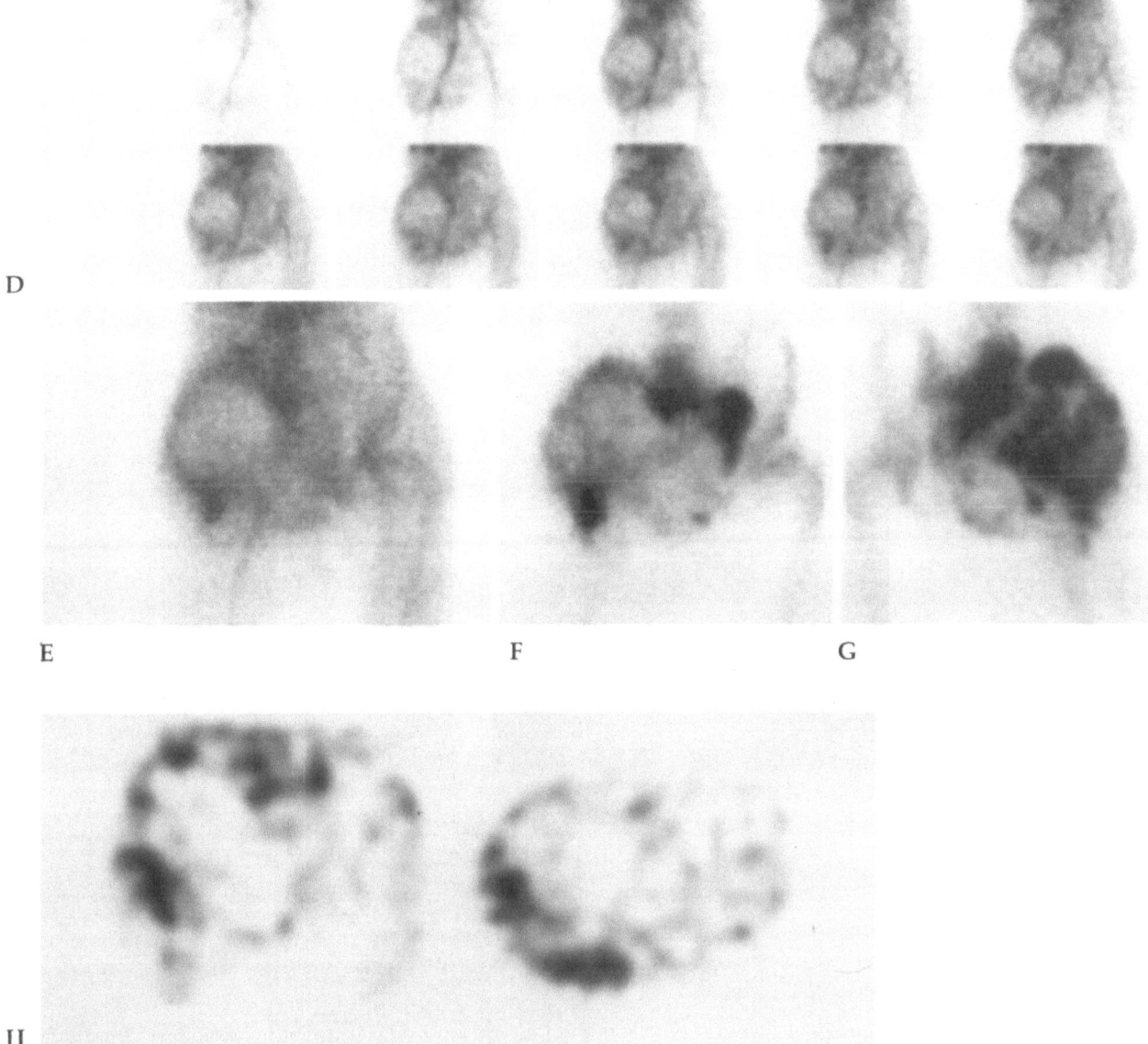

D

E   F   G

II

Figure 5.2 (*cont'd*). Radionuclide angiography (D) and tissue phase imaging (E) show increased tracer localization about the periphery of the mass, corresponding to regions where gadolinium enhancement is observed. Anterior (F) and posterior (G) skeletal phase images show intense tracer localization, particularly posteriorly. Thallium-201 SPECT (H: coronal and transverse images) demonstrates a pattern similar to that seen with tissue phase skeletal scintigraphy and gadolinium-enhanced MRI. Thallium-201 localization, indicating the location of viable tumor, typically correlates well with areas of increased vascularity.

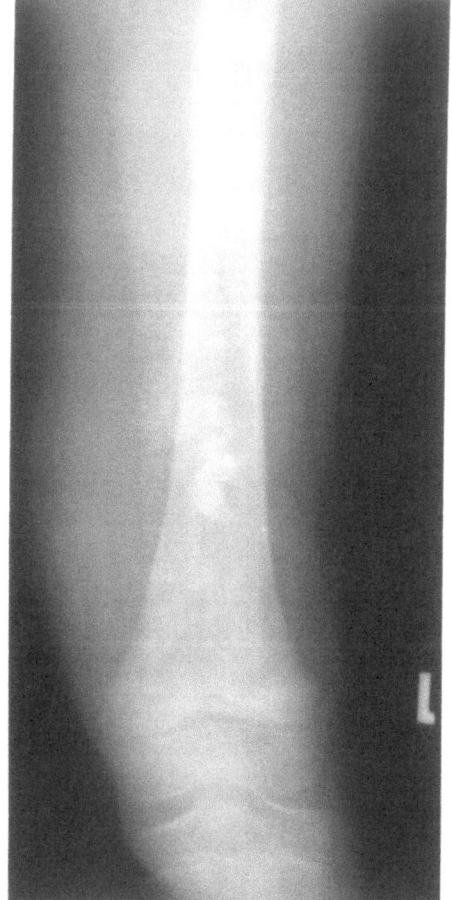

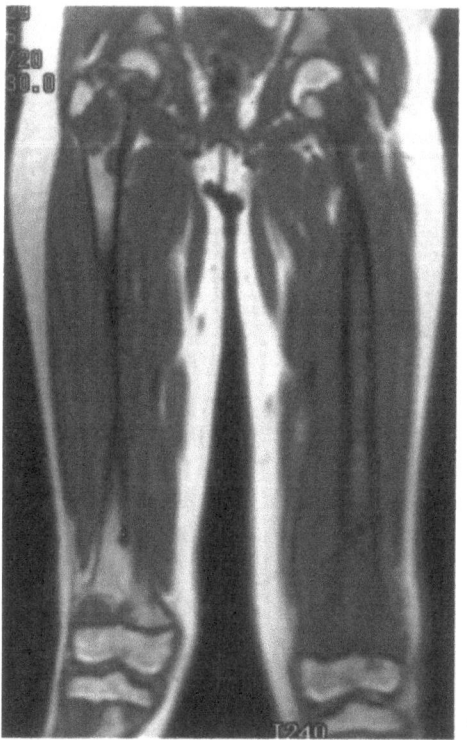

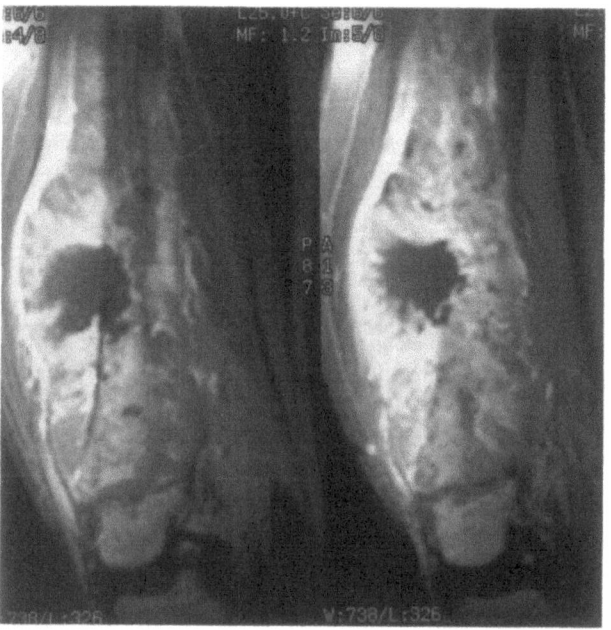

Figure 5.3. Multifocal osteosarcoma. A radiograph (A) of a 7-year-old girl who presented with a history of progressive limp and left leg pain over a 2- to 3-month period reveals a predominantly intraosseous, mixed sclerotic and lytic lesion of the distal left femoral metaphysis and diaphysis. An aggressive laminated periosteal reaction and fluffy calcification in the soft tissues indicates a diagnosis of osteosarcoma. Coronal T1-weighted images of both femurs demonstrate abnormal signal intensity throughout the left femur, including the distal epiphysis but sparing the proximal epiphysis. Focal regions of low T1 signal, consistent with metastatic deposits, are present in the proximal and distal right femoral metaphyses as well as the proximal metaphysis of the right tibia (B). Postgadolinium T1-weighted imaging (C) shows the distal left femur to be surrounded by an enhancing subperiosteal mass with a central nonenhancing osseous or necrotic region.

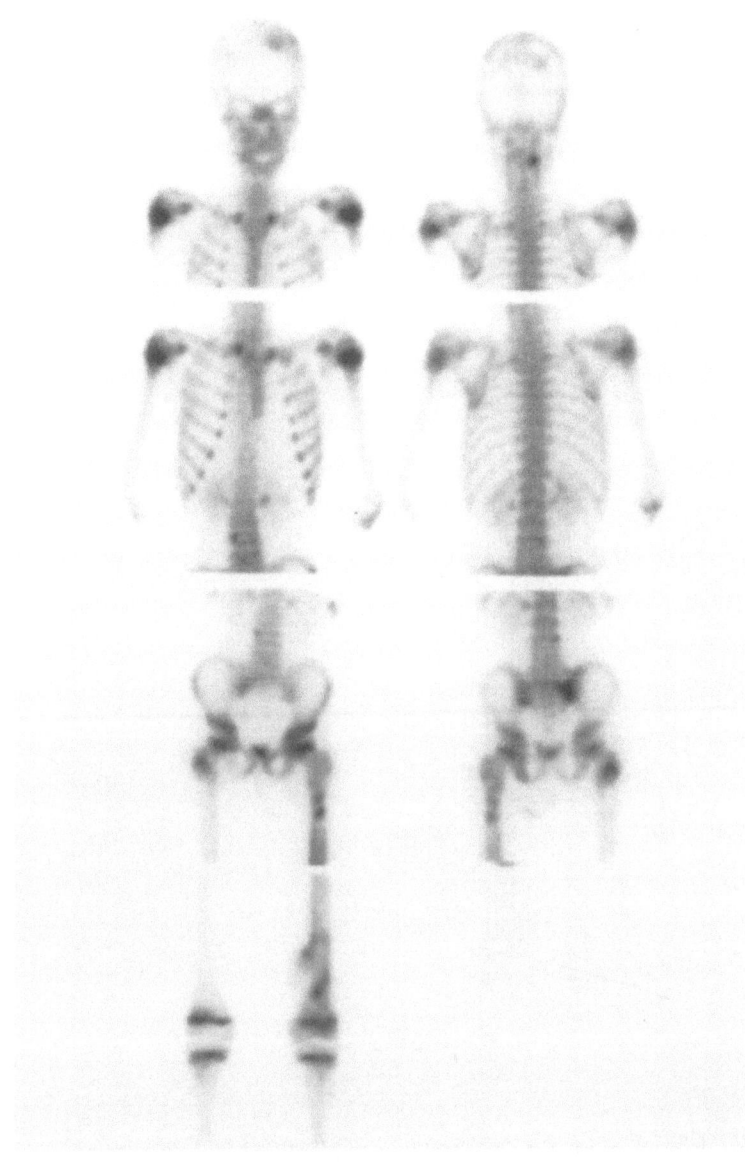

D

Figure 5.3 (*cont'd*). Skeletal scintigraphy (D) demonstrates the left femoral tumor as well as metastatic sites in the left proximal tibial metaphysis, the right intertrochanteric femur, the right distal femoral and proximal tibial metaphyses, the left ischium, the sacrum, L4, C2, the left third rib, and the calvarium. A thoracic CT had revealed no evidence of pulmonary metastases. Sagittal T2-weighted images of the spine (E,F) reveal evidence of more extensive metastatic disease than suggested by planar skeletal scintigraphy. Areas of abnormal signal are present in C2 (E), T11, L1, L4, L5, and S1 (F).

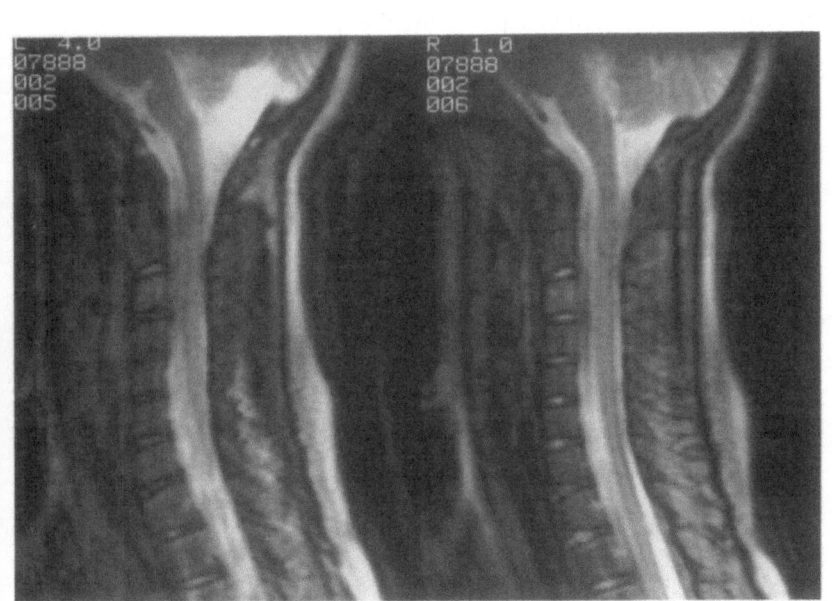

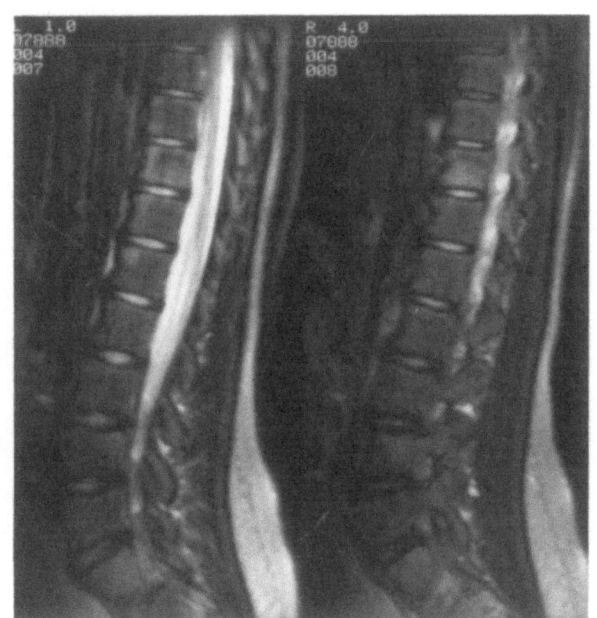

F

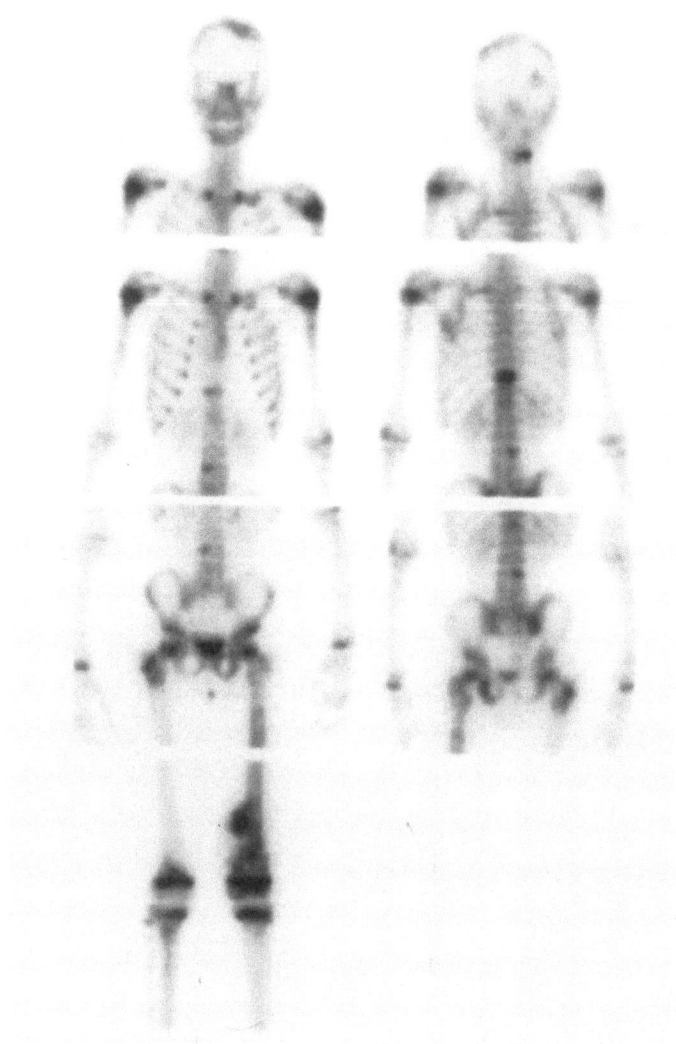

G

Figure 5.3 (*cont'd*). During chemotherapy, the vertebral lesions identified by MRI became manifest scintigraphically (G) and the previously demonstrated lesions showed a greater degree of tracer localization. While this pattern could represent either a flare phenomenon or progressive disease, the latter was indicated by a poor clinical response.

Local extent of the tumor in bone and soft tissue is well defined with magnetic resonance imaging (MRI) (Figs. 5.1 and 5.2). At our institution,[50] this examination begins with coronal T1-weighted images using a large field of view to estimate intramedullary tumor extent, to detect skip metastases,[84] and to serve as a localizer for further imaging sequences. Short tau inversion recovery (STIR) sequences are useful to further define the extent of marrow abnormality and to help differentiate hematopoietic marrow from intramedullary tumor. The relationship of the tumor to adjacent structures and the patency of adjacent vessels are assessed with axial proton-density or T2-weighted images and axial gradient-recalled echo (GRE) images. Gadolinium-enhanced T1-weighted images assist in differentiating viable from necrotic tumor.

The tumor mass typically appears as low signal intensity on T1-weighted images and high signal intensity on T2-weighted images. Areas with abundant neoplastic bone formation demonstrate low signal intensity on all sequences. Intraosseous areas of intermediate T1-weighted signal intensity and streaky regions of high T2-weighted signal intensity with poorly defined margins in the soft tissues and muscles are likely to represent peritumoral edema.[8] Any area of abnormal signal intensity within bone is assumed, however, to be involved by the neoplasm. This may result in overestimation of actual tumor extent but is preferable to underestimating the margins needed for excision. Fluid-fluid levels in the cystic spaces of telangiectatic osteosarcomas are well demonstrated with MRI (Fig. 5.6). Transphyseal extension of tumor into the epiphysis has been identified with MRI in 80% of cases.[82] Articular involvement is rare as articular cartilage generally serves as an effective barrier to tumor extension. Spread does occur, however, along the cruciate ligaments in some cases.[106] Demonstration of the relationship of the tumor to adjacent vascular or neural structures is an especially important contribution of MRI to surgical planning as limb-sparing procedures are generally contraindicated when there is major neurovascular involvement.[1]

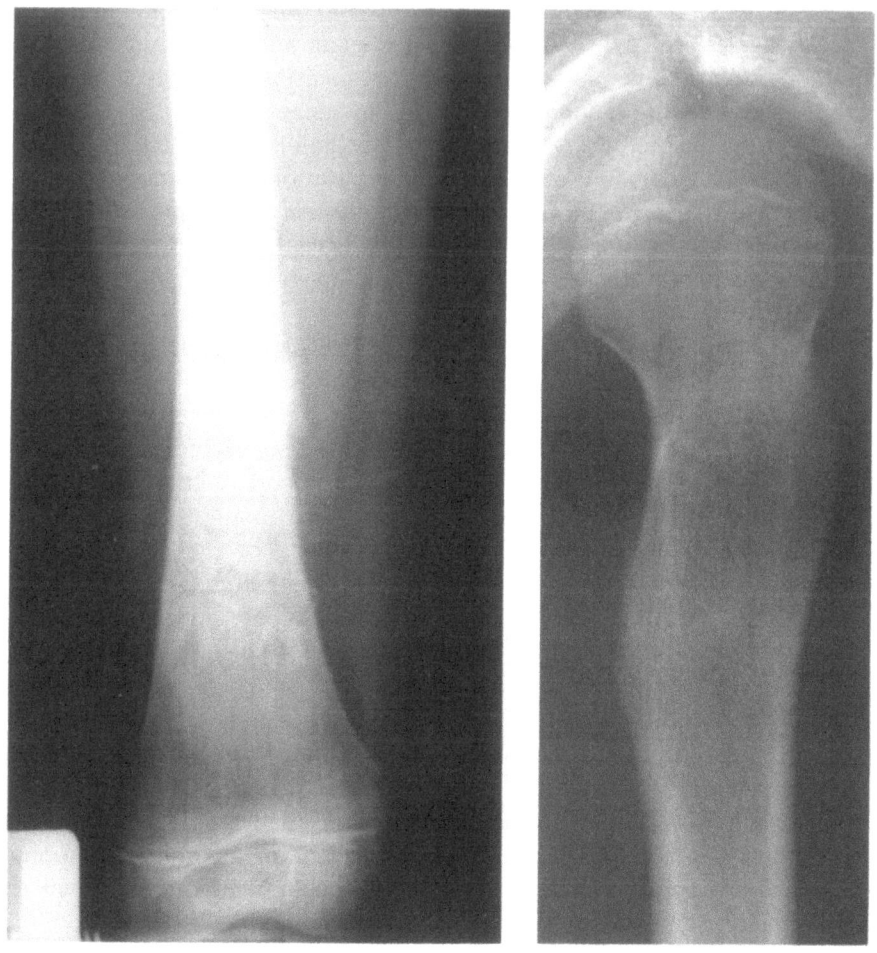

A   B

Figure 5.4. Osteosarcoma with skip metastases. A radiograph (A) shows an extensive permeative lytic and sclerotic lesion involving the right femoral diaphysis and distal metaphysis with neoplastic ossification extending into the soft tissues. Pathologic transverse fracture has occurred in the distal diaphysis. A subtle 5-mm sclerotic lesion is demonstrated radiographically at the level of the lesser trochanter (B).

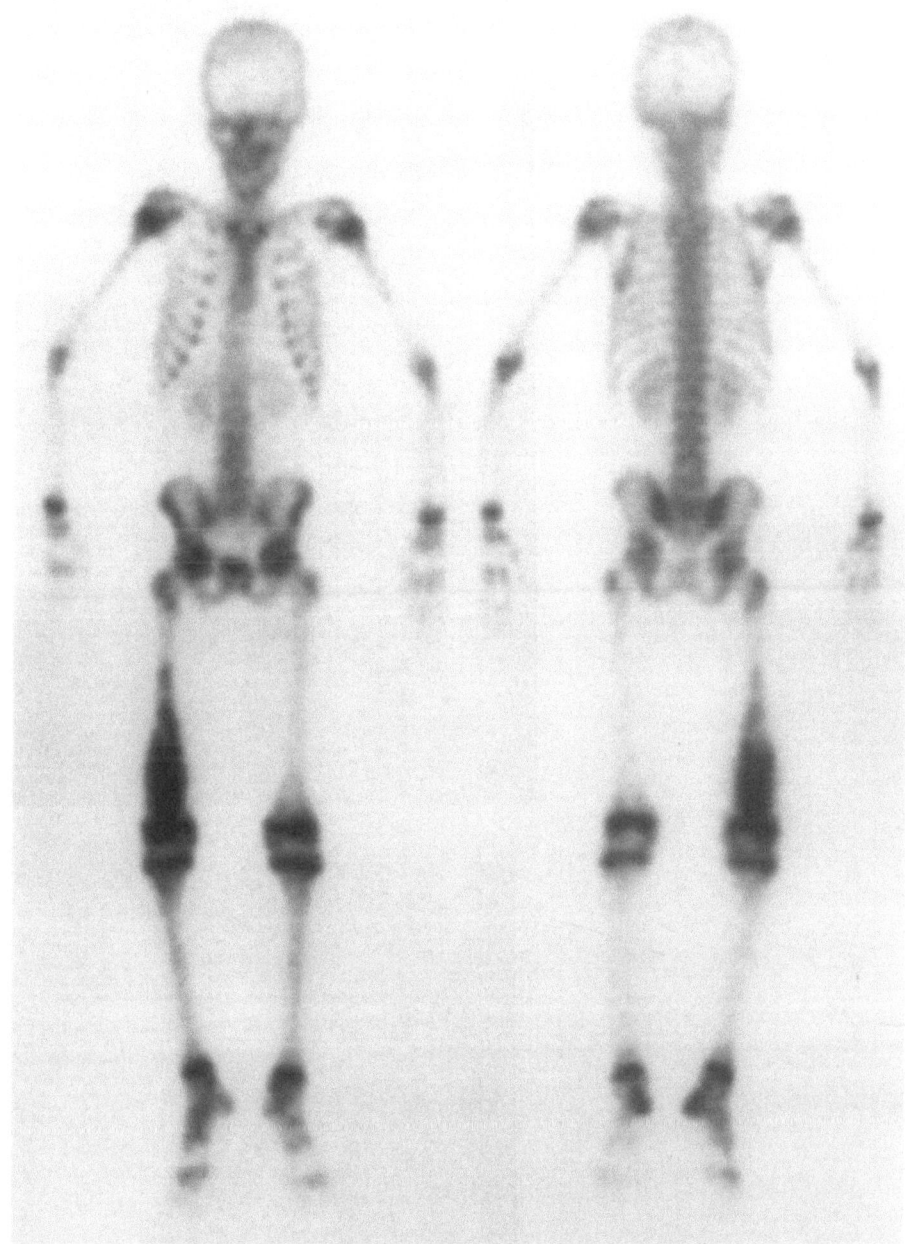

C

Figure 5.4 (cont'd). Anterior and posterior whole-body skeletal scintigrams (C) show intense tracer localization in a right femoral osteosarcoma. Separate foci of increased ^{99m}Tc-MDP localization in the mid-diaphysis and at the level of the lesser trochanter are indicative of skip metastases, with the latter abnormality correlating to the subtle radiographic finding.

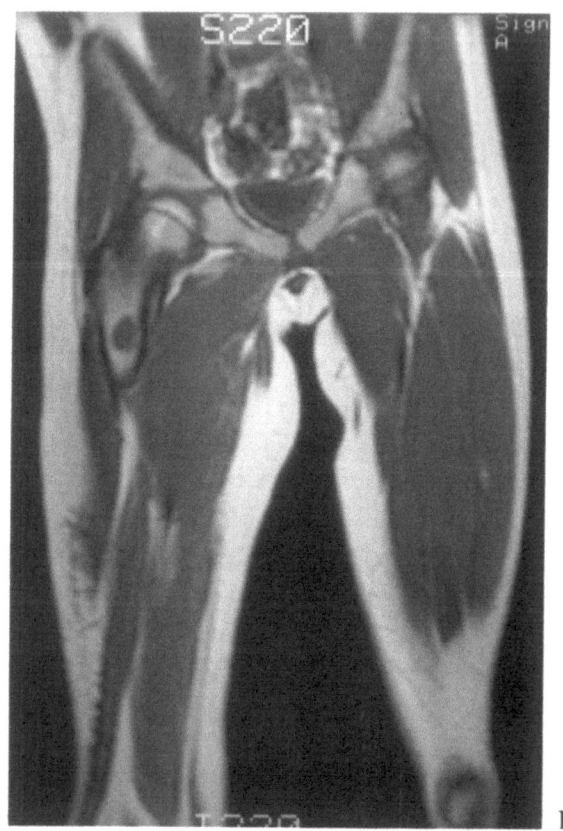

D

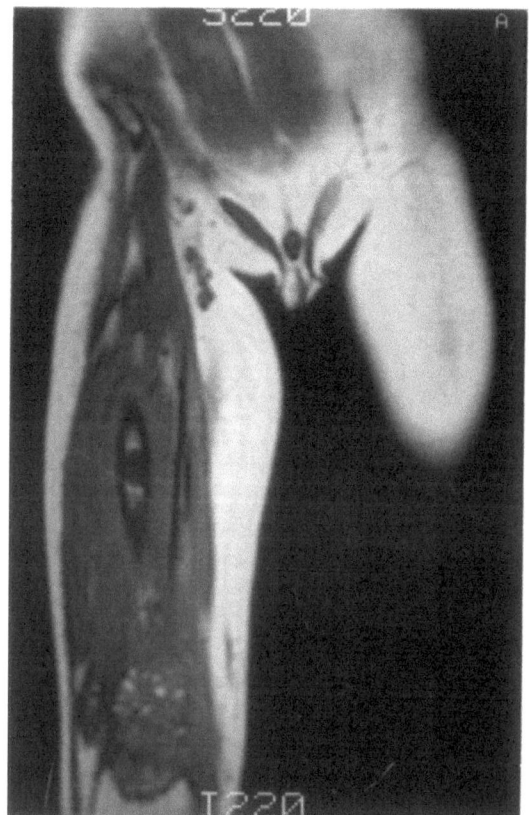

E

Figure 5.4 (*cont'd*). Coronal T1-weighted images (D,E) define two low signal intensity skip metastases in the right femur, proximal to the distal metadiaphyseal osteosarcoma.

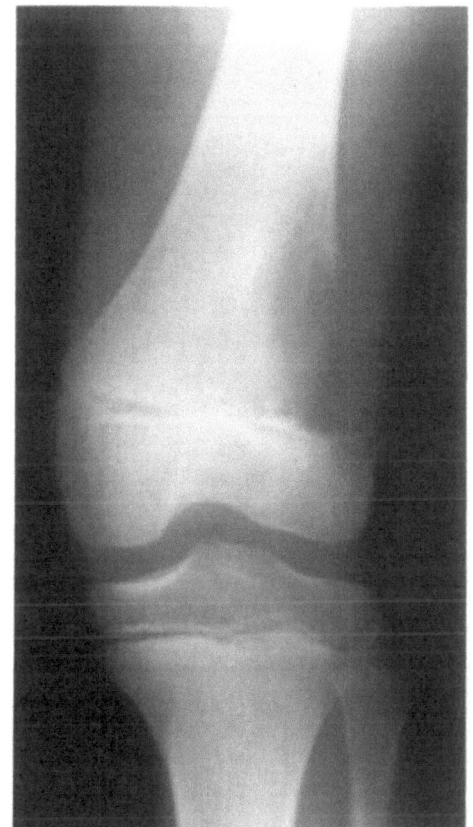

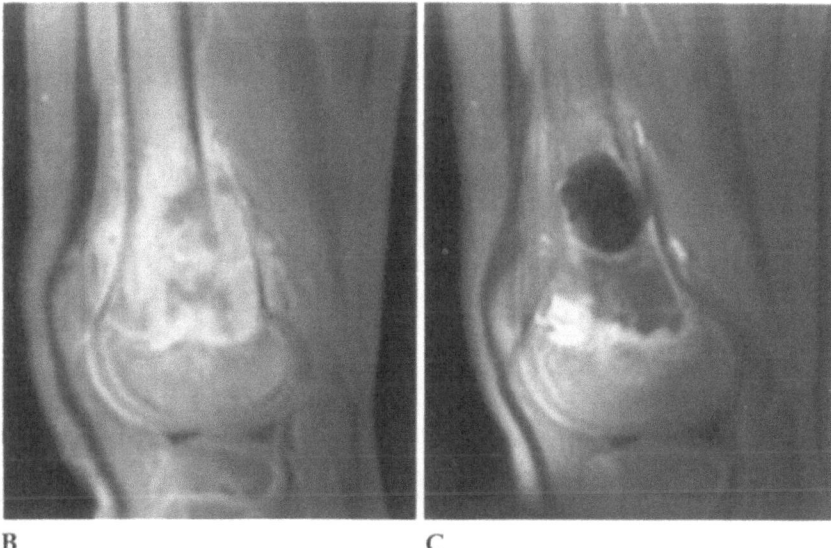

B

C

Figure 5.5. Osteosarcoma. A radiograph shows a predominantly lytic lesion originating in the lateral distal left femoral metaphysis and extending into the epiphysis (A). Sagittal T1-weighted gadolinium-enhanced images are depicted (B,C). At diagnosis (B), there is a large enhancing distal femoral tumor with physeal extension, periosteal breakdown, cortical disruption, and an associated soft tissue mass. Following biopsy and chemotherapy (C), decreased enhancement suggests a favorable chemotherapeutic response. The ovoid signal-void represents a methacrylate plug placed during biopsy.

A

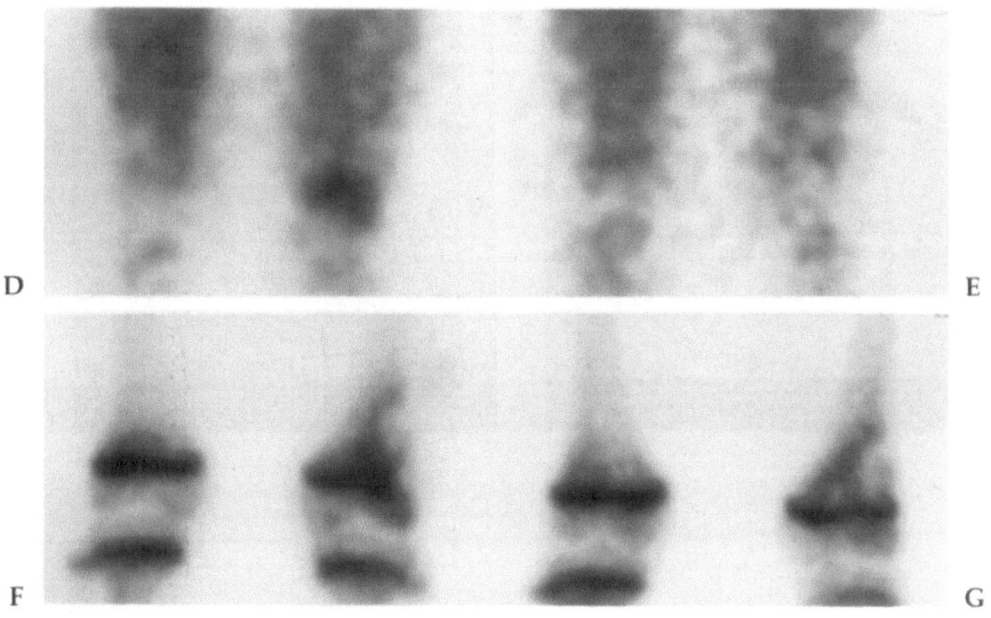

D

E

F

G

Figure 5.5 (cont'd). Thallium-201 uptake noted in the tumor at diagnosis (D) resolved following chemotherapy (E). The T/C ratio decreased from 8.7 to 0.9. Histologically, greater than 95% tumor necrosis was noted. Skeletal scintigraphy at diagnosis (F) and after therapy (G) revealed increased tracer localization along the periphery of the lytic lesion seen radiographically and in the epiphysis.

Figure 5.6. Telangiectatic osteosarcoma. A radiograph shows a destructive lesion involving the medial distal left femoral metaphysis and adjacent diaphysis (A). Neoplastic bone formation is faintly visualized in the adjacent soft tissues. At diagnosis, coronal (B) and transaxial (C) T1-weighted gadolinium-enhanced images show eccentric cortical destruction associated with a lobulated soft tissue mass that heterogeneously enhances. The transaxial image reveals a fluid-fluid level within the tumor.

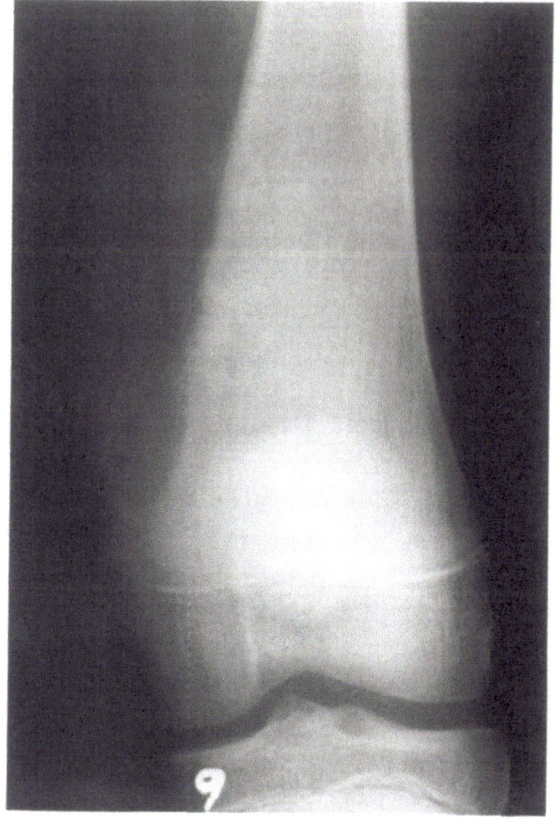

A

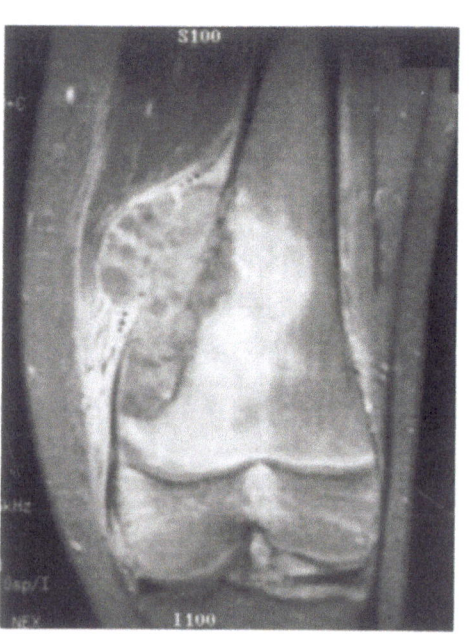

B

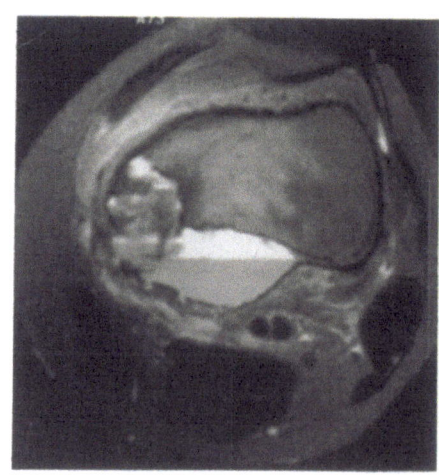

C

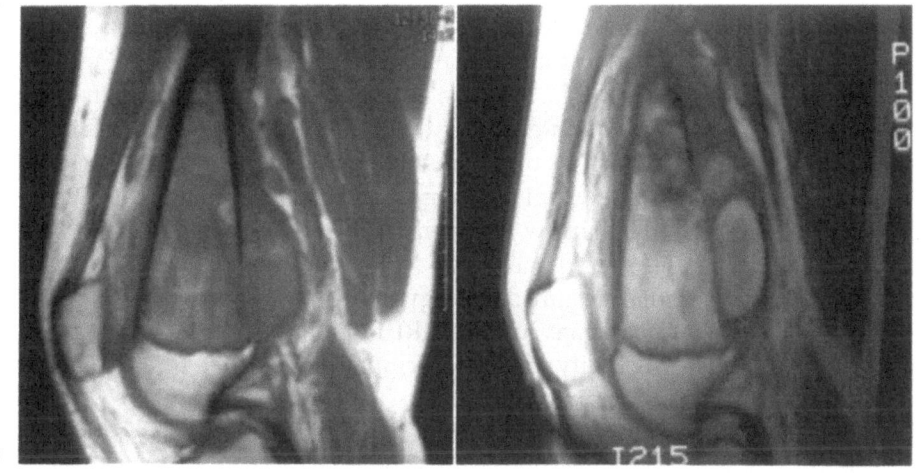

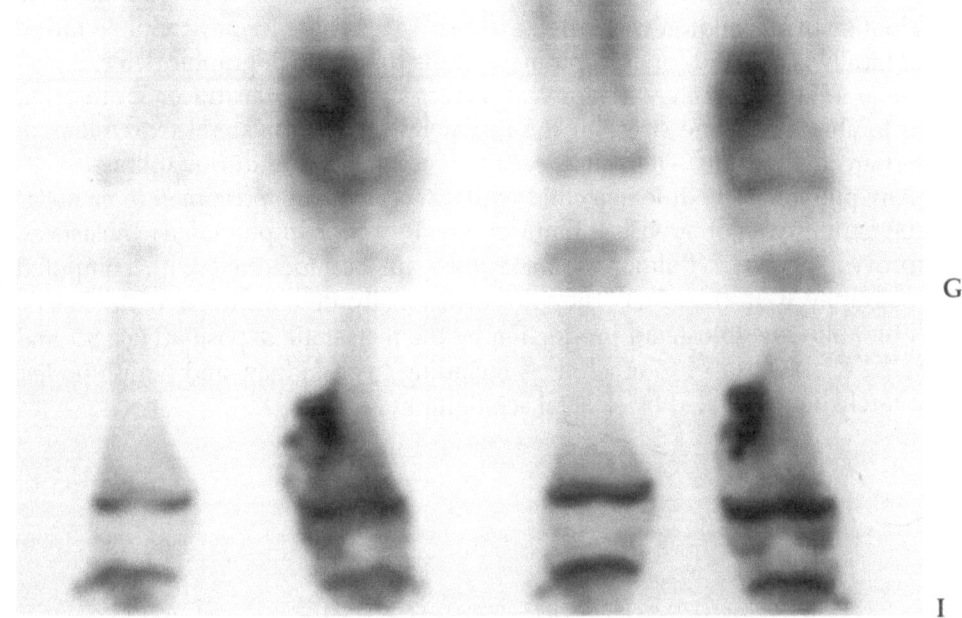

Figure 5.6 (*cont'd*). A sagittal T1-weighted image at diagnosis shows extensive metaphyseal and diaphyseal involvement with periosteal elevation and a large soft tissue mass (D). Following chemotherapy, improvement is suggested by a more normal-appearing marrow signal and a change in the signal characteristics of the soft tissue mass (E). At diagnosis, a [201]T1 study (F) shows intense uptake in the tumor. The T/C ratio was 17.1. Following chemotherapy, persistence of marked [201]T1 uptake is seen in this child whose T/C ratio increased to 20.1 (G). By pathologic examination, there was less than 25% tumor necrosis at the time of the second [201]T1 study. On skeletal scintigraphy, the tumor appears as areas of increased tracer localization within the femur with abnormal tracer localization extending into the soft tissues on images obtained at diagnosis (H) and after therapy (I).

The primary tumor typically demonstrates marked tracer localization on skeletal scintigraphy (Figs. 5.1–5.6). Regions of decreased tracer localization within viable nonossified tumor and necrotic tumor are also frequently present (Figs. 5.2, 5.3, 5.5, and 5.6). Increased tracer localization often extends beyond the pathologic confines of the tumor.[14,34,119] The intensity of this localization varies from faint to marked. This "extended pattern" typically involves bone in immediate contiguity with, or immediately across the joint adjacent to, the tumor. Rarely, it affects the entire ipsilateral extremity. Marrow hyperemia, medullary reactive bone, and periosteal new bone have been demonstrated in some cases that exhibited this pattern.[14] In other cases, the presumed etiology of this pattern is increased tracer delivery secondary to hyperemia. Just as MRI is limited in determining local extent of tumor in bone, the utility of skeletal scintigraphy is, therefore, limited in defining the margins of an osteosarcoma.

Skeletal scintigraphy is most useful in detecting skeletal metastases, which appear as areas of increased tracer localization (Figs. 5.1, 5.3, and 5.4). The exact incidence of skeletal metastases at diagnosis is uncertain but is accepted to be sufficiently high for skeletal scintigraphy to be included in the initial diagnostic evaluation of all children with osteosarcoma.[16,35,45,73] These lesions are often radiographically occult and/or asymptomatic at the time of scintigraphic detection.[73,99] Skeletal scintigraphy may also reveal increased periarticular tracer localization due to abnormal bone stress in the ipsilateral and contralateral extremities of osteosarcoma patients. This can be seen at presentation and during follow-up.[9,53]

Any pulmonary nodule in a child with osteosarcoma is presumed to be metastatic until proven otherwise at thoracotomy. Resection of pulmonary metastases improves survival.[36] Pulmonary metastases are best detected with computed tomography (CT) (Fig. 5.1). They are occasionally demonstrated with skeletal scintigraphy due to osteoid production by the metastatic deposits (Figs. 5.7 and 5.8).[43,54,99,122] Metastases to other sites, including liver, kidney, and lymph nodes, are rarely demonstrated by skeletal scintigraphy.

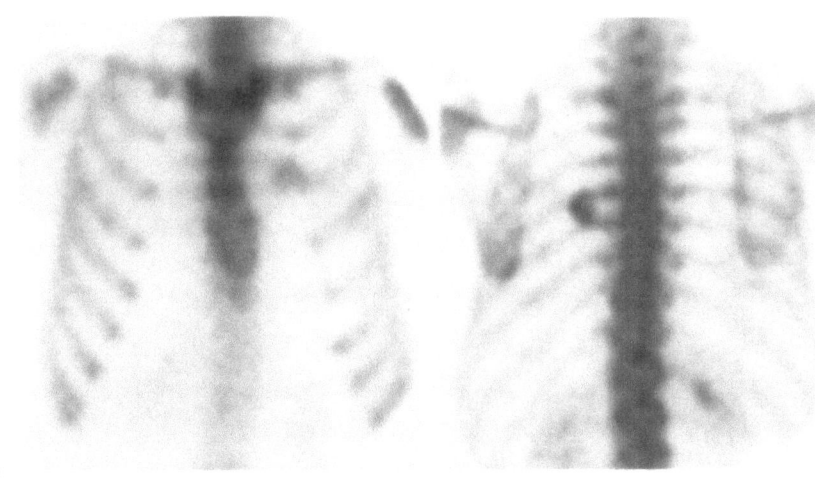

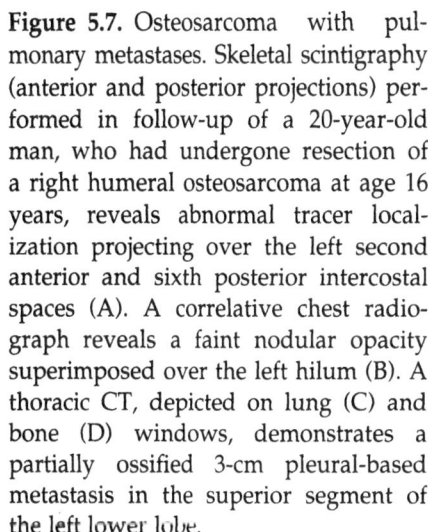

A

Figure 5.7. Osteosarcoma with pulmonary metastases. Skeletal scintigraphy (anterior and posterior projections) performed in follow-up of a 20-year-old man, who had undergone resection of a right humeral osteosarcoma at age 16 years, reveals abnormal tracer localization projecting over the left second anterior and sixth posterior intercostal spaces (A). A correlative chest radiograph reveals a faint nodular opacity superimposed over the left hilum (B). A thoracic CT, depicted on lung (C) and bone (D) windows, demonstrates a partially ossified 3-cm pleural-based metastasis in the superior segment of the left lower lobe.

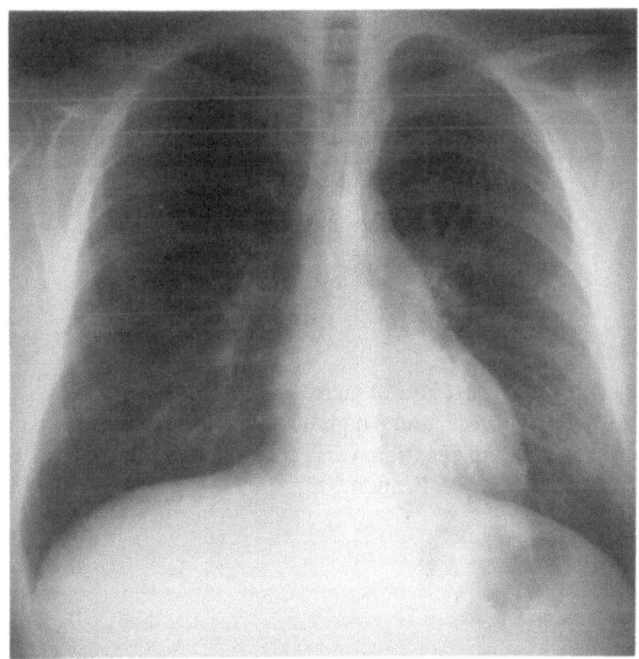

B

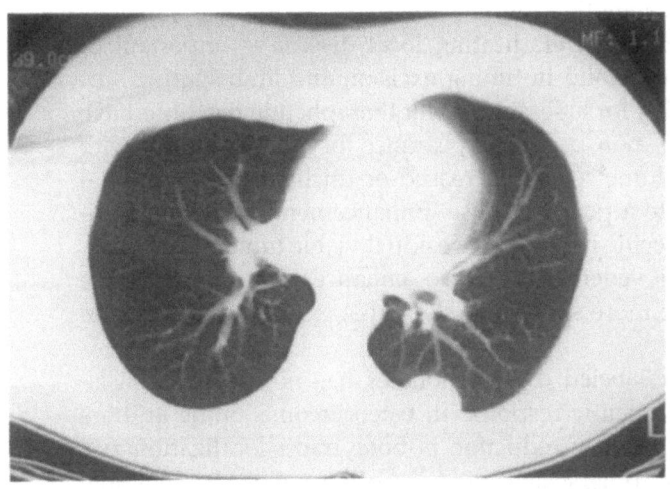

C

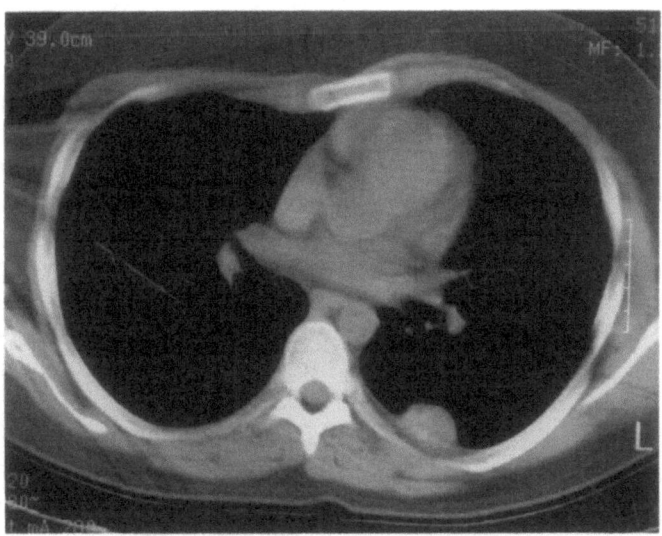

D

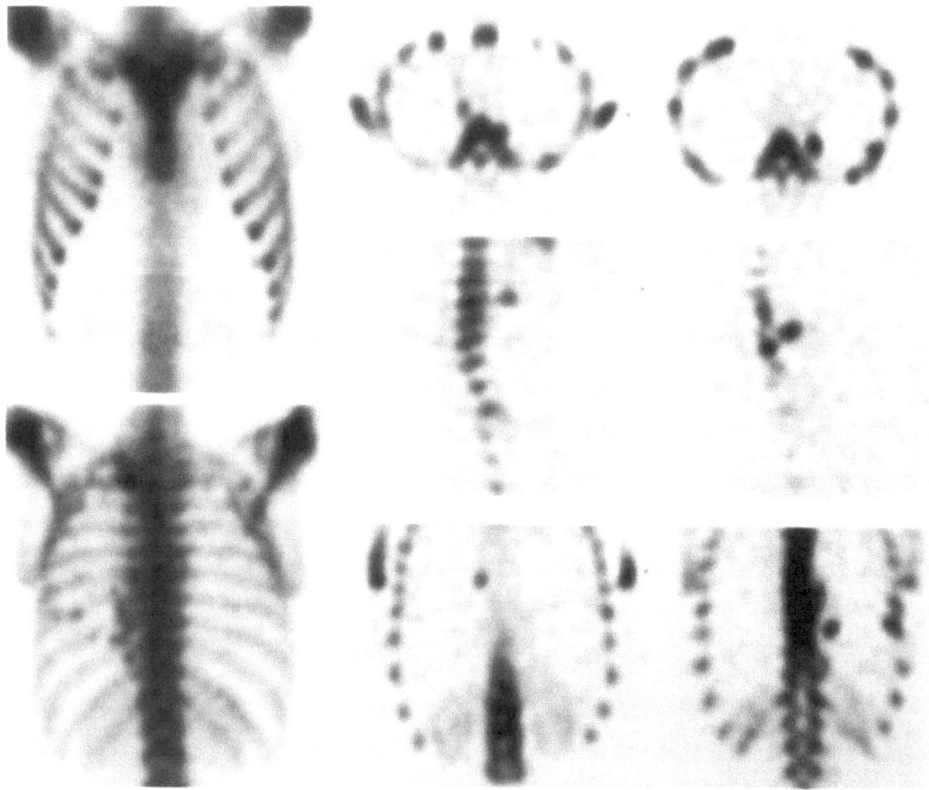

Figure 5.8. Osteosarcoma with pulmonary metastases. Foci of increased tracer localization along the left paraspinal region and related to ribs 1, 2, and 8 on the left are demonstrated with planar ^{99m}Tc-scintigraphy. Selected SPECT images (transverse, sagittal and coronal) depict bilateral peripheral pulmonary foci of tracer localization.

Evaluation of Response to Chemotherapy

Determining if preoperative chemotherapy has been successful, as defined by greater than 95% tumor necrosis, in eradicating local disease is important in adjusting chemotherapy regimens and in timing excision and limb-sparing surgery. Variable results using MRI for assessing chemotherapeutic response have been reported, reflecting the nonspecific appearance of viable tumor with MRI.[27,44,58] Increased tumor volume[44,58] and increased or unchanged peritumoral edema[44] independently indicate a poor response. Enhancement following gadolinium is a sensitive but nonspecific indicator of residual viable tumor as granulation tissue and perineoplastic edema may also enhance. The slope of the enhancement curve appears to more specific. A slope that exceeds 35% indicates viable tumor.[39]

Scintigraphy with the ^{99m}Tc-labeled diphosphonates has not proven consistently useful in assessing therapeutic response in osteosarcoma. Some authors have found good correlation between reduction in bone tracer localization and therapeutic response[55,116] while others have not.[27,96] Gallium-67 (^{67}Ga) imaging, although slightly more reliable than skeletal scintigraphy in the evaluation of therapeutic response, has also not proven to be accurate for this purpose.[96]

Scintigraphy with thallium-201 (^{201}Tl) has been shown to be valuable for the assessment of therapy in osteosarcoma.[18,61,75,85,96,103] The advantage of ^{201}Tl relative to skeletal tracers, such as ^{99m}Tc–methylene diphosphonate (MDP), results from the different mechanisms by which these tracers localize in osteosarcoma. Tumoral uptake of the [201]T1 reflects cellular viability, metabolic activity, and vascularity,[108] while ^{99m}Tc-MDP localization in osteosarcoma reflects vascularity and osteoblastic activity. Since ^{99m}Tc-MDP accumulates in both the tumor itself and adjacent reparative bone, ^{201}Tl imaging provides a more accurate depiction of viable tumor.

Osteosarcomas show intense ^{201}Tl uptake, which markedly decreases with a favorable (Fig. 5.5), but not with an unfavorable, therapeutic response (Figs. 5.6 and 5.9). This is assessed visually or quantitatively. In a pilot study of a small group of patients with osteosarcoma of the extremities, we recently found the background corrected ratio of the average counts per pixel within the tumor to the average counts per pixel within an identically sized and positioned ("mirror image") contralateral region of interest (tumor to contralateral [T/C] ratio) to be a

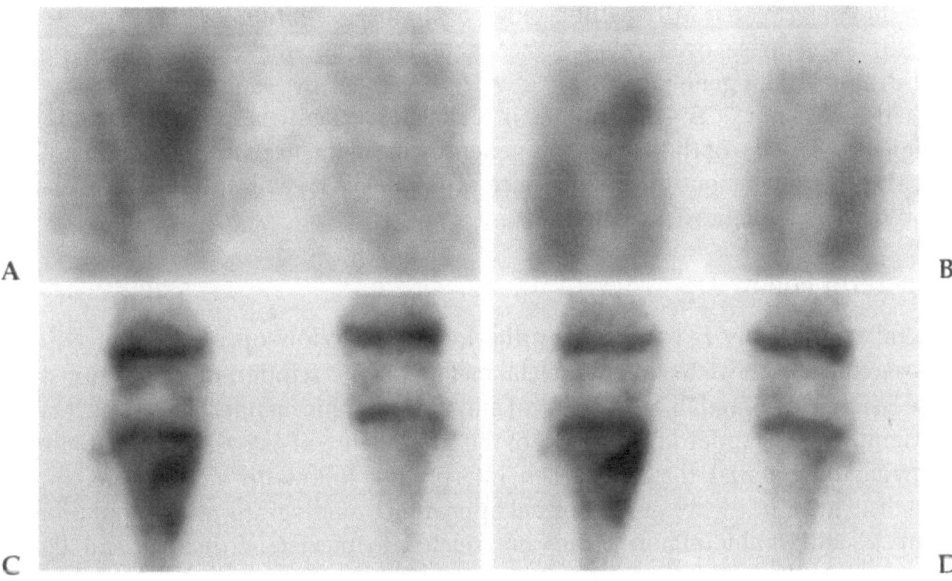

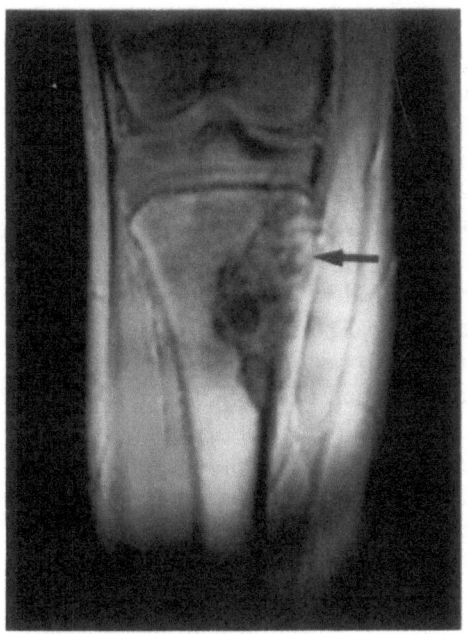

Figure 5.9. Osteosarcoma. Thallium-201 uptake in this right proximal tibial osteosarcoma decreased following chemotherapy: prechemotherapy (A), postchemotherapy (B). The focus of prominent ^{201}Tl that persisted in the tumor exhibited a T/C ratio of 2.7 following chemotherapy as compared to 3.7 pretherapy. Correlative ^{99m}Tc-MDP images, showing increasing intensity of localization are also depicted (C: prechemotherapy; D: postchemotherapy). Gadolinium-enhanced postchemotherapy MRI shows an area of enhancement corresponding to the site of persistent ^{201}Tl uptake (E: arrow).

highly significant predictor of chemotherapeutic response.[18] In cases where this ratio was less than 1.5 on the postchemotherapy study, the probability of a favorable therapeutic response has exceeded 88%. Estimated tumor necrosis based on MRI findings was less strongly predictive. Quantitative comparison of prechemotherapy and postchemotherapy studies has also proven valuable in our experience and that of others. Both the percent change in the ratio of tumor to contralateral ^{201}Tl uptake[18,61] and the percent change in tumor to background ratio of ^{201}Tl uptake[85] are useful. Although it must be emphasized that the T/C value cited above can not be regarded as an established standard, quantitative ^{201}Tl imaging appears to be valuable for evaluating therapeutic response.

Localization of ^{99m}Tc-hexakis-2methoxyisobutylisonitrile (^{99m}Tc-MIBI), a lipophilic cation, in osteosarcoma has been reported.[12,13] Although ^{99m}Tc-MIBI provides information regarding tumor viability similar to that available with ^{201}Tl, ^{99m}Tc-MIBI studies of tumors must be interpreted in light of the multidrug resistance phenomenon that develops after the use of certain chemotherapeutic agents. One mechanism by which this resistance develops is through a membrane glycoprotein (P glycoprotein) that serves to transport lipophilic compounds, including ^{99m}Tc-MIBI as well as chemotherapeutic agents, out of cells.[52,91] More studies are needed to determine if ^{99m}Tc-MIBI is either a suitable substitute for ^{201}Tl in assessing tumor response or a reliable means of assessing the expression of the multidrug resistant gene in vivo.

Neither ^{201}Tl nor ^{99m}Tc-MIBI uptake in a skeletal lesion has proven specific for malignancy. Uptake of these tracers is generally more intense, however, in malignant than benign lesions.[13,97] The absence of uptake of these tracers in a skeletal lesion renders a diagnosis of osteosarcoma unlikely.

Long-Term Follow-Up

Skeletal scintigraphy is employed in the long-term follow-up of children with osteosarcoma for the detection of skeletal metastases. As scintigraphic detection of these lesions often predates their clinical and radiographic manifestations, skeletal scintigraphy is a standard component of the surveillance of osteosarcoma patients following their initial therapy. When interpreting follow-up studies, imaging specialists must be aware of the normal appearance of allografts and amputation stumps, scintigraphic abnormalities not related to metastatic disease, and the occurrence of the "flare phenomenon" in osseous metastatic deposits.

Allografts

Transplantation of a cadaveric bone allograft is frequently performed as part of a limb-sparing procedure. The goal is to preserve function. Intercalary allografts reestablish a segment of a long bone exclusive of the epiphysis and articulating surfaces, which are not resected, while osteoarticular allografts include these structures.

Allografts are incorporated into the skeleton by a process referred to as creeping substitution. Host capillaries initially invade the allograft. Host osteocytes then deposit new bone on the allograft matrix and resorb the allogeneic bone. Remodeling takes place as dictated by mechanical strains.[3,30,67] A study on retrieved cadaveric bone allografts shows that this process is limited to the allograft ends and superficial layers and involves no more than 20% of the allogeneic bone by 5 years.[26] Mechanical strength and the functional integrity of allografts, however, do not appear to be related to the degree of incorporation.

Allografts have a characteristic scintigraphic appearance that reflects their incorporation process (Figs. 5.10–5.12).[7] Increased tracer localization is typically seen at the junction between host and allograft bone, where host bone unites with the allograft by callus formation, and at sites of plate and screw fixation. The allograft itself is visualized as an area of decreased tracer localization with its periphery

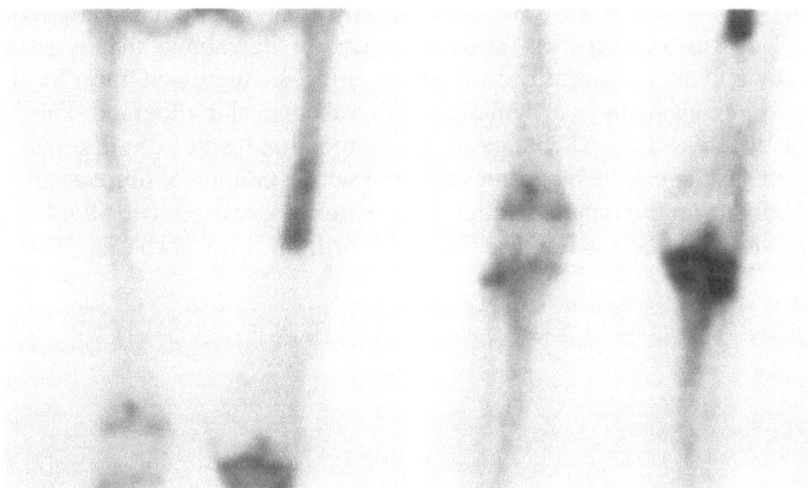

Figure 5.10. Osteoarticular allograft. The distal left femoral osteoarticular allograft appears as an area of decreased tracer localization. Its periphery is outlined by a rim of tracer localization slightly greater than that in adjacent soft tissues. Increased tracer localization in the left midfemoral diaphysis is due to a plate and screw fixation device. Increased tracer localization is demonstrated in the articulating surfaces of the left tibia.

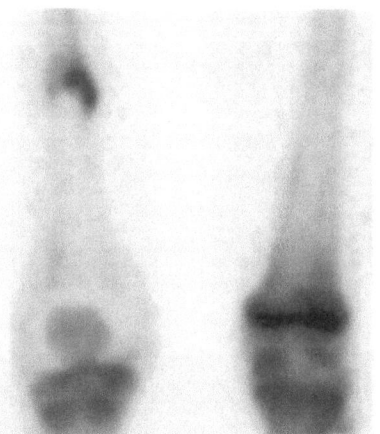
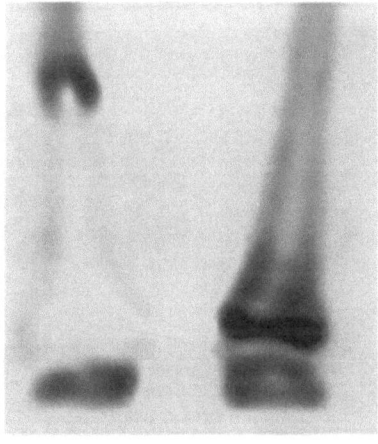

Figure 5.11. Osteoarticular allograft. Increased tracer localization is present at the junction with native bone of the right femur and in the right tibial plateau. Faint tracer localization outlining the allograft is seen with planar imaging (left panel) and SPECT (right panel).

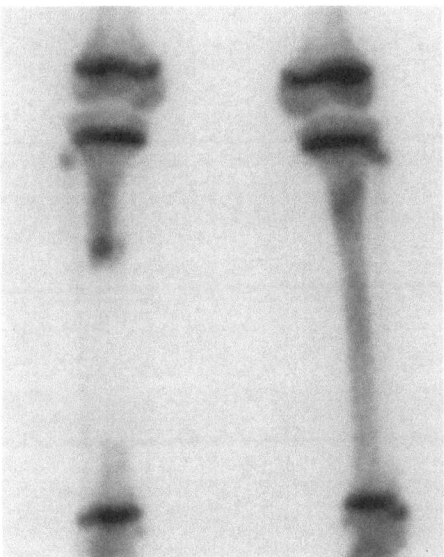

Figure 5.12. Intercalary allograft. Tracer localization is increased at the proximal junction with the native right tibia.

outlined by a rim of tracer localization that is slightly greater than that in adjacent soft tissues. This rim corresponds to a thin seam of new bone that is seen macroscopically and microscopically on allograft surfaces.[26] Increased tracer localization is noted in joint surfaces articulating with osteoarticular allografts. This is accounted for by stress-induced changes in host joints that result from degeneration of allograft cartilage, which becomes covered with a pannus of fibrovascular tissue.[26] Deviation from the typical scintigraphic pattern associated with allografts suggests complication, such as fracture (Fig. 5.13) or local recurrence (Fig. 5.14).

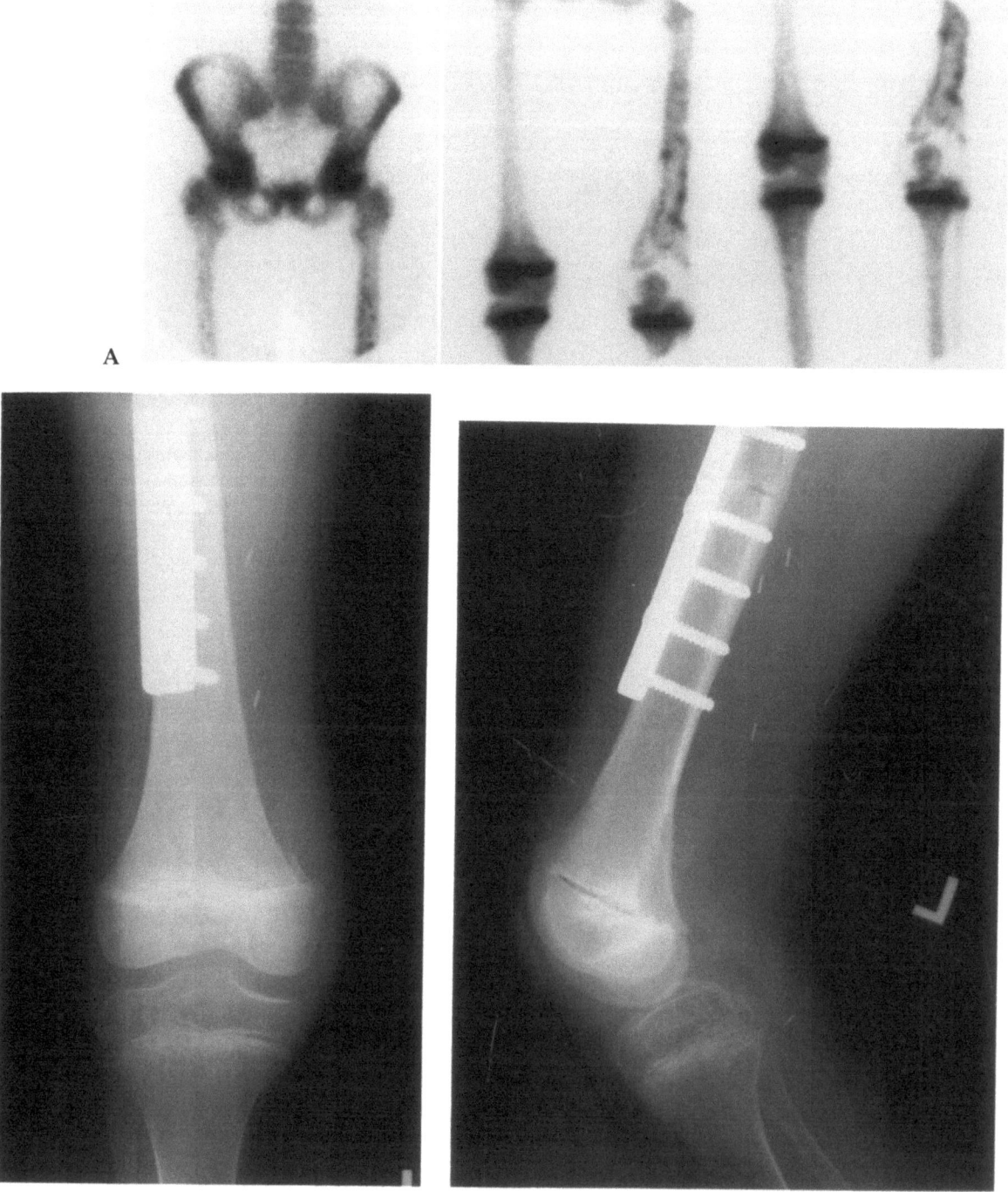

A

B   C

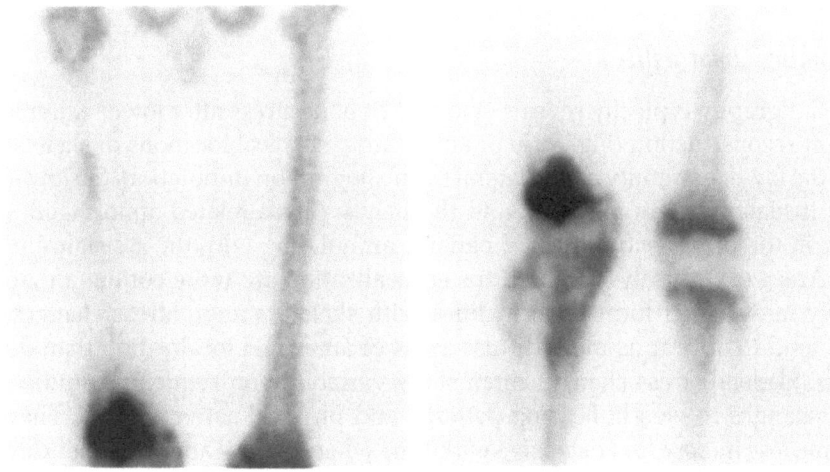

A

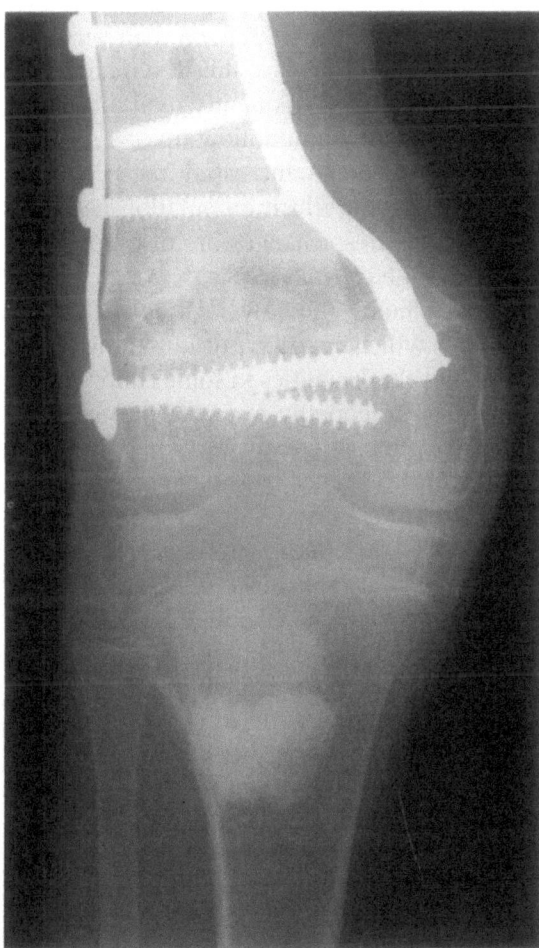

B

Figure 5.14. Local recurrence and metastases following allograft. Increased tracer localization in the right distal femur and proximal tibia is secondary to recurrent and metastatic disease in a child who had undergone allograft reconstruction following excision of a right femoral osteosarcoma (A). Increased localization proximally in the right femur relates to a plate and screw fixation device. An radiograph shows a mixed sclerotic and permeatively lytic lesion involving the right tibial metaphysis (B).

←————

Figure 5.13. Allograft fracture. This 9-year-old girl had an osteosarcoma of her left distal femur, which was resected. A skeletally immature allograft was used for limb salvage. Skeletal scintigraphy (A) shows tracer localization within the allograft that is variably of lesser and greater intensity to that in native bone. An anteroposterior radiograph (B) reveals separation of the allograft epiphysis and a small metaphyseal fracture fragment medial to the distal femur. The graft host junction is visible as an area of lucency on the lateral radiograph between the upper two visualized fixation screws (C).

237

Nonmetastatic Abnormalities

Skeletal scintigraphy typically reveals evidence of bone stress after lower extremity allograft reconstruction (Fig. 5.15) or amputation. Typical locations of skeletal stress are the lower extremity contralateral to an allograft or amputation, the lower extremity ipsilateral to an allograft, and the pelvis. Stress-related abnormalities also occur in the upper extremities of patients ambulating with the assistance of crutches. Areas of diffusely increased tracer localization are more common than are sharply marginated focal abnormalities with skeletal stress. Stress changes, therefore, tend to appear as more diffuse areas of abnormal localization than do metastases. Skeletal stress changes often show variability on sequential studies, reflecting changes in weight-bearing patterns and physical activity levels. They may become less intense and extensive with time whereas focal abnormalities due to metastases tend to show more intense tracer localization and tend to enlarge. When focal abnormalities are noted in the skull or spine, metastatic disease is likely.[9] On a single study, the distinction between skeletal stress and metastatic disease can be difficult, leaving individual practitioners to rely on their previous experience. A high level of suspicion for metastatic disease must be maintained and further imaging with radiography, CT, or MRI is frequently required. Some uncertainties are resolved only with clinical and imaging follow-up.

Following amputation and the fitting of a prosthesis, increased tracer localization is usually seen at the tip of the bone through which amputation has been performed.[9] With tibiofemoral rotationplasty, stress changes are also apparent, particularly in the foot and ankle that act on the prosthesis (Fig. 5.16).

Chemotherapeutic regimens for osteosarcoma frequently include the use of methotrexate. Use of this folic acid analogue, which impedes purine synthesis and DNA biosynthesis, is associated with skeletal abnormalities in some children. The typical radiographic findings of methotrexate osteopathy resemble those seen in scurvy: severe osteopenia, dense zones of provisional calcification, transverse metaphyseal bands, and metaphyseal fractures. The mechanism of skeletal injury is postulated to result from osteoblast suppression and osteoclast recruitment induced by methotrexate.[71] Initially described in children receiving low-dose, long-term, oral maintenance methotrexate for acute leukemia,[80,95,107,117] this complication also develops in some children with osteosarcoma who undergo high-dose, short-term, intravenous methotrexate therapy.[24] Methotrexate osteopathy should be considered as a possible etiology for metaphyseal abnormalities seen on skeletal scintigrams of children receiving, or who have recently received, this agent. Correlation with radiographs permits the diagnosis to be reached and methotrexate to be discontinued (Fig. 5.17). This is important as rapid improvement is seen after discontinuation of the drug,[80,117] whereas nonunion and angulation may occur at fracture sites despite adequate immobilization when methotrexate therapy is continued.[117] Compression fractures of the spine and a sacral insufficiency fracture have also been noted secondary to methotrexate osteopathy.[24]

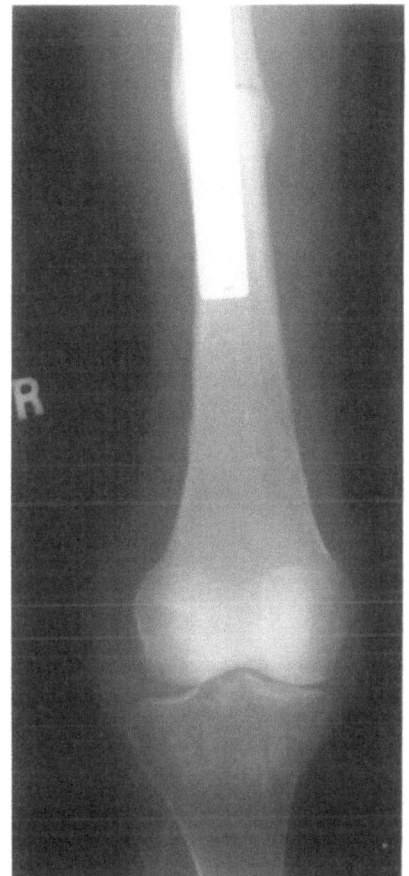

A

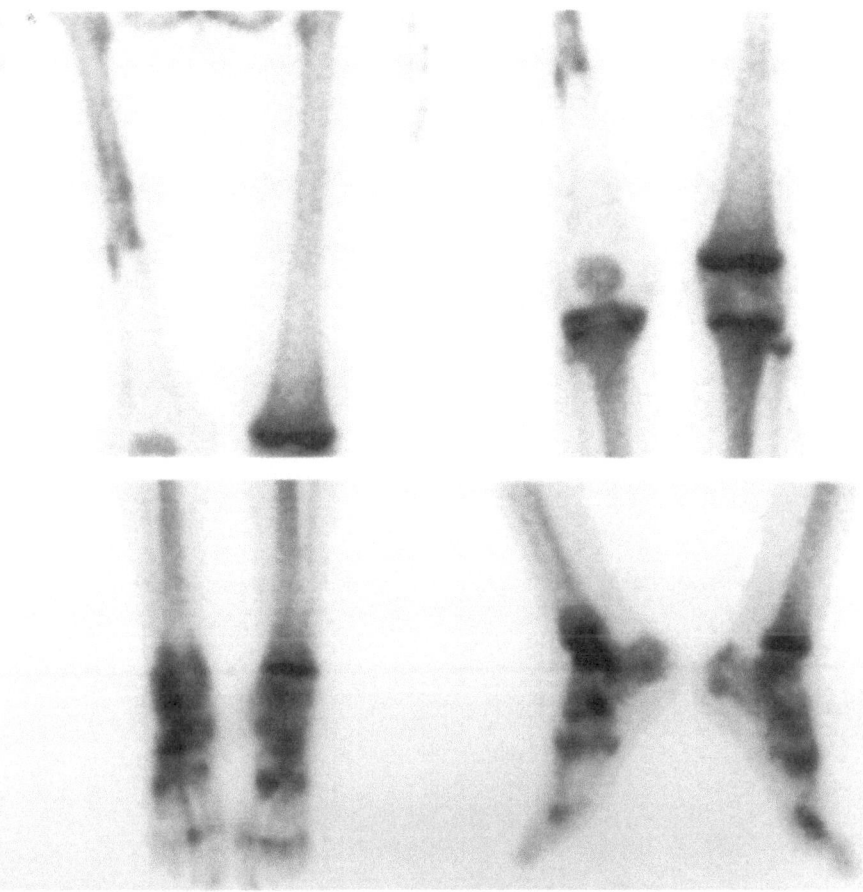

B

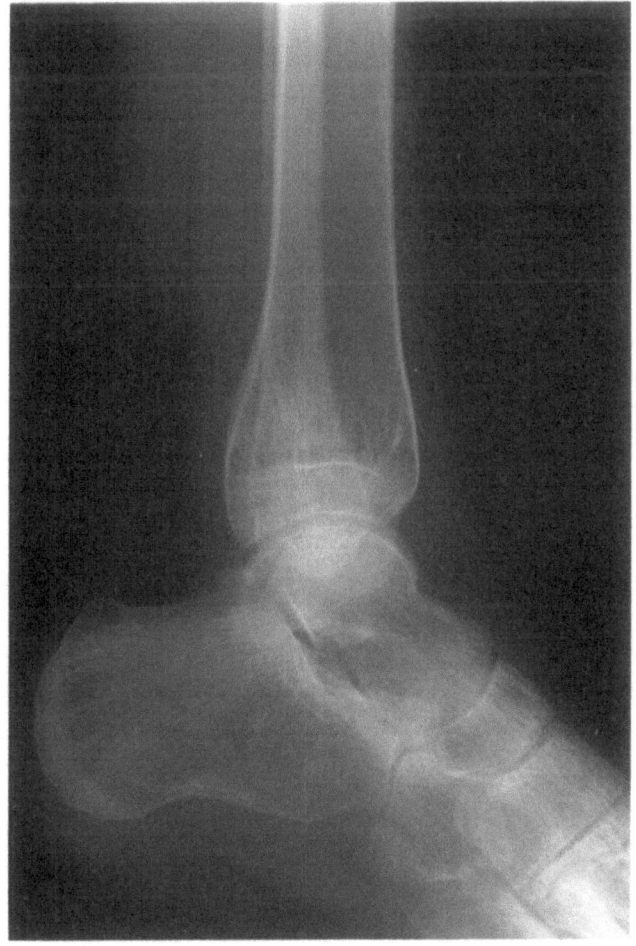

C

Figure 5.15. Skeletal stress following limb salvage surgery. The patient is status post–distal right femoral osteoarticular allograft for osteosarcoma. Radiographically, callus is visible at the junction of the allograft and native bone (A). The allograft is traversed by an anteriorly located plate and multiple cortical screws. Relative to native bone, the allograft appears dense. On skeletal scintigraphy (B), the allograft appears as a photon-deficient area outlined by a faint rim of tracer localization. Immediately related to the allograft, increased tracer localization is seen corresponding to callus at the allograft-host junction, along the right femur related to the fixation hardware, in the right patella, and in the right tibial articulating surfaces. Increased tracer localization in the right medial and lateral malleoli, in the right talus and cuboid, in the right third metatarsal, and at the first tarsometarsal joints bilaterally indicates skeletal stress. A lateral radiograph of the right ankle (C) shows generalized demineralization. Alternating linear areas of sclerosis and lucency in the distal tibia and in the calcaneus are consistent with disuse osteopenia and stress changes. They are not suggestive of metastatic disease.

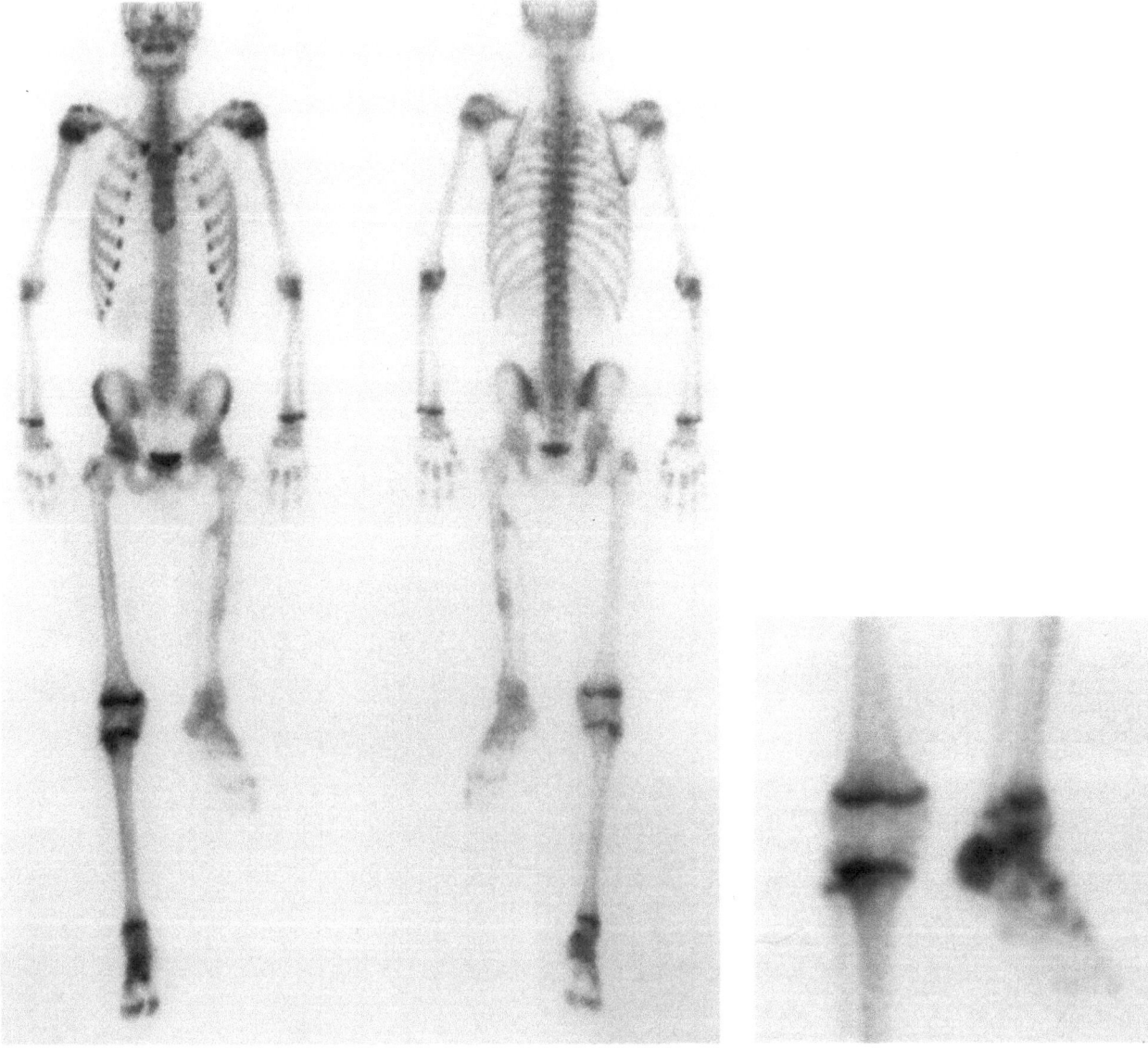

A   B

Figure 5.16. Femorotibial rotationplasty. Whole-body images of a 15-year-old following left femorotibial rotationplasty (A). One year later, there is diffusely increased tracer localization in the left calcaneus secondary to fracture (B).

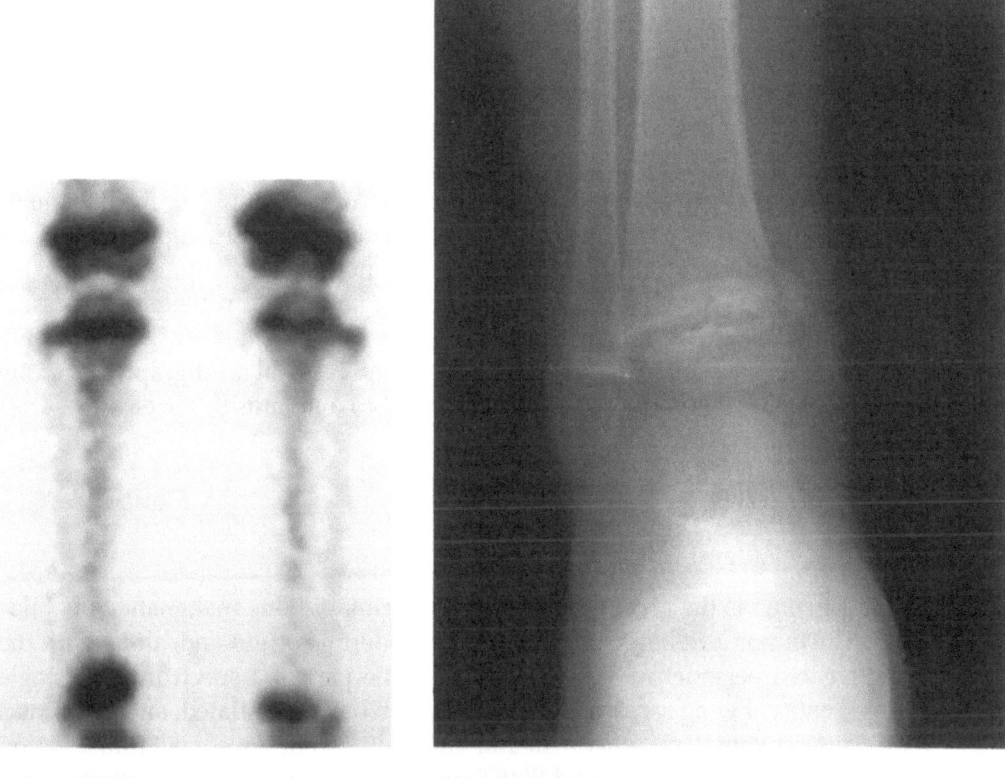

A   B

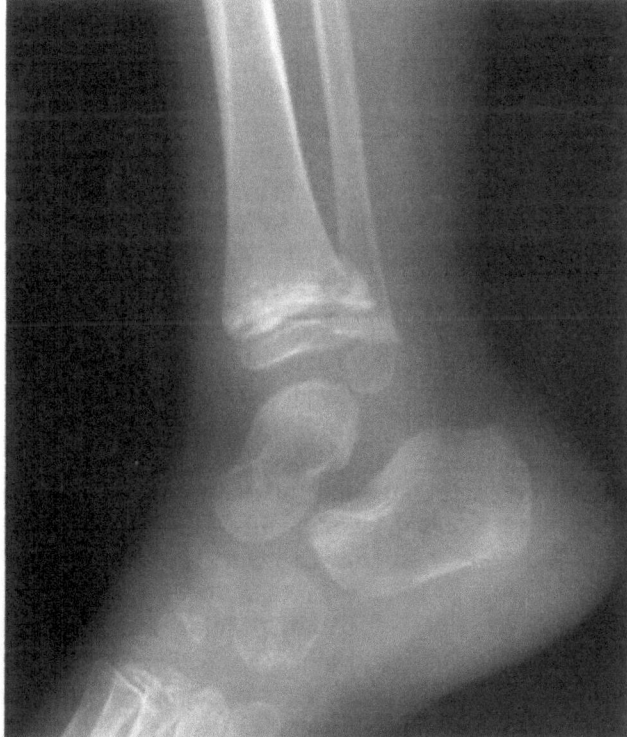

C

Figure 5.17. Methotrexate osteopathy. Skeletal scintigraphy (A) of a 5-year-old boy with left maxillary osteosarcoma whose chemotherapy included methotrexate, reveals focally increased tracer localization in the left distal femoral and right distal tibial metaphyses. The scintigraphic findings corresponded to right distal tibial (B,C) and left distal femoral metaphyseal fractures. Radiographically, the right distal tibial and fibular metaphyses are sclerotic and irregular with a flared appearance and the bones appear demineralized. These findings are consistent with methotrexate osteopathy.

Flare Phenomenon

Osteosarcoma metastases may demonstrate the scintigraphic flare phenomenon during therapy.[42] This pattern is characterized by increasing intensity of tracer localization at sites of known metastases or the appearance of new foci of increased tracer localization on a study obtained within months of a therapeutic intervention, despite a patient's apparent clinical improvement.[92] It is likely due to bone repair. The flare phenomenon should be considered when the appropriate findings are observed, especially within 2 months of initiating therapy, in patients who appear to be responding well clinically. Excluding disease progression remains the primary concern, particularly when new abnormalities are detected. Close correlation with clinical and other imaging paramenters, therefore, is essential (Figs. 5.1 and 5.3). Unfortunately, a patient's subsequent clinical and imaging course are the only reliable arbiters in some cases. Skeletal scintigraphy typically shows regression of a flare phenomenon over 4 to 6 months.[92]

Ewing Sarcoma

Clinical Considerations

Ewing sarcoma is the second most common primary bone malignancy of childhood. The tumor is believed to be of neuroectodermal origin and, along with the primitive neuroectodermal tumor (PNET), to be part of a spectrum of a single biologic entity. Ewing sarcoma is regarded as an undifferentiated, and PNET as a more differentiated, peripheral neural tumor.[120] A chromosomal translocation expressed in Ewing sarcoma and PNET suggests that oncogenes contribute to the development of these tumors.[19,46]

The tumor is composed of small round cells. Absence of lobular rosettes, neuron-specific enolase, and neurosecretory granules helps differentiate Ewing sarcoma from PNET.[68] In some cases, it can be difficult to distinguish the histologic features of Ewing sarcoma from those of other small round cell tumors of childhood, such as neuroblastoma, leukemia, and lymphoma.[19,46]

The incidence of Ewing sarcoma is highest in the second decade of life. Almost all cases occur between the ages of 5 and 30 years. Caucasians are predominantly affected.[48,57,100,118]

Pain and swelling are the most common symptoms at presentation. A palpable mass is often present. The patient may be febrile. Hematologic analysis reveals elevation of the erythrocyte sedimentation rate, leukocytosis, and anemia in some cases. The constellation of clinical and hematologic findings occasionally suggests a diagnosis of osteomyelitis.[48,57,100,118]

Ewing sarcoma occurs in both the long bones and the flat bones. In patients younger than 20 years of age, Ewing sarcoma most often affects the appendicular skeleton, particularly the femur, tibia, and humerus. Ewing sarcoma of the long bones is centered in the metaphysis slightly more often than the diaphysis (Figs. 5.18–5.20). Metaphyseal lesions are typically eccentrically positioned and tend to extend into the diaphysis. Pelvic, rib, and vertebral lesions (Fig. 5.21) predominate in patients older than 20 years of age.[57,89] Skeletal metastases often precede pulmonary metastases and are present in 10% to 20% of patients at diagnosis.[118]

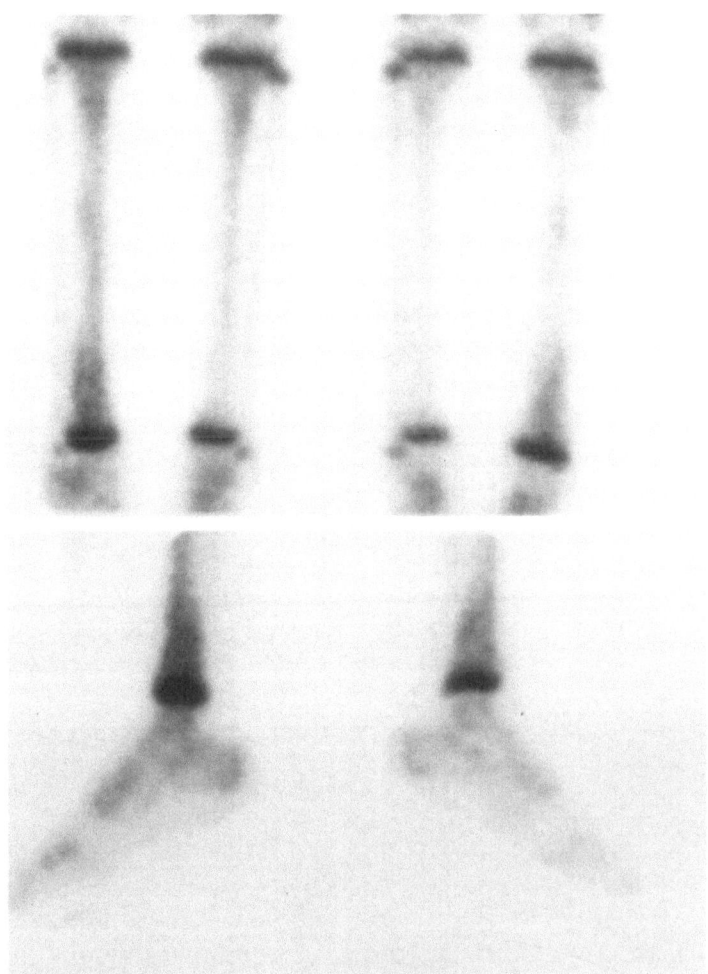

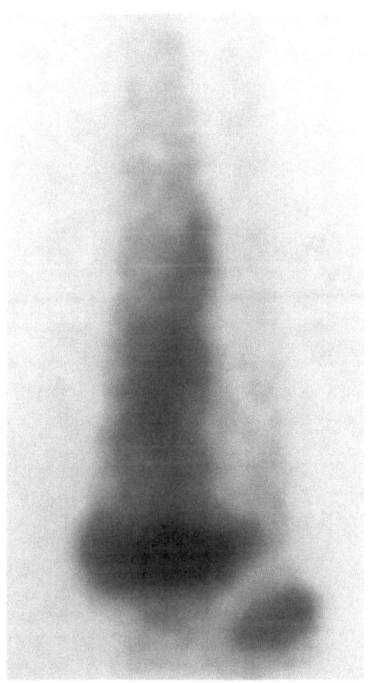

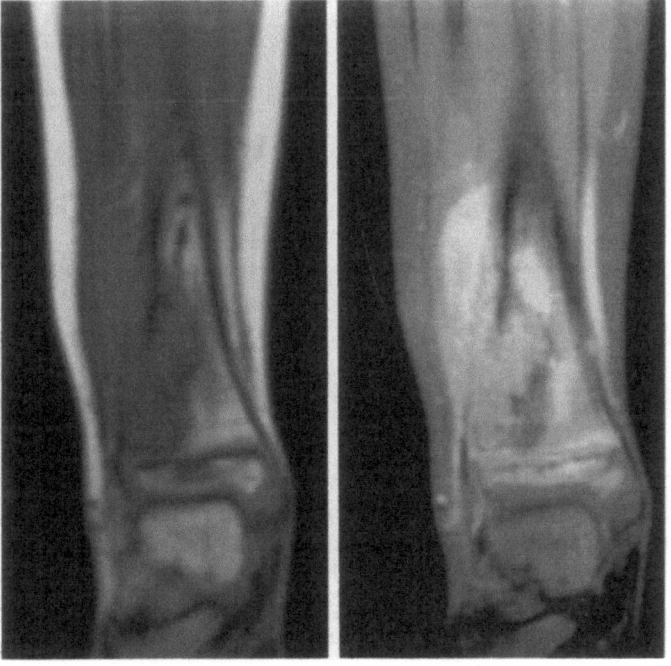

Figure 5.18. Ewing sarcoma. Skeletal scintigraphy (A) shows increased tracer localization in the distal right tibial metaphysis and diaphysis (upper row: anterior and posterior images; lower row; medial and lateral images of right tibia). The extent of the scintigraphic abnormality is depicted with pinhole imaging (B: posterior projection). Coronal T1-weighted MRI (C) reveals extensive signal abnormality involving the metadiaphysis, epiphysis, and adjacent soft tissues. A large soft tissue mass is more conspicuous following gadolinium administration (D).

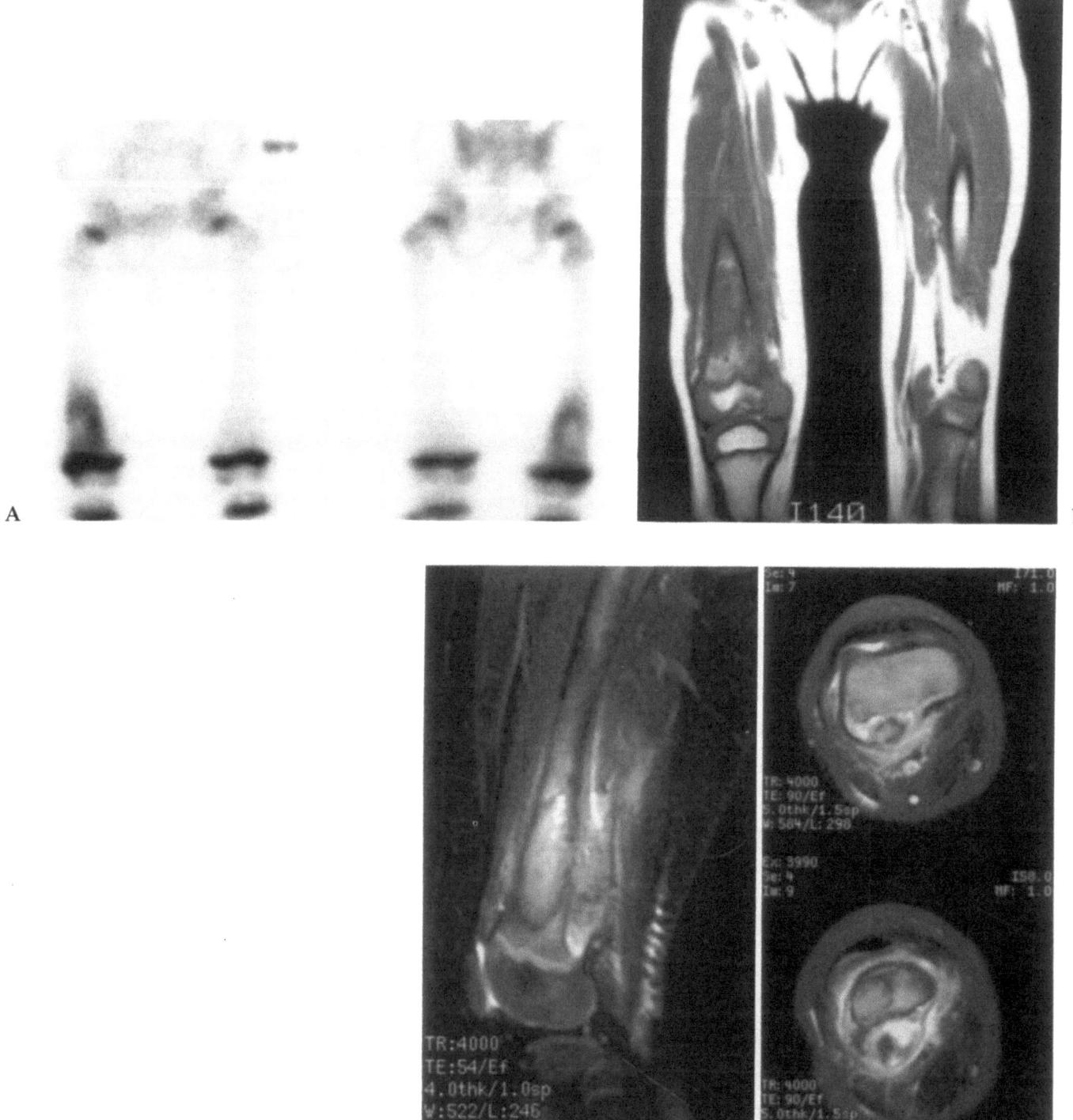

Figure 5.19. Ewing sarcoma. Skeletal scintigraphy (anterior and posterior projections) demonstrates an area of increased ^{99m}Tc-MDP localization involving the metaphysis and distal diaphysis of the right femur (A). T1-weighted coronal (B) and sagittal (C) and T2-weighted fat suppressed transaxial (D) MR images show extensive medullary edema, cortical destruction, a soft tissue mass, and edema within muscles adjacent to the tumor. The soft tissue mass is seen to abut the neurovascular bundle on the axial images.

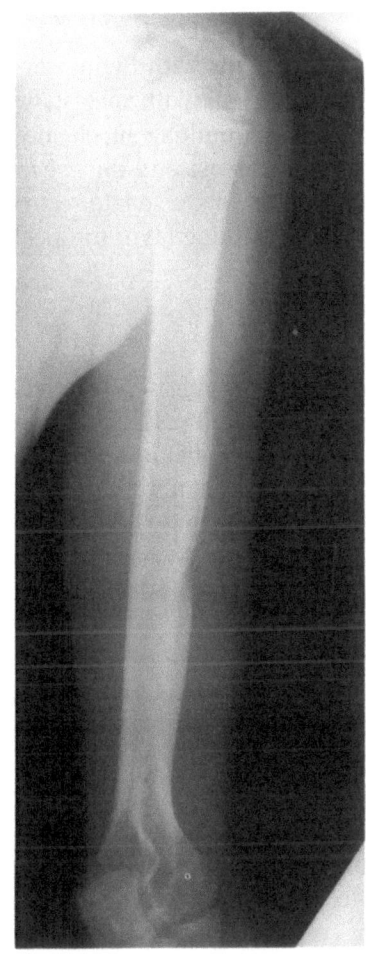

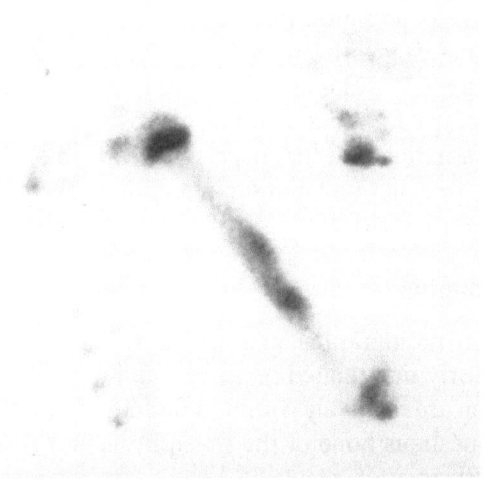

Figure 5.20. Ewing sarcoma. A radiograph of a 13-year-old boy's left humerus reveals a destructive lesion affecting the diaphyseal cortex laterally (A). Skeletal scintigraphy demonstrates increased tracer localization surrounding an area of cortical excavation corresponding to the radiographic appearance of the lesion (B).

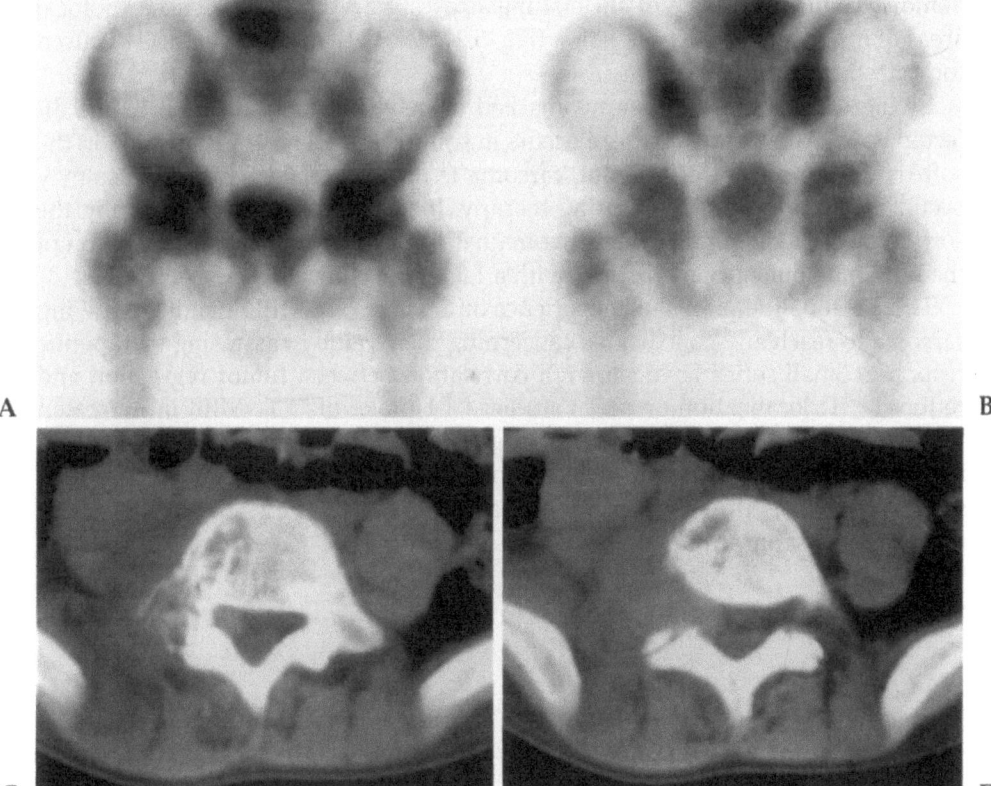

Figure 5.21. Ewing sarcoma. Skeletal scintigraphy—anterior (A), posterior (B)—depicts marked increased tracer localization at L5. Computed tomography (C,D) shows permeative osteolysis of the right L5 pedicle and the right side of the L5 vertebral body. A soft tissue component extends into the right L5–S1 neural foramen (D).

Depending on the series, the 5-year survival rate of patients with Ewing sarcoma ranges from 54% to 74%. It is less than 30% in patients with metastatic disease.[46,83] Therapy for Ewing sarcoma entails the use of multiagent chemotherapy for eradication of microscopic or overt metastatic disease and the use of irradiation and/or surgery for control of the primary lesion. Because late recurrence is not uncommon, resection of the primary tumor is gaining favor for local disease control.[83]

Imaging

The radiographic manifestations of Ewing sarcoma are variable. Permeative, poorly marginated osteolysis and a thin, laminated or spiculated periosteal reaction are relatively common findings. Reactive bone is common in flat bones and in cancellous bone of the metaphysis and ribs. Sclerosis is occasionally intermixed with areas of osteolysis. Ewing sarcoma rarely appears predominantly sclerotic. A soft tissue mass that is often large in size is frequently present. Ewing sarcoma may be entirely or predominantly within the soft tissues and erode a bone's cortical surface (cortical saucerization).[48,57,89,118]

Medullary involvement and the soft tissue component of Ewing sarcoma are well evaluated with MRI.[31] These tumors have the typical MRI appearance of bone tumors (low signal intensity on T1-weighted images and high signal intensity on T2-weighted images). Persistence of medullary signal abnormalities and variable changes in the signal associated with the soft tissue component following therapy renders MRI unreliable for the assessment of tumor viability.[31,59,64] It has been suggested, however, that an increase in T2 signal intensity to one similar to that of water indicates a favorable response and is due to marrow replacement by a hypocellular myxoid matrix with small amounts of collagen.[59] Viable tumor has not been differentiated from reactive changes following therapy with gadolinium-enhanced MRI.[31]

The primary role of skeletal scintigraphy in patients with Ewing sarcoma is to demonstrate the presence of skeletal metastases, as typically evidenced by focal areas of increased tracer localization (Fig. 5.22). As with osteosarcoma, CT is used for detection of pulmonary metastases.

Ewing sarcoma usually shows marked skeletal tracer localization in the affected bone. An extended pattern occurs in some cases.[48] Tracer localization in the soft tissue component of a Ewing sarcoma is rarely seen. A flare response may occur in skeletal metastases during therapy. Increasing tracer localization in the soft tissue component of Ewing sarcoma has been reported as a manifestation of the flare phenomenon in a patient with a favorable clinical response.[76]

There is too little published experience on ^{201}Tl or ^{99m}Tc-MIBI imaging of Ewing sarcoma to reach any conclusions concerning their value in assessing therapeutic response. Small series have shown a correlation between tumor regression and reduced ^{201}Tl localization on serial studies.[75,96] Uptake of ^{99m}Tc-MIBI in untreated Ewing's sarcoma is highly variable,[13] suggesting a limited role for ^{99m}Tc-MIBI in assessing treatment. As with osteosarcoma, neither ^{67}Ga imaging nor skeletal scintigraphy has proven consistently accurate in defining tumor extent or therapeutic response.[79,96,114]

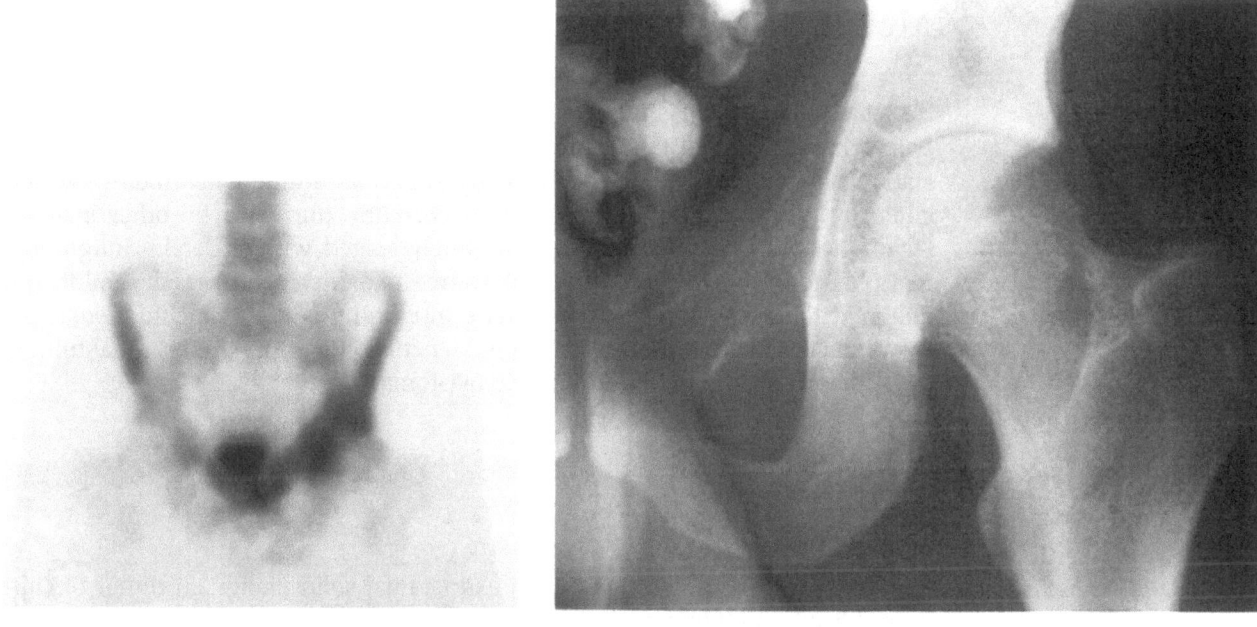

A   B

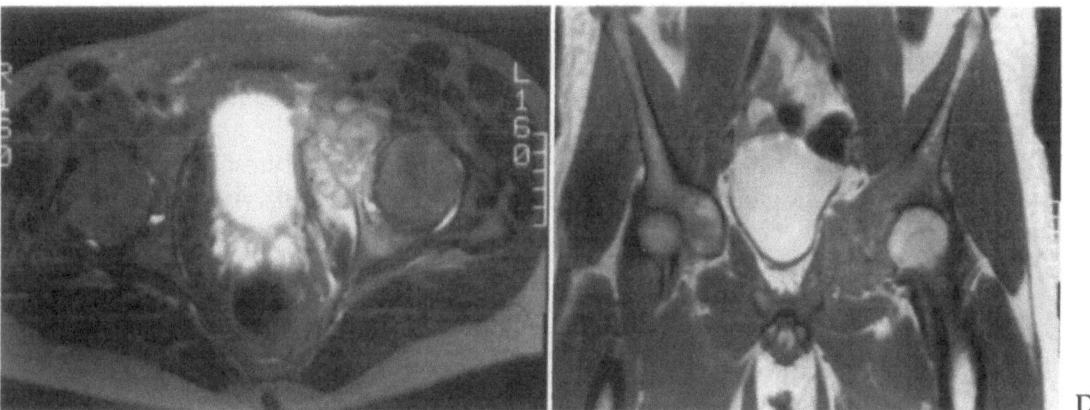

C   D

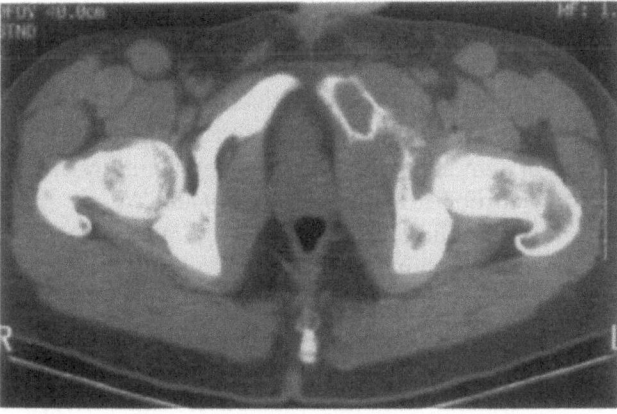

E

Figure 5.22. Relapsed Ewing sarcoma. These images are of a 21-year-old man who presented at the age of 14 years with Ewing sarcoma of the left eleventh rib. He underwent left
rib resection and received chemotherapy and postoperative radiation to the surgical site.
After noticing left inguinal pain associated with a hockey injury, skeletal scintigraphy (A)
revealed increased ^{99m}Tc-MDP localization in the left acetabulum and superior pubic ramus.
The scintigraphic finding correlates with radiographic demonstration of lysis and cortical
destruction (B). Transaxial T2-weighted FSE (C) and coronal T1-weighted gadolinium-
enhanced (D) MR images reveal abnormal signal within the left ilium, acetabulum, and
pubis associated with a heterogeneous soft tissue mass and abnormal signal within the
left pelvic floor musculature. Computed tomography (E) also demonstrates the osseous
destruction and soft tissue mass with enlargement of the pelvic muscles.   **247**

Metastatic Disease

Skeletal scintigraphy is highly useful in the staging and follow-up of a number of pediatric extraskeletal malignancies. The ability of scintigraphy to detect metastatic disease of bone with a whole-body survey at a time when metastases are clinically and radiographically occult is currently unrivaled by other imaging techniques. Of the tumors that are routinely staged with skeletal scintigraphy, neuroblastoma is the most frequent source of bone metastases in childhood. Other malignancies for which skeletal scintigraphy is useful include leukemia, lymphoma, rhabdomyosarcoma, primitive neuroectodermal tumor, renal tumors other than Wilms' tumor, and medulloblastoma.

Neuroblastoma

Clinical Considerations

Neuroblastoma is the most common extracranial solid malignant tumor of children. Of all childhood malignancies, only leukemia, lymphoma, and primary brain tumors occur more frequently.[10] The tumor is predominantly encountered in the very young. The mean age of patients at presentation is 20 to 30 months.[16] A significant percentage of cases come to diagnosis during the first year of life. Patients older than 10 years at the time of diagnosis account for less than 10% of cases.[10]

Neuroblastoma originates from the embryonal neural crest anywhere along the sympathetic ganglion chain or within the adrenal medulla. Approximately 70% of tumors are located in the abdomen or pelvis. The most common location of the primary tumor is the adrenal gland, where 40% to 50% of neuroblastomas originate. Other abdominal sites of origin include the paravertebral and presacral sympathetic chain and the organ of Zuckerkandl. Thoracic tumors, which are usually located in the posterior mediastinal sympathetic ganglia, and cervical tumors, which arise from sympathetic plexuses in the lower neck, account for 15% and 5% of tumors, respectively. A primary tumor is not detected in as many as 10% of patients, who present with disseminated disease.[10]

Histologically, neuroblastoma is characterized by small round cells that contain neurofilaments and form tumor rosettes in bone marrow and blood. Gross or microscopic calcification is often present in the tumor. Neuroblastomas are typically solid masses. Their size varies. Abdominal tumors tend to be larger than those in the thorax or neck. Areas of hemorrhage or necrosis are frequently present in larger tumors. A purely cystic neuroblastoma is highly unusual.[10,16]

Two related neural crest tumors, ganglioneuroma and ganglioneuroblastoma, have been described. Ganglioneuroma contains mature ganglion cells. Some neuroblastomas spontaneously regress or mature into this benign tumor. The peculiar capacity of neuroblastoma to mature into a histologically benign tumor or, in occasional cases to regress completely, is a unique aspect of this malignancy. The unpredictability and apparent infrequency of these occurrences and the consequences of delaying therapy militate that treatment be instituted at diagnosis, however. Ganglioneuroblastoma is a malignant tumor that contains both undifferentiated neuroblasts and mature ganglion cells. Its histologic differentiation from neuroblastoma is somewhat arbitrary and subject to sampling variations.[16]

The clinical manifestations of neuroblastoma are truly protean in scope. Many children present with nonspecific signs and symptoms including fever, weight loss, irritability, an elevated erythrocyte sedimentation rate, and anemia. The tumor may produce a palpable mass or produce symptoms due to invasion or compression of adjacent structures.

Signs and symptoms may result from distant metastases. Bone pain or refusal to move an extremity resulting from skeletal metastases may be the presenting complaint. In some cases where this occurs, the initial clinical impression is osteomyelitis.[2] Paraneoplastic syndromes associated with tumoral hormone production and other undetermined, perhaps immunologic, mechanisms are also well known. Although most neuroblastomas secrete hormones, this is clinically evident in only a small percentage of cases. Hypertension related to catecholamine secretion and watery diarrhea, hypokalemia, and achlorhydria due to vasoactive intestinal peptide secretion each occur in approximately 10% of cases. Excess urinary excretion of catecholamine metabolites (vanillymandelic acid [VMA], homovanillic acid [HVA], norepinephrine, and dopamine), as determined by 24-hour urine collections, are detected in approximately 80% of cases.[10,38] An immunologic cross-reaction between tumor antigens and cerebellar tissue has been proposed to explain an association between neuroblastoma and infantile myoclonic encephelopathy (IME), a rare clinical syndrome that potentially includes opsoclonus, myoclonus, and cerebellar ataxia. Neuroblastoma is present in 50% of children with IME, but IME occurs in less than 2% of children with neuroblastoma.[10]

Disseminated disease is present in up to 70% of cases at diagnosis. This most commonly involves cortical bone and bone marrow, but also involves liver, skin, and occasionally lung. The distribution of metastases varies with the age of the child at diagnosis. Through 1 year of age, metastatic involvement is frequently confined to the bone marrow, liver, and skin. In infants, the bone marrow is often sparsely involved and hepatic metastases tend to be diffusely infiltrative. Despite dissemination, infants with this pattern of disease have a favorable prognosis and often require only excision of the primary tumor for treatment. In children who are older at diagnosis, metastases usually involve cortical bone, bone marrow, liver, and lymph nodes. The marrow is often extensively infiltrated and liver metastases are commonly well-defined single or multiple lesions in these older children.[16] This pattern of metastatic disease carries a poor prognosis.

Three different systems are used in staging neuroblastoma (Tables 5.1–5.3).[10,11,16] Strengths and weaknesses of each staging system have resulted in much debate and controversy. Regardless of which system is used, certain factors effect prognosis independently of the initial staging. A karyotype analysis of a neuroblastoma revealing either deletion of the short arm of chromosome 1, amplification of the N-*myc* oncogene, or both, indicates a poor prognosis. More differentiated tumors exhibit relatively greater synthesis of norepinephrine and VMA, both of which require dopamine β-hydroxylase, than less differentiated tumors. This suggests that urinary VMA/HVA levels carry some prognostic significance in patients with neuroblastoma.[140] Classification of tumors as stroma rich or stroma poor, differentiated or undifferentiated, and an estimation of the number of cells per 5,000 cells undergoing mitosis or nuclear fragmentation with consideration given to patient age at diagnosis constitutes the Shimada classification, a useful prognostic indicator.[110] Elevated serum ferritin and elevated serum neuron-specific enolase indicate an unfavorable prognosis.[16] As a general rule, patients younger than 1 year of age at diagnosis have a better prognosis than older children, although age may not be an independent prognostic indicator.

Table 5.1. Evans staging system for neuroblastoma.

Stage	Description
I	Tumor confined to organ of origin (totally excised)
II	Tumor extension beyond the organ of origin
	Tumor does not cross the midline
	Regional lymph nodes may be involved
III	Tumor extension across midline with encroachment on contralateral tissues
IV	Distant metastases (skeletal, other organs, soft tissues, distant lymph nodes)
IV-S	Localized primary tumor not crossing midline
	Remote disease confined to liver, subcutaneous tissues, and bone marrow
	Cortical bone not involved

Table 5.2. International neuroblastoma staging system.

Stage	Description
1	Localized tumor, complete gross resection, with or without microscopic residual disease; nonadherent lymph nodes microscopically negative for tumor
2A	Localized tumor, incomplete gross resection; nonadherent lymph nodes microscopically negative for tumor
2B	Localized tumor, complete or incomplete gross resection; nonadherent lymph nodes microscopically positive, contralateral lymph nodes microscopically negative for tumor
3	Unresectable unilateral tumor, infiltrating across midline with or without regional nodal involvement
	OR
	Localized unilateral tumor with contralateral nodal involvement
	OR
	Midline tumor with bilateral infiltration or nodal involvement
4	Any tumor with dissemination to distal lymph nodes, bone, bone marrow, liver, skin, and/or other organs (except as defined for stage 4S)
4S	Localized primary tumor with dissemination limited to skin, liver, and/or marrow with marrow involvement <10% by biopsy or aspirate; MIBG should be negative in the marrow; limited to infants <1 year of age

Table 5.3. Pediatric Oncology Group staging system for neuroblastoma.

Stage	Description
A	Localized primary tumor, completely resected
B	Incomplete resection of primary tumor
	Lymph nodes and liver uninvolved
C	Complete or incomplete resection of primary tumor
	Lymph nodal involvement, liver uninvolved
D	Disseminated metastatic tumor

Imaging of Skeletal Metastases

Radiography and scintigraphy with various radiopharmaceuticals are used for detection of neuroblastoma metastatic to cortical bone and bone marrow.

Radiography

Metastases to cortical bone are usually lytic, but are partially or completely sclerotic in some instances. Cortical bone metastases are typically multiple and most commonly involve the long bones, spine, pelvis, calvarium, periorbital facial bones, and ribs. Involvement of the long bones is characteristically metaphyseal and occasionally diaphyseal. The distribution of long bone metastases is usually asymmetric but symmetrically positioned lesions are frequently encountered. Vertebral involvement may result in vertebral body collapse. Calvarial metastases demonstrate permeative osteolysis, often associated with areas of sclerosis or cortical thickening. Vertical osseous striations may extend from the outer table ("hair on end" appearance). Sutural diastasis suggests increased intracranial pressure secondary to dural-based metastases. Local tumor extension can produce enlargement of an intervertebral foramen, widening of an interpedicular distance or an intercostal space, and erosive changes. Calcification is demonstrated radiographically in approximately 15% of thoracic and 66% of abdominal tumors.[16]

Skeletal Scintigraphy

Cortical metastases are detected earlier with skeletal scintigraphy than with radiography. For the detection of cortical metastases, skeletal scintigraphy has been shown to be superior to radiography both on the basis of the number of cases of metastatic disease detected and the number of lesions demonstrated.[6,10,47,93] Proper positioning of the child, high-resolution imaging, and familiarity with the normal distribution of skeletal tracer in the growing skeleton are essential. Pinhole magnification assists in evaluating suspicious areas. Experience in interpreting pediatric scintigrams is especially important for identifying findings that are merely an accentuation of, or a slight alteration in, normal tracer distribution. With strict attention to detail and experience, only very rarely is skeletal scintigraphy interpreted as normal in a child with radiographic evidence of cortical bone metastases. Conversely, it is common for skeletal scintigraphy to depict metastases that are occult radiographically.[41,47,93]

Cortical bone metastases typically appear as areas of high tracer localization on bone scintigraphy (Figs. 5.23–5.28). Occasionally decreased tracer localization is demonstrated with highly aggressive bone destruction or ischemia (Figs. 5.23 and 5.26).[6,10,47,93] When multifocal disease in the characteristic distribution described above is noted, skeletal scintigraphy is highly specific for cortical bone metastases.

Skeletal scintigraphy demonstrates tracer localization at the primary disease site in 40% to 85% of patients (Figs. 5.23–5.26 and 5.29–5.31).[47,69,93,115,127] This is postulated to reflect active calcium metabolism by viable tumor.[69] The likelihood of skeletal tracer localization in neuroblastoma increases with tumor size but does not carry prognostic significance[69] or correlate with the demonstration of calcification by radiography or computed tomography.[93] Skeletal tracer also concentrates in some hepatic, pulmonary, and nodal metastases.[17,65]

Metaiodobenzylguanidine (MIBG) Imaging

Scintigraphy with MIBG has a sensitivity of greater than 85% for detecting neuroblastoma.[28] Absence of the type 1 uptake mechanism described in Chapter 1 (see Fig. 1.38), rapid washout of MIBG, and small tumor size account for the absence of demonstrable MIBG uptake in some neuroblastomas.[109]

Metastases to the skeleton are demonstrated with MIBG imaging (Figs. 5.23, 5.24, 5.27, and 5.28). Definitive differentiation between cortical and marrow metastases is not possible with MIBG, as both cortical and marrow metastases appear as areas of MIBG localization within the skeleton.

For detecting metastatic disease with iodine-123 (^{123}I)-MIBG, single photon emission computed tomography (SPECT) may increase the number of lesions detected[105] or, at least, increase the certainty of interpretation.[32] We perform SPECT 24 hours following tracer administration in cases where detection of additional sites of disease to those shown with planar imaging is of clinical importance and in cases where an uncertainty persists after planar imaging is completed. Supplementing 24-hour planar images with additional planar imaging at 48 hours does not appear to increase the sensitivity of the examination,[105] although it provides improved visualization of some lesions.[87]

The overall sensitivities for detecting metastatic disease with skeletal and MIBG scintigraphy in a given patient do not significantly differ.[37] Either study may reveal metastases of neuroblastoma when the other does not, reflecting the different mechanisms by which these agents localize in neuroblastoma. For neuroblastoma patients whose skeletal and MIBG scintigrams both reveal metastases, MIBG imaging more accurately depicts the extent of disease by revealing more sites of skeletal involvement.[111] Unlike skeletal tracers, MIBG does not localize at sites of bone repair associated with healing metastases, bone marrow biopsy and harvest sites, or other trauma.[25,86,111] This renders MIBG imaging more useful than skeletal scintigraphy for evaluating therapeutic response in patients whose primary lesion localized MIBG (Fig. 5.24). An additional advantage that MIBG scintigraphy offers relative to skeletal scintigraphy is that less experienced observers more confidently and accurately interpret MIBG studies for metastatic neuroblastoma.[88] This results from any localization of MIBG in the skeleton being abnormal, whereas metastases occasionally produce relatively little alteration in skeletal tracer localization (Fig. 5.28). The inability to distinguish cortical from marrow metastases with MIBG is often cited as a limitation of MIBG scintigraphy. It has been suggested, however, that the prognostic implications of cortical metastases and marrow infiltration that is sufficiently extensive to allow its detection with MIBG scintigraphy are identical.[11] We believe that MIBG imaging and skeletal scintigraphy are complementary studies for assessing neuroblastoma. Individual practitioners should design their imaging approach based on the impact each study has on the staging system used at their institution and on their experience in interpreting pediatric examinations.

Somatostin Receptor Imaging

Indium-111 (^{111}In)-pentetreotide, a somatostatin analogue, localizes to neuroblastoma with a reported sensitivity of greater than 80%.[56] This reflects the presence of somatostatin receptors on some neuroblastoma cells. Experience with this radiopharmaceutical is too limited to allow its role relative to skeletal or MIBG scintigraphy to be accurately assessed. Early reports indicate that some tumors that accumulate ^{111}In-pentetreotide do not accumulate MIBG but some that do not accumulate ^{111}In-pentetreotide accumulate MIBG. Based on a small number of cases, it has been suggested that ^{111}In-pentetreotide uptake may be greater in well-differentiated and aneuploid tumors,[66] raising the possibility for this tracer to be of some value in prognostic stratification.[23,56,66]

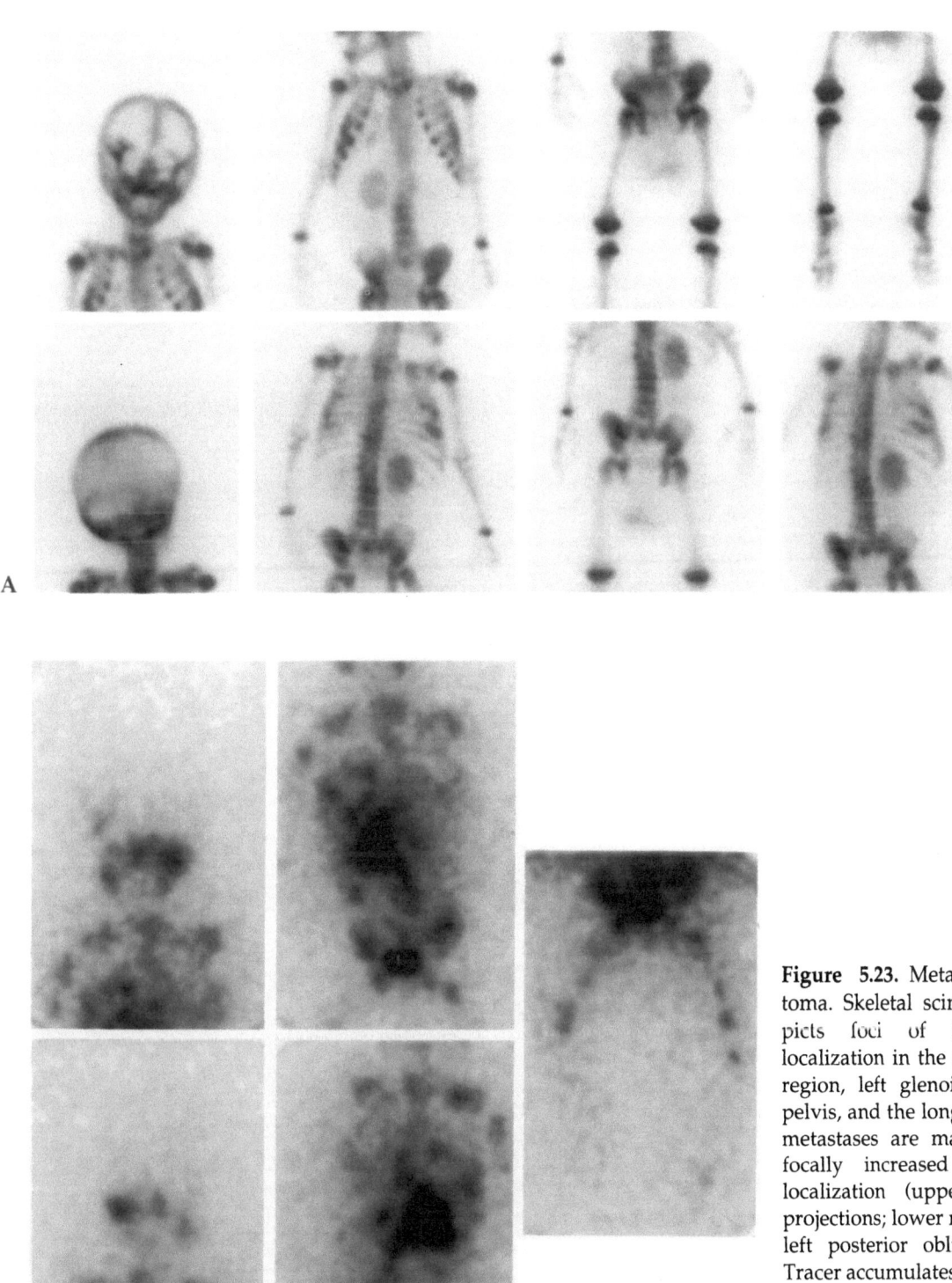

Figure 5.23. Metastatic neuroblastoma. Skeletal scintigraphy (A) depicts foci of increased tracer localization in the right supraorbital region, left glenoid, multiple ribs, pelvis, and the long bones. Vertebral metastases are manifested as both focally increased and decreased localization (upper row: anterior projections; lower row: posterior and left posterior oblique projections). Tracer accumulates in a right adrenal primary. The extent of disease is also shown with ^{131}I-MIBG imaging (B, upper row: anterior; lower row. posterior projection; extremities: anterior projection).

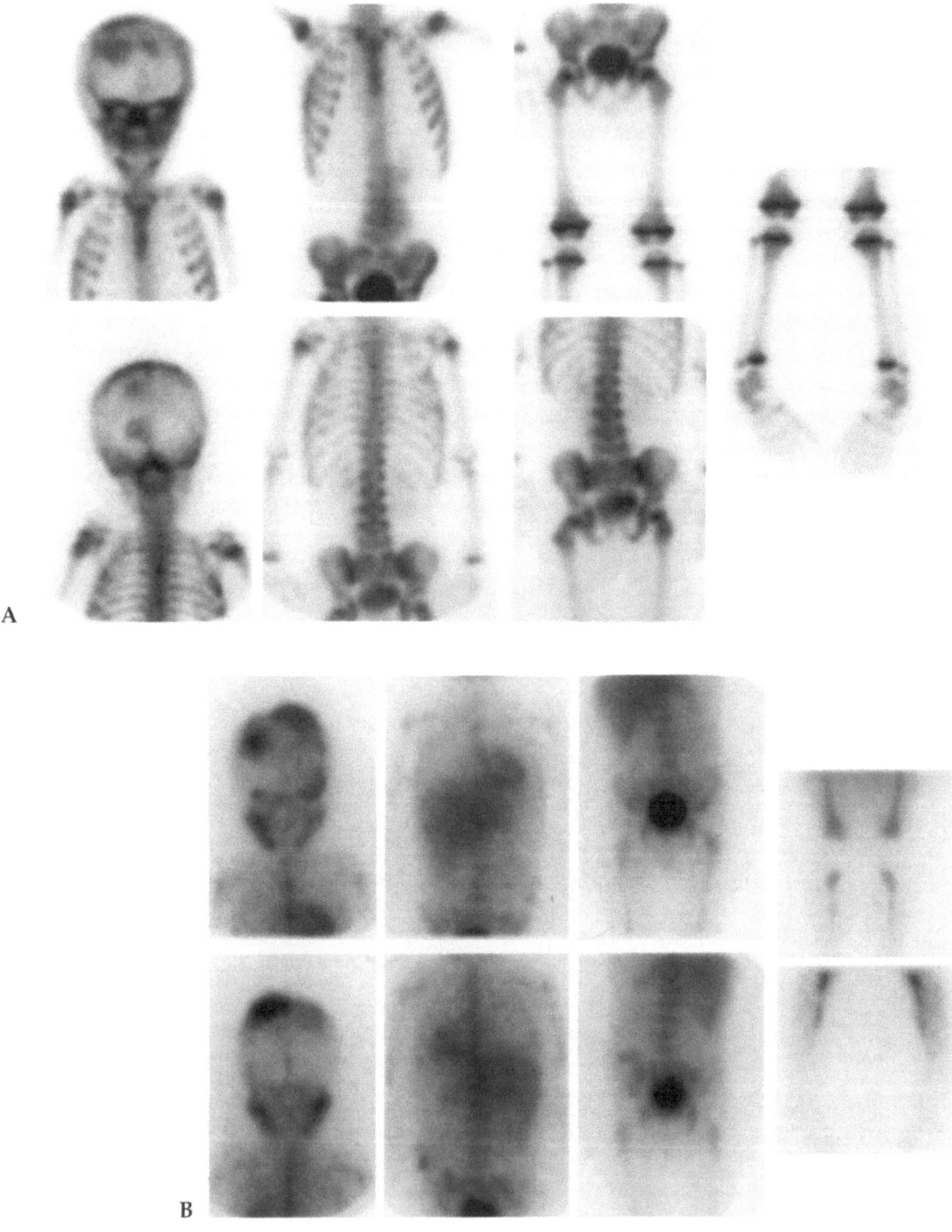

Figure 5.24. Metastatic neuroblastoma. Skeletal scintigraphy (A) reveals tracer localization in the soft tissues to the left of the lumbar spine (upper row: anterior projection; lower row: posterior projection; tibiae: anterior projection). Multiple foci of increased tracer localization are depicted in the calvarium, periorbital facial bones, spine, pelvis, and long bone metaphyses. The abnormal foci of ^{99m}Tc-MDP localization correspond to sites of abnormal ^{123}I-MIBG localization (B) in this child with a paraortic neuroblastoma and widespread metastases.

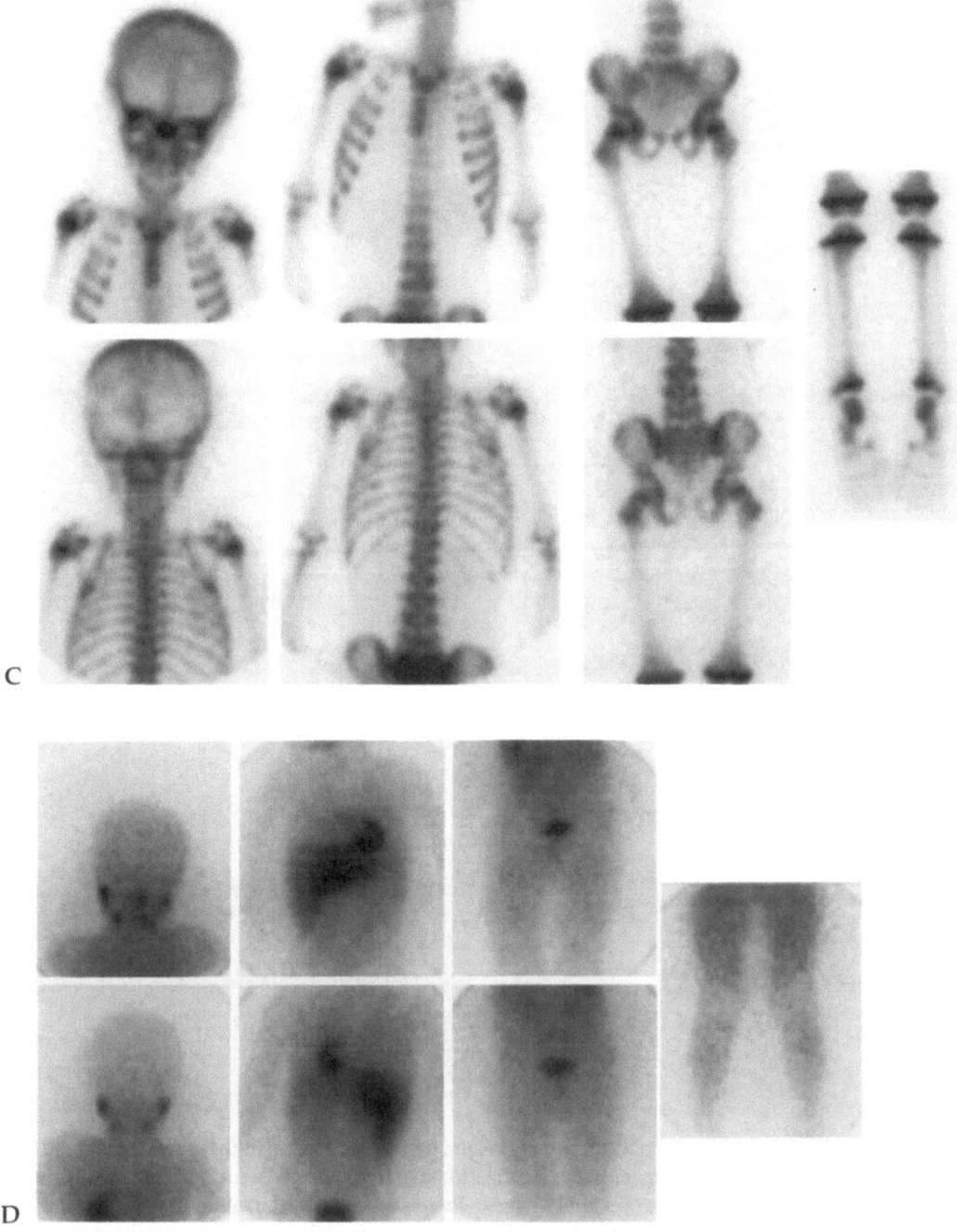

Figure 5.24 (cont'd). Following therapy, skeletal scintigraphy remained abnormal (C), while ^{123}I-MIBG imaging showed normal tracer distribution (D).

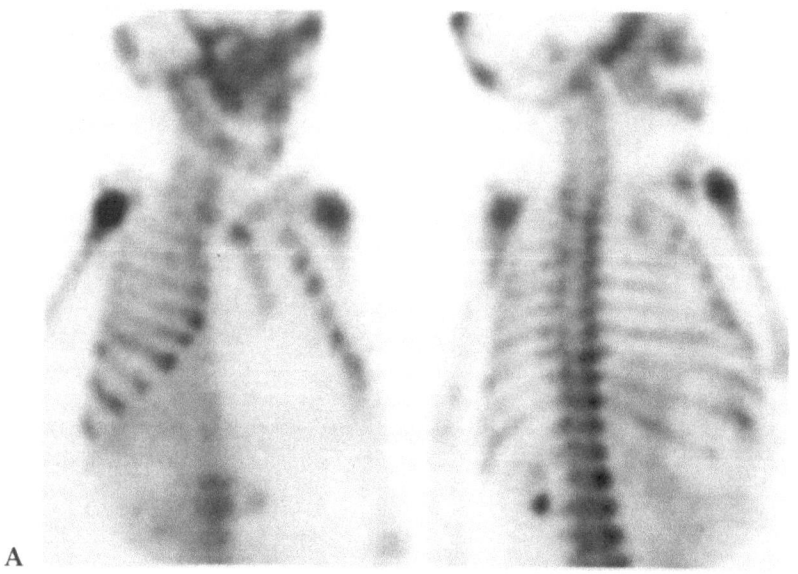

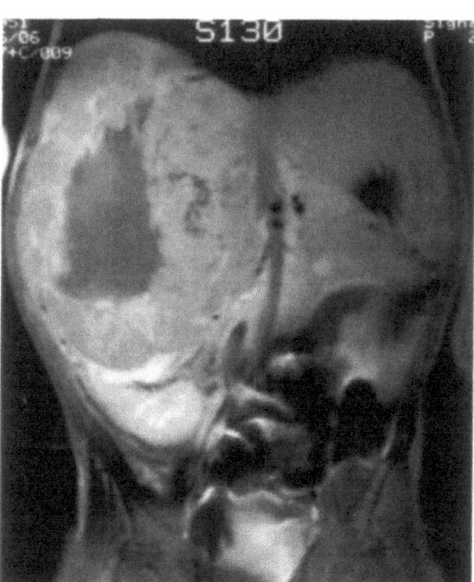

Figure 5.25. Neuroblastoma. Abnormal skeletal tracer localization in the right upper quadrant outlines a region of lower tracer localization in a right adrenal neuroblastoma (A, right anterior and right posterior oblique images). Increased tracer localization in the spine and proximal right humeral metaphysis corresponded to metastatic disease. T1-weighted imaging following gadolinium (B) shows peripheral enhancement of a large right suprarenal mass that displaces the liver and inferior vena cava superiorly and the right kidney inferiorly. It extends to the diaphragm and just crosses the midline. The mass has a central area of decreased signal suggestive of necrosis correlating to its appearance on skeletal scintigraphy.

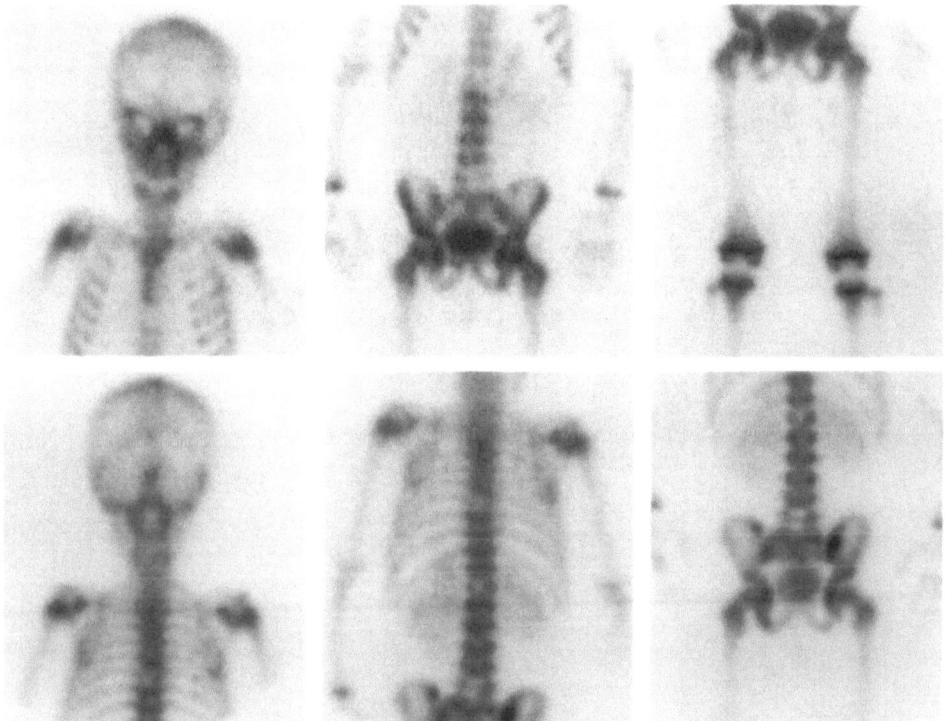

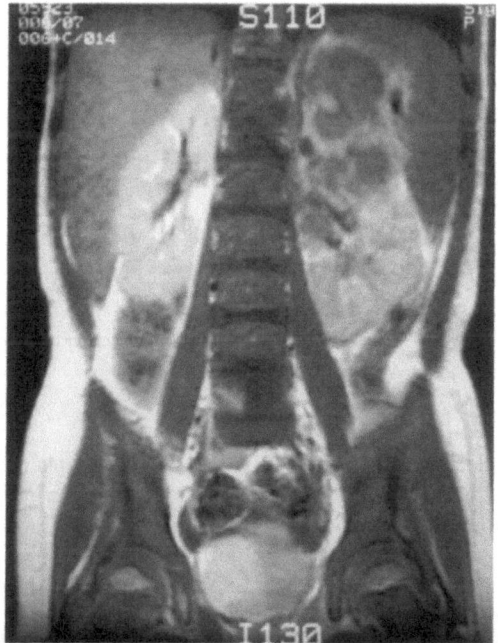

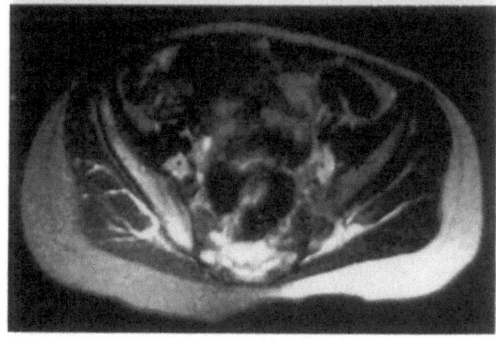

Figure 5.26. Metastatic neuroblastoma. Metastases to the spine are manifested as both increased and decreased ^{99m}Tc-MDP localization in this child with widespread skeletal metastases (A, upper row: anterior projections; lower row: posterior projections). The left adrenal primary is faintly visualized. Coronal T1-weighted imaging following gadolinium shows a left adrenal neuroblastoma and vertebral metastases (B). Transaxial T2-weighted FSE fat suppressed imaging shows extensive metastatic involvement of the left ilium (C).

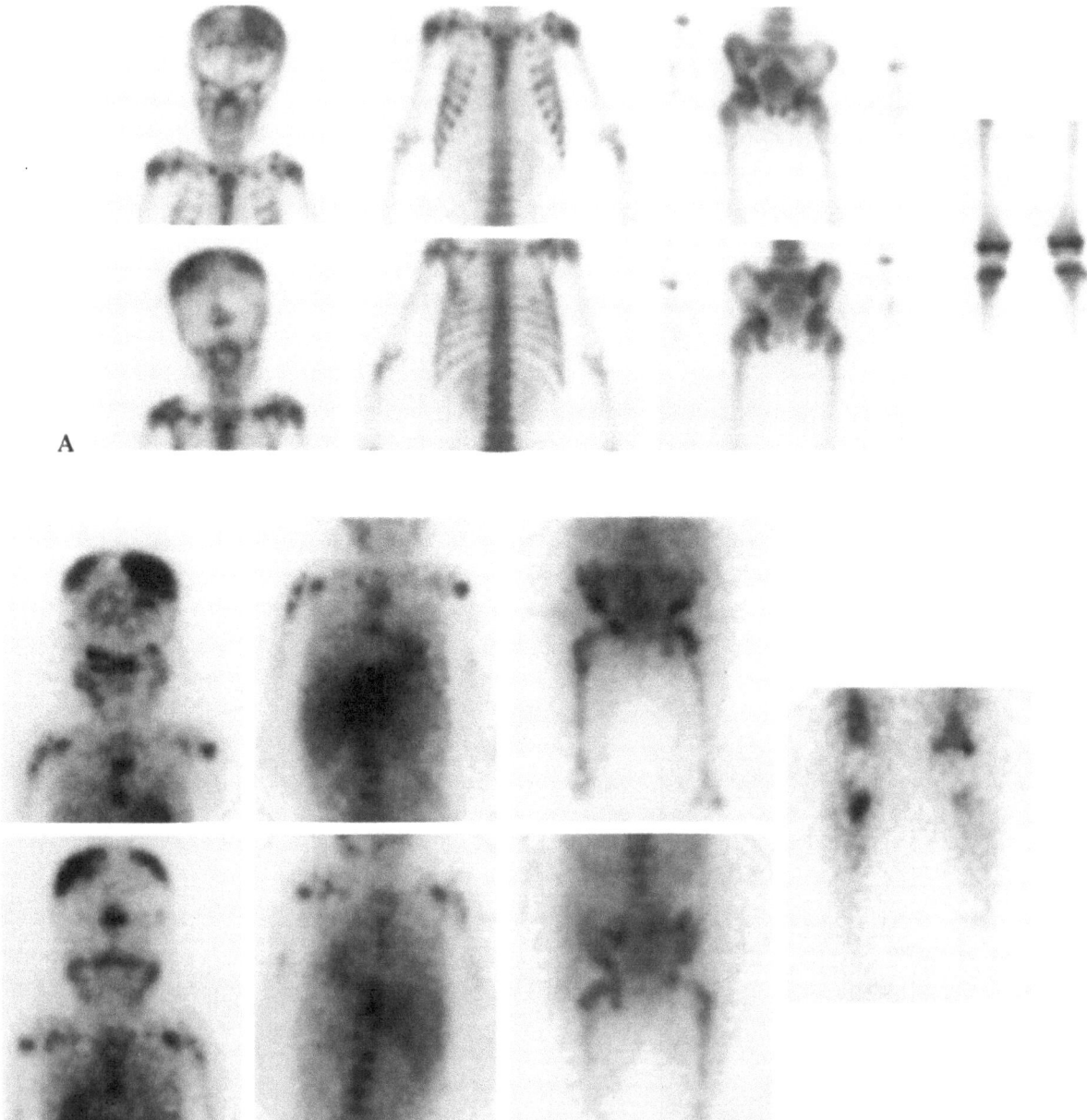

Figure 5.27. Metastatic neuroblastoma. Skeletal scintigraphy (A) shows multiple sites of increased tracer localization in the skull, spine, and pelvis as well as prominent tracer localization in the metaphyses of the femorae, tibiae, and humeri (upper row: anterior projections; lower row: posterior projections; knees: anterior projection). These correspond to sites of abnormal ^{123}I-MIBG localization (B). Ill-defined regions of sclerosis and radiolucency bilaterally correspond to the scintigraphic abnormalities in the skull (C). Sutural widening suggests dural based metastases and increased intracranial pressure. Contrast enhanced CT (D) demonstrates an extracerebral metastatic mass, abutting and possibly involving the frontal lobe and slight rightward shift of the midline markers. The primary site was not found in this 3-year-old girl.

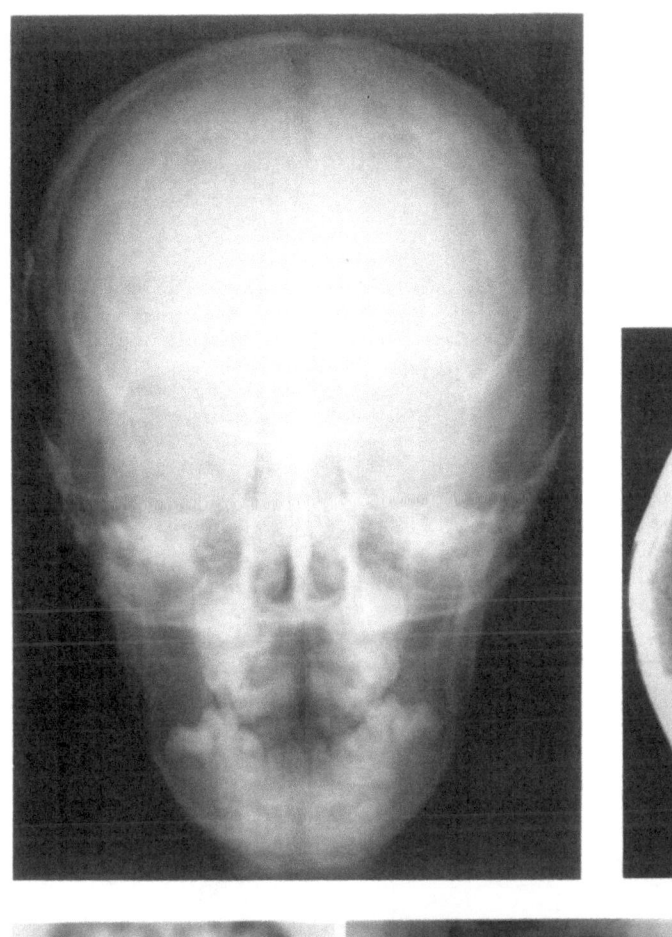

C

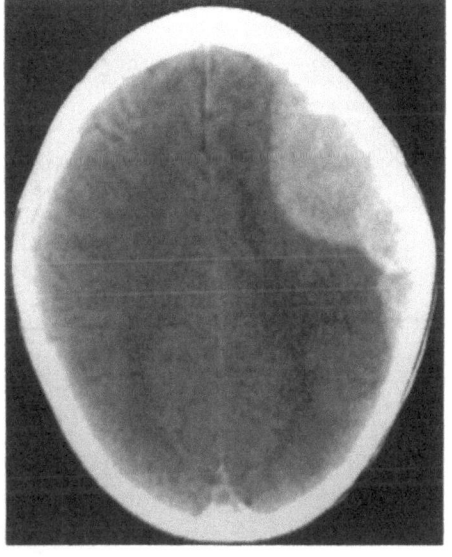

D

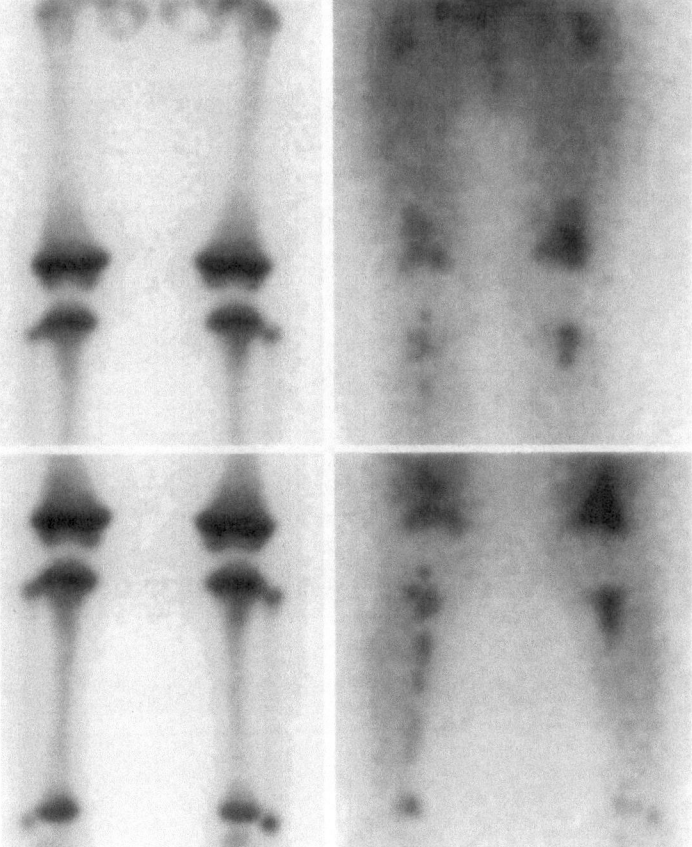

Figure 5.28. Metastatic neuroblastoma. Skeletal scintigraphy (left panels) reveals prominent tracer localization in the proximal and distal femoral and tibial metaphyses bilaterally. This is slightly asymmetric, being greater in the left than right distal femoral and proximal metaphyses. Metastatic disease is confirmed with ^{123}I-MIBG imaging (right panels). Minimal alterations of metaphyseal skeletal tracer distribution as depicted here render identification of metastases difficult and dependent on experience.

Figure 5.29. Neuroblastoma. Skeletal scintigraphy (A) shows abnormal tracer localization within the right upper quadrant (anterior, posterior, right anterior oblique and right posterior oblique projections). Gadolinium-enhanced T1-weighted coronal (B) and sagittal (C) images demonstrate a large heterogeneously enhancing right adrenal mass.

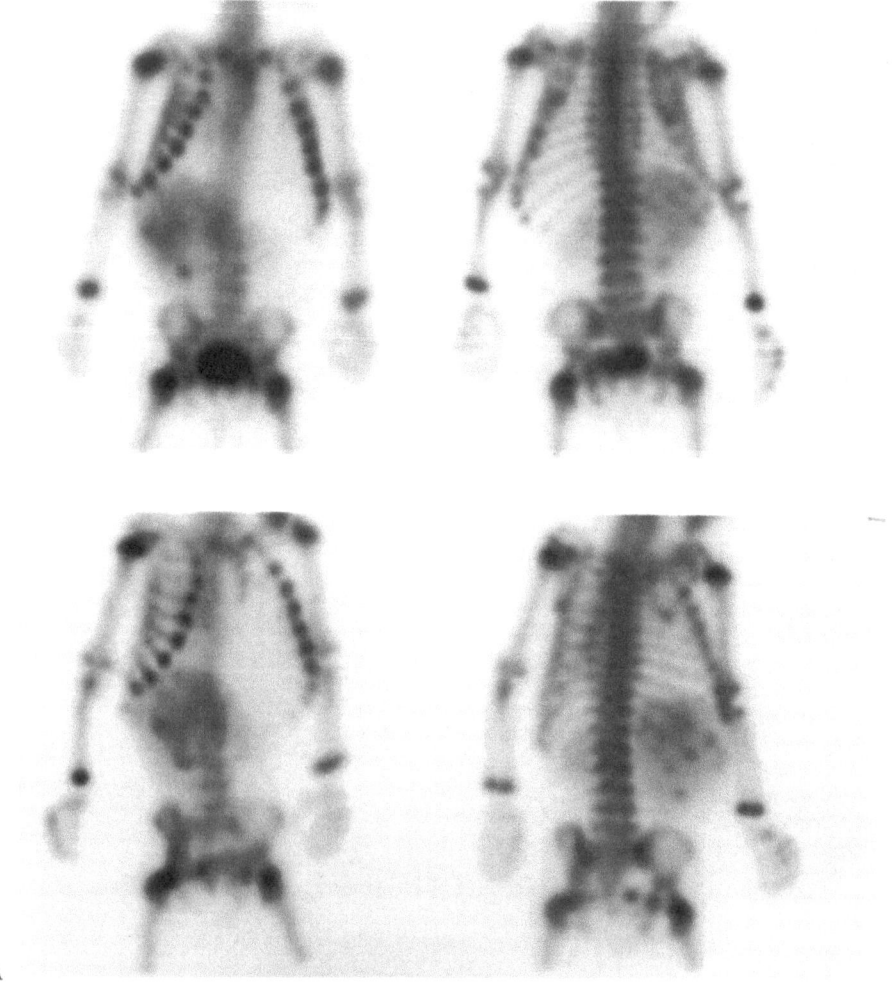

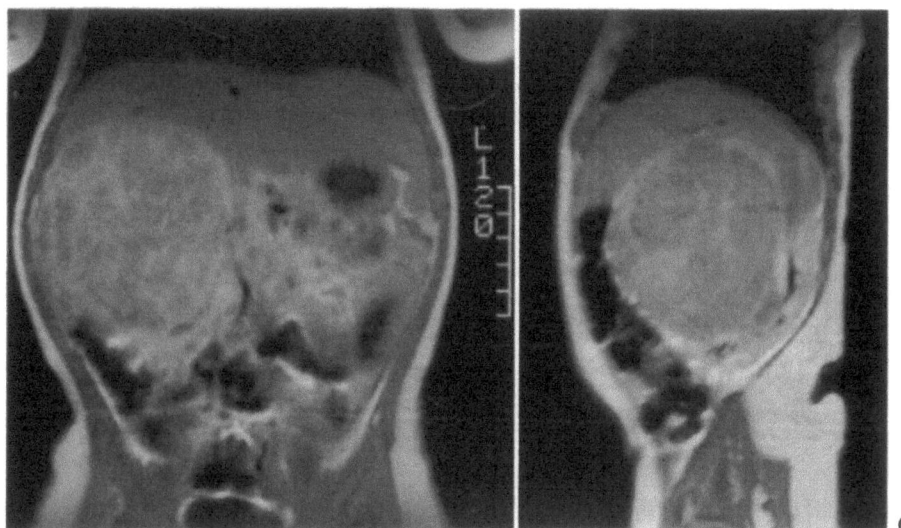

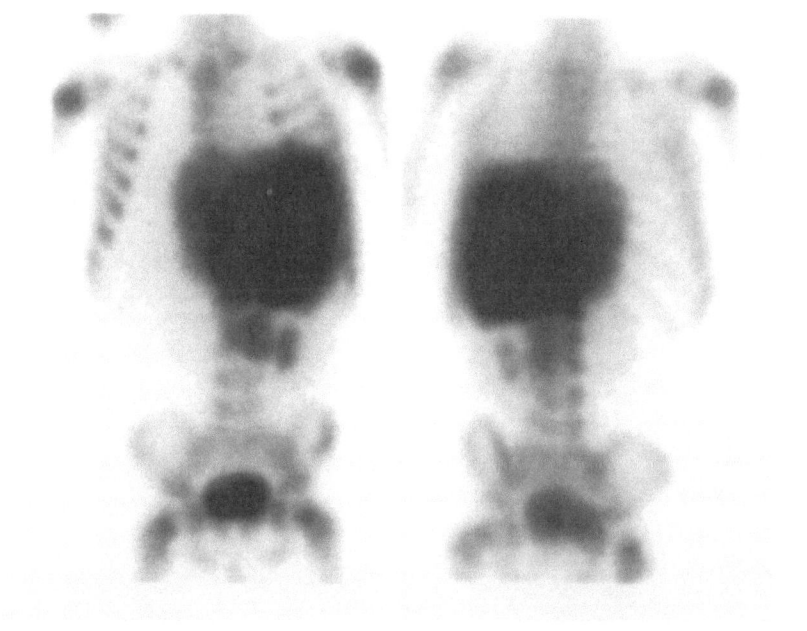

A

Figure 5.30. Neuroblastoma. Skeletal scintigraphy (A) demonstrates intense tracer localization in the soft tissues of the left upper abdomen and lower thorax (anterior and posterior projections). Coronal MR images show a left suprarenal mass that extends along the medial portion of the kidney, crosses the midline, and extends into the chest to a level just below the tracheal bifurcation (B: T1-weighted; C: T1-weighted following gadolinium). The aorta is deviated and the inferior vena cava is compressed. The spleen and left kidney are inferiorly displaced and the heart is displaced superiorly. The left renal pelvis is distended. The MR images indicate that the foci of ^{99m}Tc-MDP localization inferior to the bulk of the mass represents tumoral extension along the left kidney and tracer retention within the pelvicalyceal system.

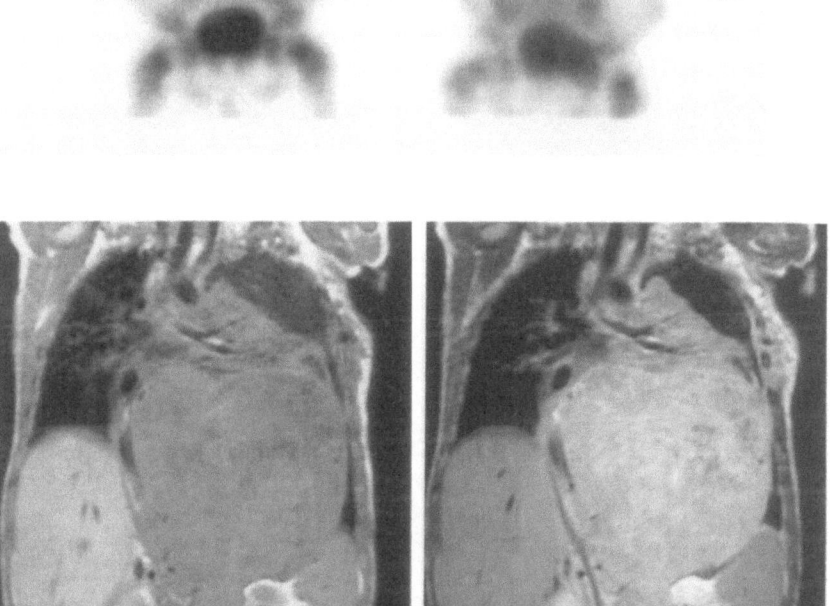

B   C

Leukemia

Leukemia, the most common malignancy of childhood, accounts for approximately one third of all pediatric cancers. Approximately 75% of all cases are acute lymphocytic leukemia (ALL). The highest incidence occurs around 4 years of age.[77]

Bone cortical abnormalities can be detected radiographically in over 40% and are symptomatic in approximately 20% of cases at diagnosis.[102] Radiographic manifestations include osteopenia, transverse metaphyseal bands, periosteal reaction, and focal lytic lesions.[16] While common, osseous disease does not have an impact on treatment or prognosis. Imaging of the skeleton, therefore, is not warranted in the absence of symptoms for children with known leukemia. It is not unusual, however, for a child with leukemia to first come to clinical attention because of skeletal symptoms.

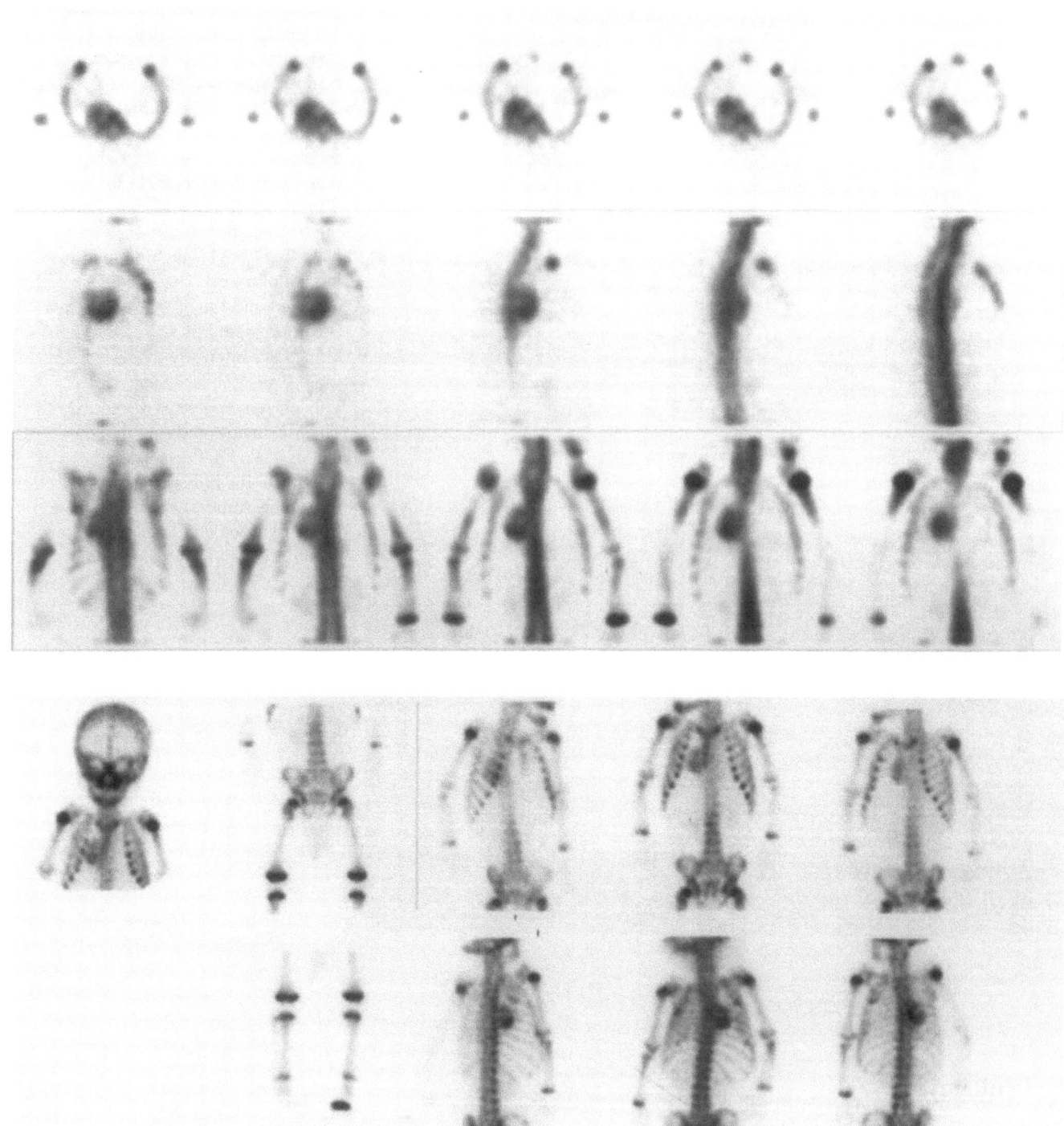

A

Figure 5.31. Neuroblastoma. Planar (bottom) and SPECT (top) images show abnormal radiotracer accumulation in the right posterior hemithorax (A). (Reprinted from Treves et al,[119a] with permission.)

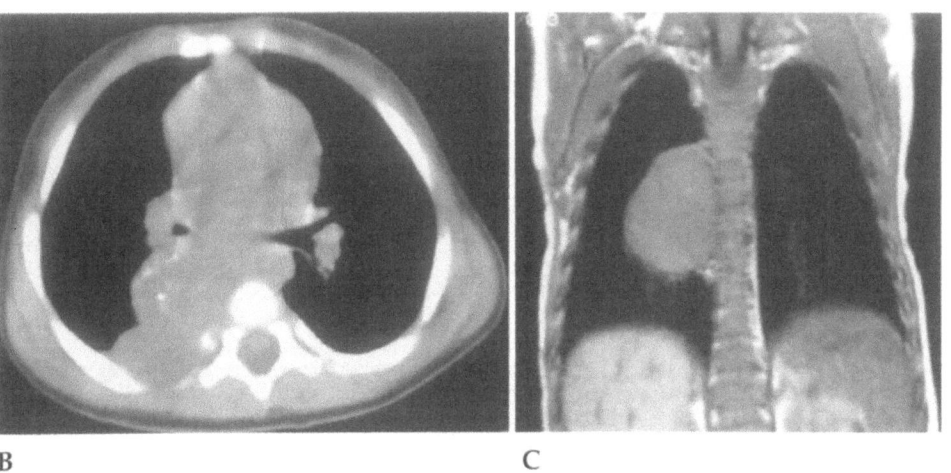

Figure 5.31 (cont'd). Computed tomography depicts a large somewhat heterogeneous mass, with speckled areas of high-density calcification, extending from the right paraspinal region to the carina (B). The craniocaudal extent of the mass is well shown with coronal MRI (C).

B   C

Skeletal scintigraphy requested when another diagnosis is suspected may reveal single or multiple areas of increased or decreased tracer localization. As many as 80% of children with leukemia have abnormalities on skeletal scintigraphy at the time of diagnosis (Figs. 5.32 and 5.33).[15] Most commonly these are metaphyseal areas of increased tracer localization or diffusely increased localization in the long bone diaphyses, the spine, and the flat bones. Regional decreased localization may occur with an aggressive lesion or due to ischemia resulting from packing of leukemic cells in the bone marrow.

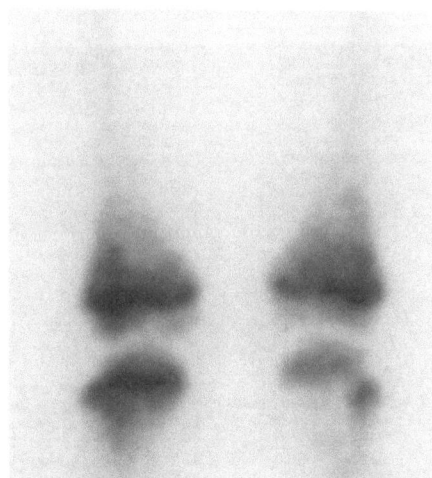

A

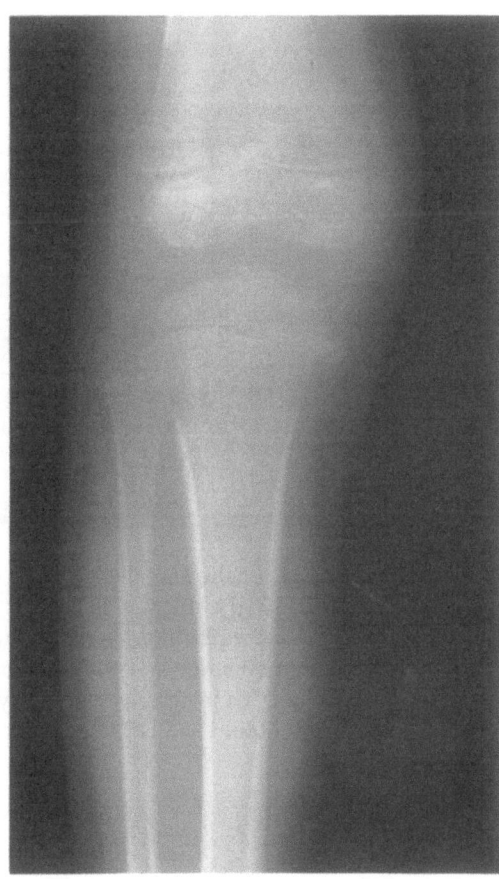

B

Figure 5.32. Leukemia. Skeletal scintigraphy demonstrates increased ^{99m}Tc-MDP localization in the distal femoral and right proximal tibial metaphyses (A). An anteroposterior radiograph (B) reveals osteopenia and lytic destruction of the proximal right tibial metaphysis and periosteal new bone along the lateral metadiaphyseal cortex.

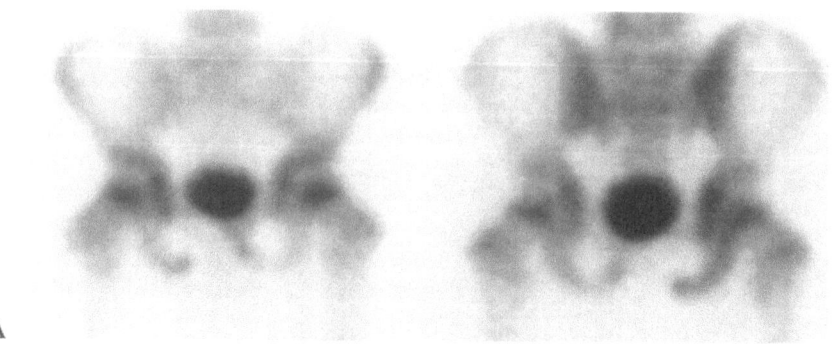

A

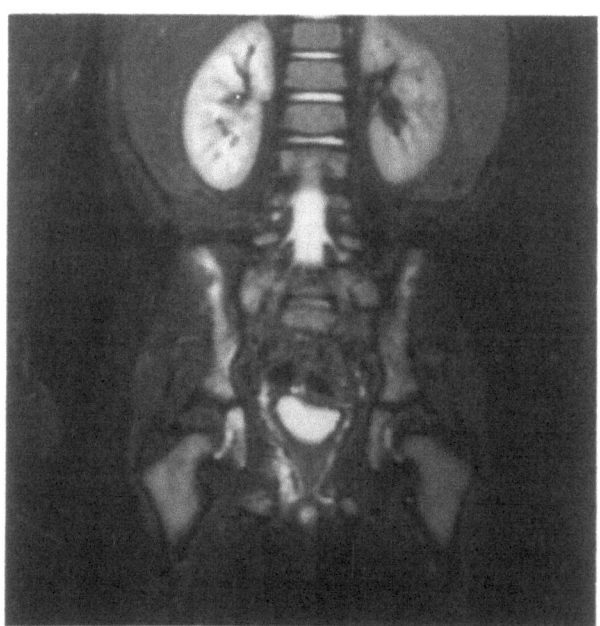

B

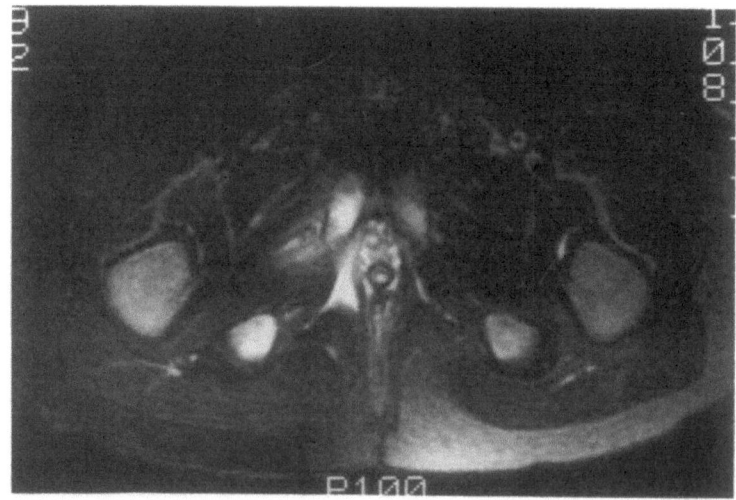

C

Figure 5.33. Leukemia. These images are of a 4-year-old boy, who presented with refusal to walk and right hip pain. Skeletal scintigraphy (A) demonstrates decreased tracer localization in the right inferior pubic ramus and increased tracer localization in the right acetabulum (anterior and posterior projections). Coronal FMPIR (B) and transaxial FSE T2-weighted (C) images reveal patchy increased T2 signal involving the entire right iliac wing, acetabulum and ischium, particularly in the region of the right ischial tuberosity.

Lymphoma

Lymphomas are the third most common pediatric malignancy. Hodgkin's disease, the incidence of which increases during the teenage years, is more frequently encountered than non-Hodgkin's lymphoma. Prior to 10 years of age, non-Hodgkin's lymphoma is more common than Hodgkin's disease.

Bone cortical abnormalities are present radiographically in as many as 20% of patients with non-Hodgkin's lymphoma, where the skeleton is occasionally the only site of disease, but in less than 1% of patients with Hodgkin's disease.[90] The absence of significant clinical importance to the identification of osseous disease in children with non-Hodgkin's lymphoma and the infrequency of cortical bone involvement with Hodgkin's disease has resulted in routine skeletal imaging not being recommended for either.[16] The presence of symptoms is variable. As with leukemia, children with lymphoma and bone involvement occasionally present with bone pain as their chief complaint.

Lymphoma involving, or arising in, bone is most often lytic but can be sclerotic or mixed sclerotic-lytic. Non-Hodgkin's lymphoma predominantly affects the axial skeleton, particularly the spine, skull, and facial bones. Skeletal involvement with Hodgkin's disease commonly involves the spine and pelvis.

Skeletal scintigraphy is a more sensitive indicator of osseous disease than ^{67}Ga scintigraphy or the radiographic skeletal survey.[16,90] Lesions are most often manifested as areas of increased tracer localization (Fig. 5.34), although decreased localization occurs on the same basis as with leukemia.

Rhabdomyosarcoma

Rhabdomyosarcoma accounts for more than 50% of all soft tissue sarcomas in children.[98] This tumor, which arises from embryonal mesenchyme, is usually situated outside of muscle. The most common locations, in decreasing order of frequency, are the head and neck, the genitourinary system, and the extremities. The highest incidence of rhabdomyosarcoma occurs between the ages of 2 and 6 years and during the late teenage years.

Metastases to cortical bone have been identified in 25% of postmortem examinations of patients who succumbed to this malignancy.[70] Skeletal scintigraphy is useful in demonstrating bone metastases, which typically appear as focal areas of increased tracer localization. Although these metastases are occasionally subtle and escape identification due to their proximity to a physis or to their inciting little osteoblastic response,[22,94] skeletal scintigraphy is the study of choice for their detection. Skeletal scintigraphy may also reveal bone involvement secondary to direct tumoral spread or may show compressive and obstructive effects of a rhabdomyosarcoma on the bladder, ureters, and kidneys.

Primitive Neuroectodermal Tumor (PNET)

Primitive neuroectodermal tumors are small round cell tumors that arise in soft tissue, bone, and the central nervous system. They occur at essentially any site. As previously noted, PNET and Ewing sarcoma are believed to be at two ends of a spectrum of tumors that arise from neural cells.[120] Skeletal scintigraphy is useful in the detection of bone metastases, which are not uncommon with these tumors.[4,68] Skeletal scintigraphy may also reveal local effects of a PNET, including high or low tracer localization due to direct bone involvement or destruction, or demonstrate tracer localization in a soft tissue PNET.

Figure 5.34. Lymphoma. Anterior and posterior skeletal scintigraphy images of this 19-year-old patient with Hodgkins disease demonstrate extensive osseous involvement (A). Foci of increased localization are present in the skull, spine, scapulae, and pelvis.

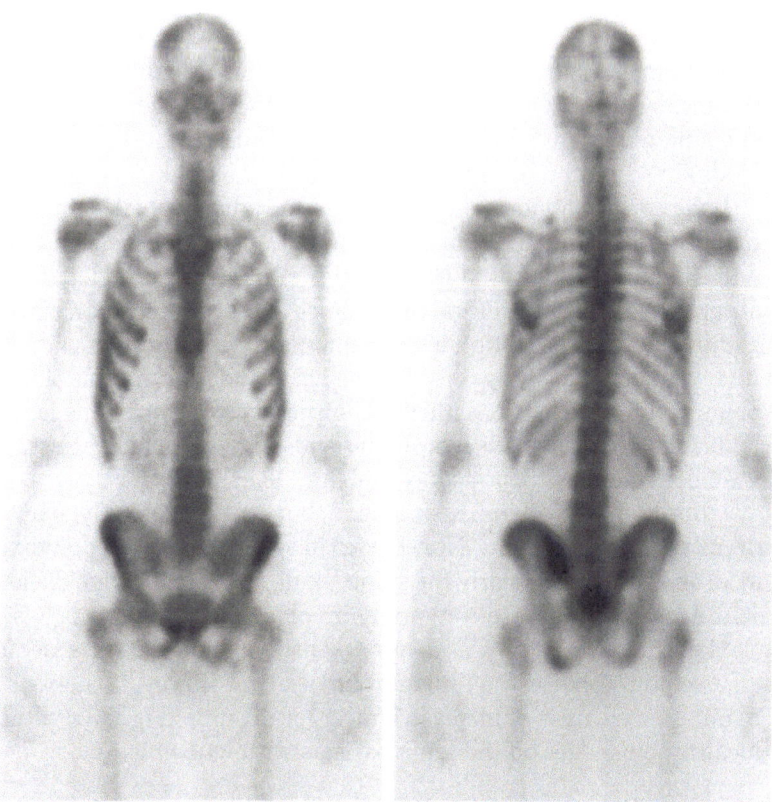

A

Renal Tumors

When biopsy of a renal mass in an infant or child reveals either clear-cell sarcoma or rhabdoid tumor, search for bone metastases with scintigraphy is important.[51,124] The incidence of bone metastases with clear-cell sarcoma has been reported as 76% in one literature review.[51] Renal-cell carcinoma is rare in childhood and typically affects older children. As is the case in adults, bone metastases occur and are manifested scintigraphically as foci of increased or decreased tracer localization. Wilms' tumor, the most common renal malignancy of childhood, metastasizes almost exclusively to regional lymph nodes, liver, and lung.[20] Skeletal scintigraphy is not routinely employed in its staging.

Medulloblastoma

Central nervous system system tumors are the most common solid tumors of childhood. Medulloblastoma, a posterior fossa tumor that accounts for 10% to 25% of pediatric intracranial tumors, is the most common brain tumor to metastasize extracranially. Bone involvement is frequent and seen in over 80% of metastatic medulloblastoma cases.[16,40] The lesions, which often appear sclerotic radiographically, typically show increased tracer localization on skeletal scintigraphy.

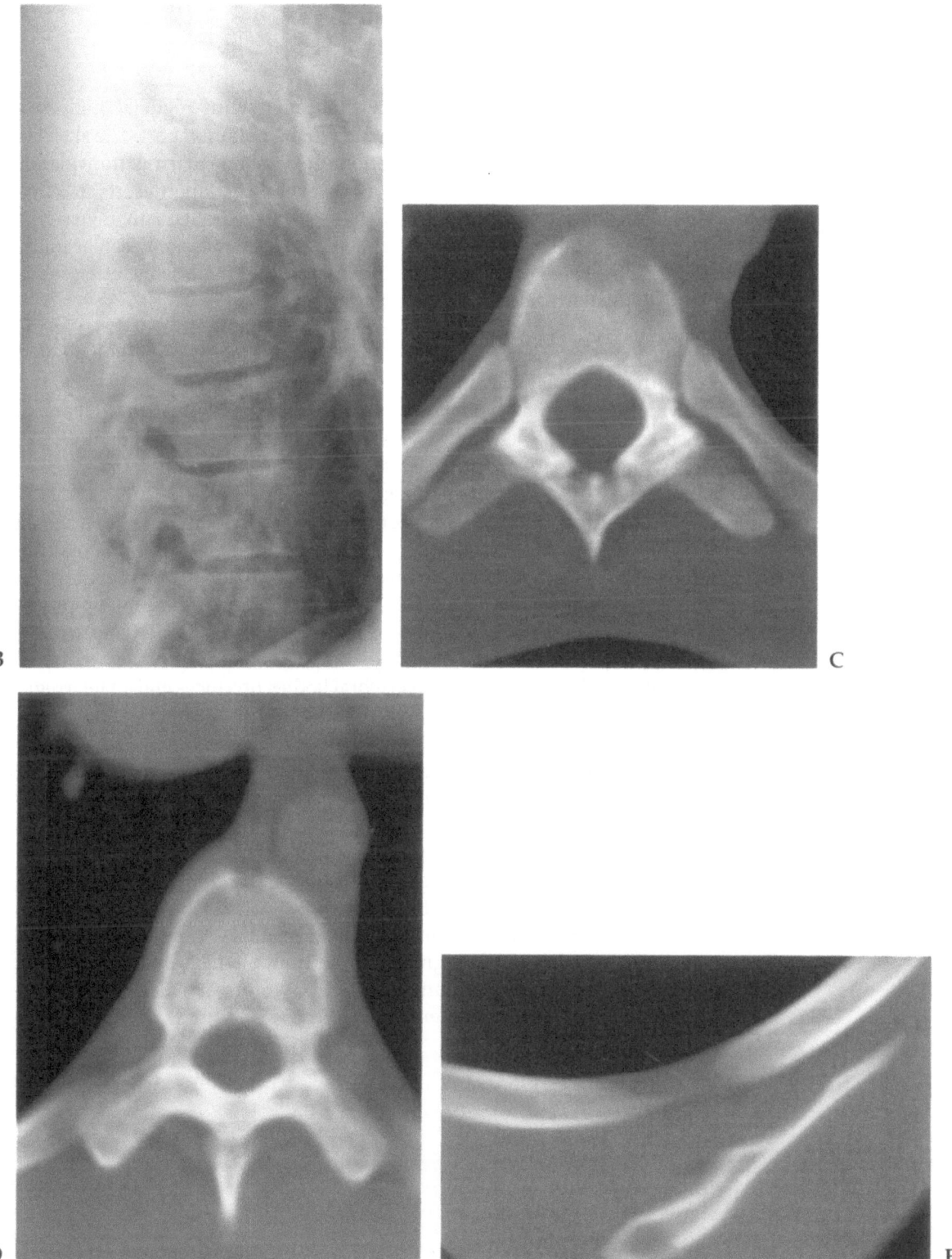

Figure 5.34 (cont'd). A correlative radiograph of the thoracic spine shows radiolucency to the anterior aspect of T5 with associated loss of vertebral body height (B). Lytic destruction of T5 is noted with CT (C). Lytic lesions of multiple other vertebrae, including T9 (D) and the scapulae (left scapula: E) were also identified by CT.

Antineoplastic Therapy: Skeletal Effects

Radiation Therapy

Radiation injury to bone is most closely associated with regional high-dose therapy, in which case the changes are confined to the radiation port. The skeleton of children, who receive total-body irradiation prior to bone marrow transplantation, is also susceptible to radiation injury, however.[29] Radiation exerts its effect primarily on osteoblasts and leads to immediate or delayed cell death, injury with recovery, arrested cellular division, abnormal repair, or neoplasia. Vascular injury also plays a role.[21] Skeletal abnormalities due to radiation therapy include growth disturbance, avascular necrosis, and neoplasia.

Growth may be disturbed in bone exposed to a radiation dose of 400 cGy and can be arrested with exposure to 1,200 to 2,000 cGy.[21,123] The risk of radiation injury is greater in the growing skeleton than in the mature adult skeleton. As this risk increases with the growth potential of bone, it is highest in young children and at sites of active growth. Whenever possible, therefore, epiphyses and physes of rapidly growing bones are excluded from a radiation port.

Radiation injury of the long bones is manifested radiographically as abnormal tubulation, premature epiphyseal fusion, physeal widening due to arrested physeal ossification, metaphyseal fraying due to impaired endochondral ossification, and metaphyseal sclerosis due to increased mineral deposition and deficient chondroclasis and osteoclasis.[57] Radiation injury of the femoral capital epiphysis radiographically simulates Legg-Calvé-Perthes disease and radiation injury to the proximal femoral physis may lead to a slipped capital femoral epiphysis (SCFE).[125] Impaired endochondral ossification in vertebral bodies produces end-plate irregularity, an altered trabecular pattern, and loss of vertebral height. Kyphosis and scoliosis may result.[21,123]

Soon after radiation therapy, there is a regional increase in tracer localization due to hyperemia and inflammation. This is followed by diffusely decreased tracer localization in the bones within the radiation port. This reflects decreased osteoblastic activity and decreased vascular patency (Fig. 5.35). Other histologically benign effects of radiation including femoral head avascular necrosis, slipped capital femoral epiphysis (SCFE), and scoliosis may also be demonstrated.

Benign or malignant neoplasms may develop secondary to radiation therapy. The most common lesion is a benign osteochondroma, which may arise in any bone subjected to radiation in the range of 1,200 cGy or greater. This lesion typically arises within 5 years of treatment.[60]

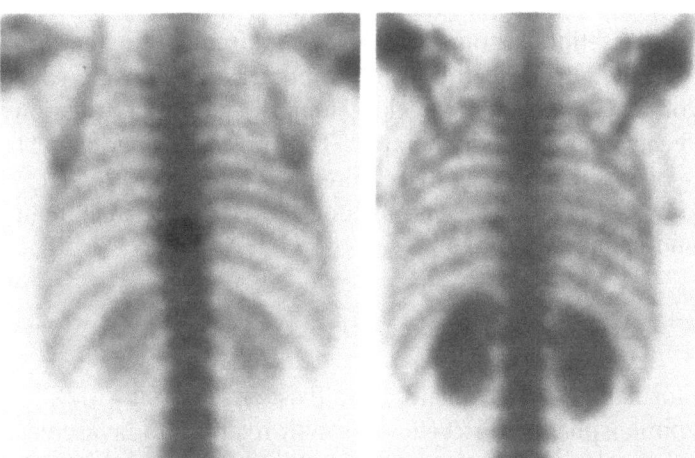

Figure 5.35. Radiation effect. Increased tracer localization is demonstrated in T8 due to Ewing sarcoma (A). Six months following radiation therapy and chemotherapy, there is decreased tracer localization in the sixth through tenth thoracic vertebrae, corresponding to the radiation port, and prominent renal tracer localization (B).

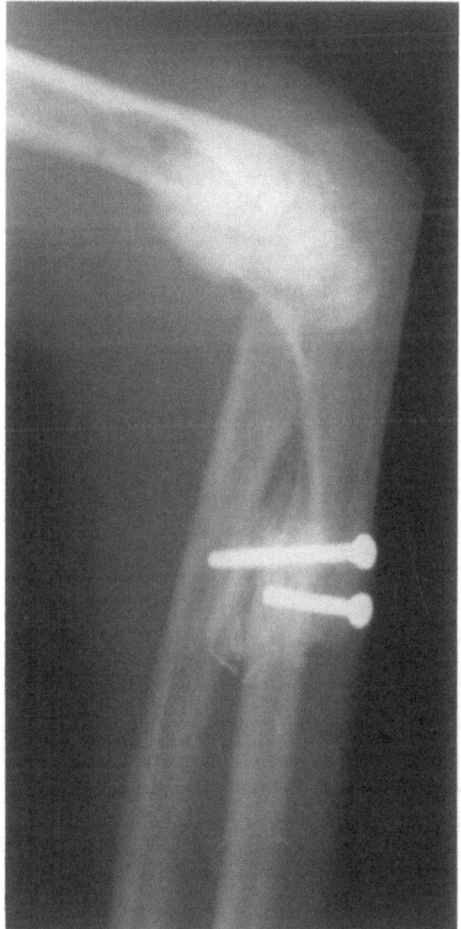

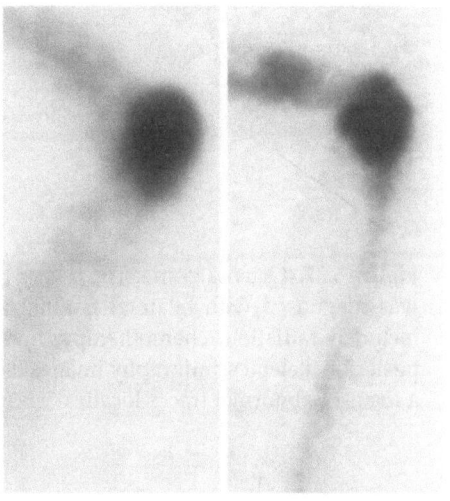

A   B   C

Figure 5.36. Osteosarcoma. This 25-year-old woman presented with a right ulnar Ewing sarcoma at 10 years of age. She was treated with chemotherapy, received 6,000 cGy of radiation therapy, and underwent tumor excision with placement of a vascularized fibular allograft. A radiograph, obtained due to recurrent pain, revealed amorphous ossification at the elbow (A). Thallium-201 (B) and Tc-99m MDP (C) intensely accumulate at this site.

Osteosarcoma may develop years after radiation therapy, most commonly for Ewing sarcoma (Fig. 5.36) or retinoblastoma (Fig. 5.37). Children with hereditary retinoblastoma are especially prone to this complication. To be considered a radiation-induced sarcoma, a tumor must develop along the path of a radiation beam no sooner than 3 years after radiation therapy.[78] The mean latent period is 11 years. A radiation dose of 3,000 cGy is usually required.[21]

Other lesions that occur in irradiated bone include fibrosarcoma, malignant fibrous histiocytoma, and chondrosarcoma.[121]

Chemotherapy

Abnormalities of bone formation, such as methotrexate osteopathy (Fig. 5.17),[24,71] ifosfamide-induced hypophosphatemic rickets,[112] growth retardation, avascular necrosis of bone, and skeletal malignancies may result from chemotherapy. A generalized decrease in skeletal tracer localization may occur with systemic chemotherapy. This may not be apparent on visual inspection of the images except when severe. The effect of chemotherapy that is most commonly encountered with skeletal scintigraphy is prominent renal retention of tracer (Fig. 5.35).[63] This is predominantly due to a nephrotoxic effect of agents such as cyclophosphamide, doxorubicin, vincristine, and amphotericin B, and may also reflect decreased tracer localization within the skeleton. Osteosarcoma also occurs as a second malignancy in children who have received chemotherapy, particularly alkylating agents (Fig. 5.38).

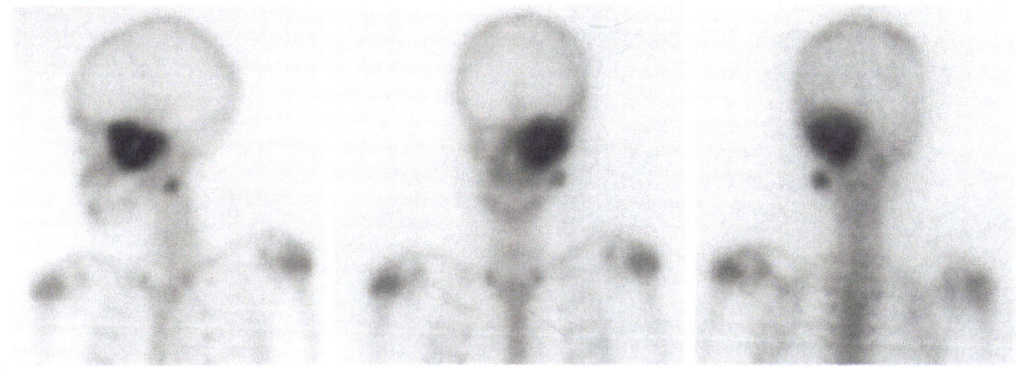

A

Figure 5.37. Osteosarcoma. The 6-year-old boy, whose imaging studies are depicted here, was diagnosed with bilateral familial retinoblastoma at 2 years of age. Treatment had included radiation, chemotherapy, and bilateral enucleation. Left lateral, anterior, and posterior skeletal scintigraphy images depict intense tracer localization in the left orbit and a focus of abnormal tracer localization related to the left mandible (A).

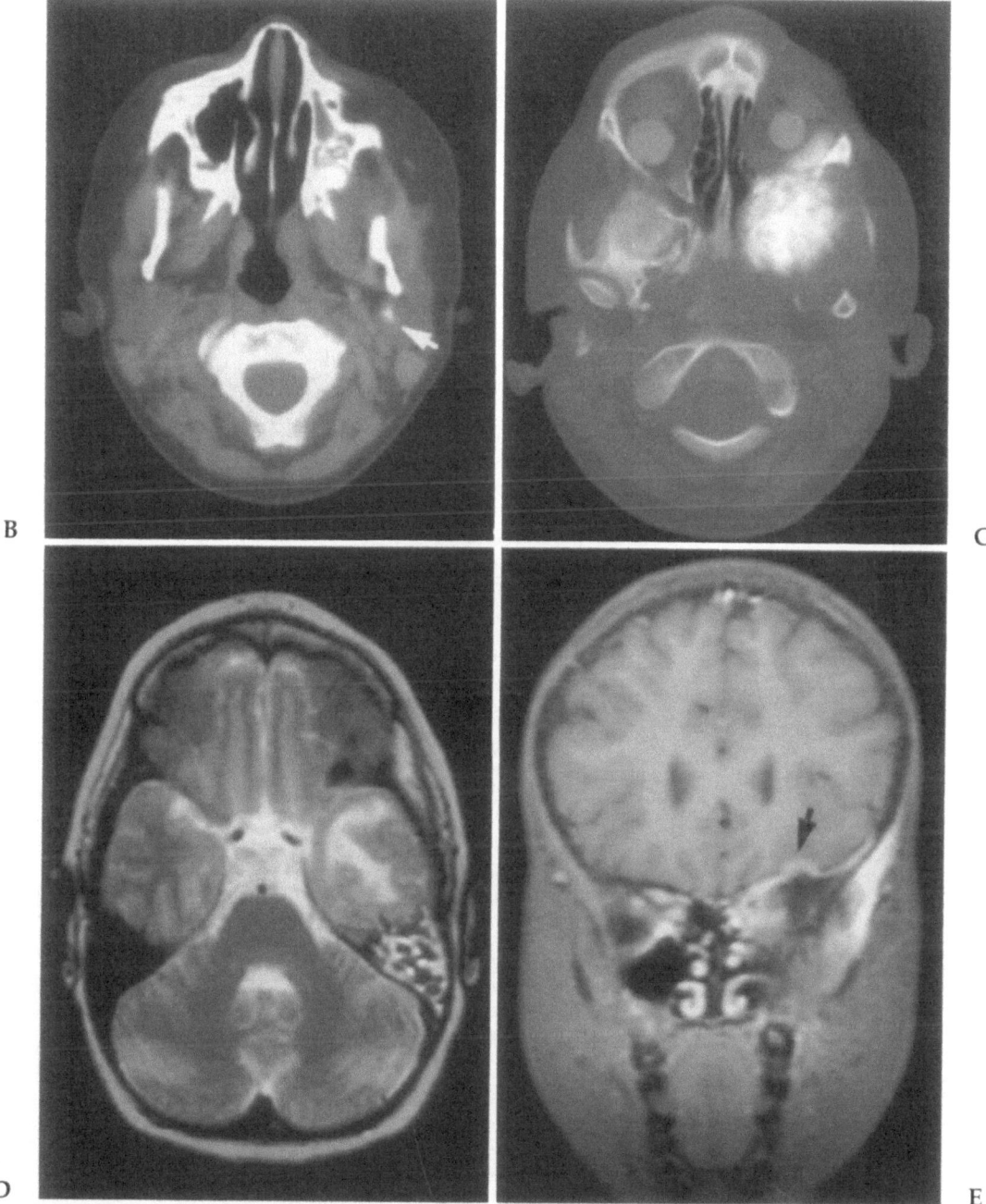

Figure 5.37 (*cont'd*). Computed tomography (B) shows this latter finding to be due to a calcified metastasis within the parotid nodal tissue (white arrow). The primary mass, which demonstrates whorl-like osseous matrix on CT (C), arises from the greater wing of the sphenoid bone and the lateral orbital wall. Note the bilateral ophthalmic prostheses. Magnetic resonance imaging performed to evaluate intracranial extension, shows edema (high T2 signal) of the inferior aspect of the left temporal lobe (D). A gadolinium-enhanced T1-weighted image (E) reveals enhancement and thickening of the left temporal meninges with a nodular component that indents, but does not invade, the left temporal lobe (black arrow).

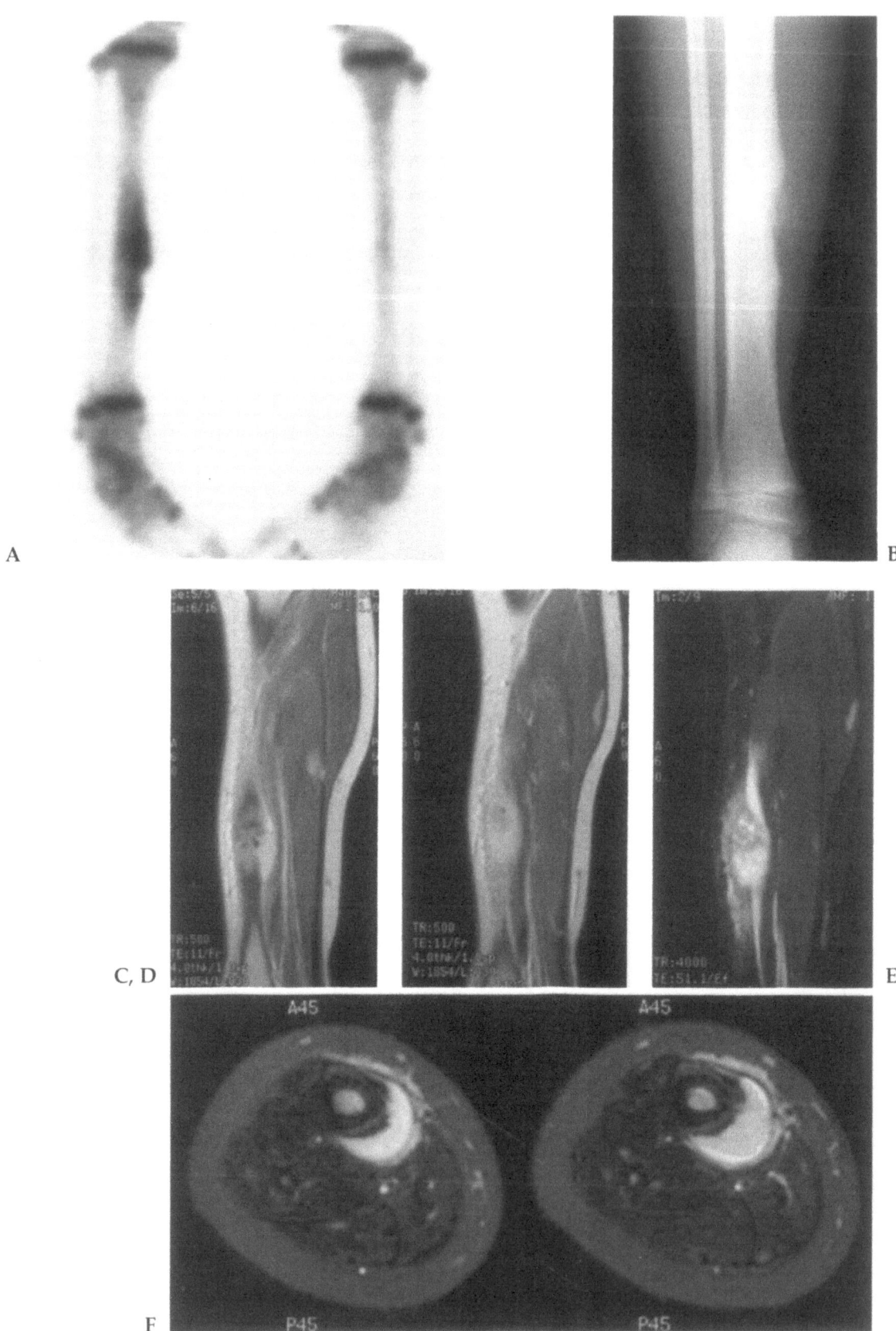

Figure 5.38. Periosteal osteosarcoma. This 7-year-old boy received chemotherapy for neuroblastoma at 6 months of age. Long-term follow-up skeletal scintigraphy revealed increased tracer localization extending over a long segment of the right tibial diaphysis with apparent cortical destruction (A). A plain radiograph confirms the presence of cortical destruction and shows cortical thickening and periosteal new bone formation (B). Sagittal T1-weighted (C) and postgadolinium T1-weighted (D) images as well as FSE T2 fat suppressed images (E: sagittal; F: transaxial) show a predominantly subperiosteal mass at the level of the mid-tibial diaphysis. The mass almost entirely enhances with gadolinium. Cortical thickening and irregularity are depicted on the transaxial images. Multiple 0.5- to 1-cm high signal lobular areas in the calf musculature represent ganglioneuromas.

References

1. Aboulafia AJ, Malawer MM. Surgical management of pelvic and extremity osteosarcoma. *Cancer* 1993;71(suppl):3358–3366.
2. Applegate KA, Connolly LP, Treves ST. Neuroblastoma presenting clinically as hip osteomyelitis: a signature diagnosis on skeletal scintigraphy. *Pediatr Radiol* 1995; 25:S93–97.
3. Aro HT, Aho AJ. Clinical use of bone allografts. *Ann Med* 1993;25:403–412.
4. Askin FB, Rosai J, Sibley RK, et al. Malignant small cell tumor of the thoracopulmonary region in childhood. A distinctive clinicopathologic entity of uncertain histogenesis. *Cancer* 1979;43:2438–2451.
5. Bacci G, Picci P, Ruggieri P, et al. Primary chemotherapy and delayed surgery (neoadjuvant chemotherapy) for osteosarcoma of the extremities. *Cancer* 1990;65:2539–2553.
6. Baker M, Siddiqui AR, Provisor A, et al. Radiographic and scintigraphic skeletal imaging in patients with neuroblastoma: concise communication. *J Nucl Med* 1983; 24:467–469.
7. Bar-Sever Z, Connolly LP, Gebhardt MC, Treves ST. Scintigraphy of lower extremity cadaveric bone allografts in osteosarcoma patients. Clin Nucl Med 1997;22:532–535.
8. Beltran J, Simon DC, Katz W, et al. Increased MR signal intensity in skeletal muscle adjacent to malignant tumors: pathologic correlation and clinical relevance. *Radiology* 1987;162:251–255.
9. Ben Ami T, Treves ST, Tumeh S, et al. Stress fractures after surgery for osteosarcoma: scintigraphic assessment. *Radiology* 1987;163:157–162.
10. Bousvaros A, Kirks DR, Grossman H. Imaging of neuroblastoma: an overview. *Pediatr Radiol* 1986;16:89–106.
11. Brodeur GM, Pritchard J, Berthold F, et al. Revisions of international criteria for neuroblastoma diagnosis, staging, and response to treatment. *J Clin Oncol* 1993; 11:1466–1477.
12. Caner B, Kitapci M, Aras T, et al. Increased accumulation of hexakis (2-methoxyisobutylisonitrile) technetium (I) [Tc-MIBI] in osteosarcoma and its metastatic lymph nodes. *J Nucl Med* 1991;32:1977–1978.
13. Caner B, Kitapci M, Unlu M, et al. Technetium-99m MIBI uptake in benign and malignant bone tumors: a comparative study with technetium-99m MDP. *J Nucl Med* 1992;33:319–324.
14. Chew FS, Hudson TM. Radionuclide bone scanning of osteosarcoma: falsely extended uptake patterns. *AJR* 1982;139:49–54.
15. Clausen N, Gotze H, Pedersen A, et al. Skeletal scintigraphy and radiography at onset of acute lymphocytic leukemia in children. *Med Pediatr Oncol* 1983;11:291–296.
16. Cohen MD. *Imaging of Children with Cancer*. St. Louis: Mosby Year Book; 1992.
17. Connolly LP, Bloom DA, Kozakewich H, et al. Localization of Tc-99m MDP in neuroblastoma metastases to liver and lung. *Clin Nucl Med* 1996;21:629–633.
18. Connolly LP, Laor T, Jaramillo D, et al. Prediction of chemotherapeutic response of osteosarcoma with quantitative thallium-201 scintigraphy and magnetic resonance imaging (abstract). *Radiology* 1996;201(P):349.
19. Crist WM, Kun LE. Common solid tumors of childhood. *N Engl J Med* 1991;324:461–471.
20. D'Angio GL, Breslow N, Beckwith JB, et al. Treatment of Wilms' tumor: results of the third National Wilms' Tumor Study. *Cancer* 1989;64:349–360.
21. Dalinka MK, Haygood TM. Radiation changes. In: Resnick D, ed. *Diagnosis of Bone and Joint Disorders*. 3rd ed. Philadelphia: W.B. Saunders; 1995:3276–3308.
22. Dillon E, Parkin GJS. The role of diagnostic radiology in the diagnosis and management of rhabdomyosarcoma in young persons. *Clin Radiol* 1978;29:53–59.
23. Dorr U, Sautter-Bihl ML, Schilling FH, et al. Somatostatin receptor scintigraphy: a new diagnostic tool in neuroblastoma? *Prog Clin Biol Res* 1994;385:355–361.
24. Ecklund K, Laor T, Goorin AM, et al. Methotrexate osteopathy in patients with osteosarcoma. *Radiology* 1997;202:543–547.

25. Englaro EE, Gelfand MJ, Harris RE, et al. I-131 MIBG imaging after bone marrow transplantation for neuroblastoma. *Radiology* 1992;182:515–520.

26. Enneking WF, Mindell ER. Observations on massive retrieved human allografts. *J Bone Joint Surg [A]* 1991;73:1123–1142.

27. Erlemann R, Sciuk J, Bosse A, et al. Response of osteosarcoma and Ewing sarcoma to preoperative chemotherapy: assessment with dynamic and static MR imaging and skeletal scintigraphy. *Radiology* 1990;175:791–796.

28. Farahati J, Mueller SP, Coennen HH, et al. Scintigraphy of neuroblastoma with radioiodinated m-iodobenzylguanidine. In: Treves ST, ed. *Pediatric Nuclear Medicine.* 2nd ed. New York: Springer-Verlag; 1995:528–545.

29. Fletcher BD, Crom DB, Krance RA, et al. Radiation-induced bone abnormalities after bone marrow transplantation for childhood leukemia. *Radiology* 1994;191:231–235.

30. Friedlaender GE. Bone grafts. Current concepts (review). *J Bone Joint Surg [A]* 1987;69:786–790.

31. Frouge C, Vanel D, Coffre C, et al. The role of magnetic resonance imaging in the evaluation of Ewing sarcoma—a report of 27 cases. *Skeletal Radiol* 1988;17:387–392.

32. Gelfand MJ, Elgazzar AH, Kriss VM, et al. Iodine-123-MIBG SPECT versus planar imaging in children with neural crest tumors. *J Nucl Med* 1994;35:1753–1757.

33. Glasser DB, Lane JM, Huvos AG, et al. Survival, prognosis, and therapeutic response in osteogenic sarcoma: the Memorial Hospital experience. *Cancer* 1992;69:698–708.

34. Goldman B, Braunstein P. Augmented radioactivity on bone scans of limbs bearing osteosarcomas. *J Nucl Med* 1978;16:423–424.

35. Goldstein H, NcNeil BJ, Zufall E, et al. Changing indications for bone scintigraphy in patients with osteosarcoma. *Radiology* 1980;135:177–180.

36. Goorin AM, Shuster JJ, Baker A, et al. Changing pattern of pulmonary metastases with adjuvant chemotherapy in patients with osteosarcoma: results from the Multi-institutional Osteosarcoma Study. *J Clin Oncol* 1991;9:600–605.

37. Gordon I, Peters AM, Gutman A, et al. Tc-99m bone scans are more sensitive than I-123 MIBG scans for bone imaging in neuroblastoma. *J Nucl Med* 1990;31:129–134.

38. Grosfeld JL, Baehner RL. Neuroblastoma: an analysis of 160 cases. *World J Surg* 1980;4:29–38.

39. Hanna SL, Parham DM, Fairclough DL, et al. Assessment of osteosarcoma response to preoperative chemotherapy using dynamic FLASH gadolinium-DTPA-enhanced magnetic resonance imaging. *Invest Radiol* 1992;27:367–373.

40. Heideman RL, Packer RJ, Albright LA, et al. Tumors of the central nervous system. In: Pizzo PA, Poplack DG, eds. *Principles and Practice of Pediatric Oncology.* 2nd ed. Philadelphia: JB Lippincott; 1993:633–682.

41. Heisel MA, Miller JH, Reid BS, et al. Radionuclide bone scan in neuroblastoma. *Pediatrics* 1983;71:206–209.

42. Herrlin K, Willen H, Wiebe T. Flare phenomenon in osteosarcoma after complete remission. *J Nucl Med* 1995;36:1429–1431.

43. Hoefnagel CA, Bruning PF, Cohen P, et al. Detection of lung metastases from osteosarcoma by scintigraphy using ^{99m}Tc-methylene diphosphonate. *Diagn Imaging* 1981;50:277–284.

44. Holscher HC, Bloem JL, Vanel D, et al. Osteosarcoma: chemotherapy-induced changes at MR imaging. *Radiology* 1992;182:839–844.

45. Hopper KD, Moser RP, Haseman DB, et al. Osteosarcomatosis. *Radiology* 1990;175:233–239.

46. Horowitz ME, DeLaney TE, Malawer MM, et al. Ewing's sarcoma family of tumors: Ewing's sarcoma of bone and soft tissue and the peripheral primitive neuroectodermal tumors. In: Pizzo PA, Poplack DG, eds. *Pediatric Oncology.* 2nd ed. Philadelphia: JB Lippincott; 1993:795–821.

47. Howman-Giles RB, Gilday DL, Ash JM. Radionuclide skeletal survey in neuroblastoma. *Radiology* 1979;131:497–502.

48. Hudson TM. *Radiologic-Pathologic Correlation of Musculoskeletal Lesions.* Baltimore: Williams & Wilkins; 1987.

49. Jaffe HL. *Tumor and Tumorous Conditions of the Bones and Joints.* Philadelphia: Lee & Febiger; 1958.

50. Jaramillo D, Laor T, Gebhardt M. Pediatric musculoskeletal neoplasms. Evaluation with MR imaging. *MRI Clin North Am* 1996;4:1–22.

51. Kagan RA, Steckel RJ. Clear cell sarcoma of the kidney: a renal tumor of childhood that metastasizes to bone. *AJR* 1986;146:64–66.

52. Kartner N, Riordan JR, Ling V. Cell surface P-glycoprotein associated with multidrug resistance in mammalian cell lines. *Science* 1983;221:1285–1288.

53. Keller SM, Rosenbaum RC, Rosenberg SA. The significance of bone scan abnormalities in patients with primary osteogenic sarcoma. *J Surg Oncol* 1984;26:122–129.

54. Kirks DR, Cook TA, Merten DF, et al. The value of radionuclide bone imaging in selected patients with osteosarcoma metastatic to lung. *Pediatr Radiol* 1980;9:139–143.

55. Knop J, Dellin G, Heise U, et al. Scintigraphic evaluation of tumor regression during preoperative chemotherapy of osteosarcoma: correlation of Tc-99m methylene diphosphonate parametric imaging with surgical histopathology. *Skeletal Radiol* 1990;19:165–172.

56. Krenning EP, Kwekkeboom DJ, Bakker WH, et al. Somatostatin receptor scintigraphy with [In-111-DTPA-D-Phe1] and [123I-Tyr3]-octreotide: the Rotterdam experience with more than 1,000 patients. *Eur J Nucl Med* 1993;20:716–731.

57. Laor T, Jaramillo D, Oestrich A. Skeletal system. In: Kirks DR, ed. *Practical Pediatric Imaging. Diagnostic Radiology of Infants and Children.* 3rd ed. Philadelphia: Lippincott-Raven; 1997:327–510.

58. Lawrence JA, Babyn PS, Chan HS, et al. Extremity osteosarcoma in childhood: prognostic value of radiologic imaging. *Radiology* 1993;189:43–47.

59. Lemmi MA, Fletcher BD, Marina NM, et al. Use of MR imaging to assess results of chemotherapy for Ewing sarcoma. *AJR* 1990;155:343–346.

60. Libshitz HI, Cohne MA. Radiation-induced osteochondromas. *Radiology* 1982;142:643–647.

61. Lin J, Leung WT. Quantitative evaluation of thallium-201 uptake in predicting chemotherapeutic response of osteosarcoma. *Eur J Nucl Med* 1995;22:553–555.

62. Link MP, Eilber F. Osteosarcoma. In: Pizzo PA, Poplack DG, eds. *Pediatric Oncology.* 2nd ed. Philadelphia: JB Lippincott; 1993:841–866.

63. Lutrin CL, McDougall IR, Goris ML. Intense concentration of technetium-99m pyrophosphate in the kidneys of children treated with chemotherapeutic drugs for malignant disease. *Radiology* 1978;128:165–167.

64. MacVicar AD, Olliff JFC, Pringle J, et al. Ewing sarcoma: MR imaging of chemotherapy-induced changes with histologic correlation. *Radiology* 1992;184:859–864.

65. Mandell GA, Heyman S. Extraosseous uptake of technetium-99m MDP in secondary deposits of neuroblastoma. *Clin Nucl Med* 1986;11:337–341.

66. Manil L, Edeline V, Lumbroso J, et al. Indium-111-pentetreotide scintigraphy in children with neuroblast-derived tumors. *J Nucl Med* 1996;37:893–896.

67. Mankin HJ, Springfield DS, Gebhardt MC, et al. Current status of allografting for bone tumors. *Orthopedics* 1992;15:1147–1152.

68. Marina NM, Etcubanas E, Parham DM, et al. Peripheral primitive neuroectodermal tumor (peripheral neuroepithelioma) in children. A review of the St. Jude experience and controversies in diagnosis and management. *Cancer* 1989;64:1952–1960.

69. Martin-Simmerman P, Cohen MD, Siddiqui A, et al. Calcification and uptake of Tc-99m diphosphonates in neuroblastomas: concise communication. *J Nucl Med* 1984; 25:656–660.

70. Maurer HM. Rhabdomyosarcoma. *Curr Probl Cancer* 1978;2:3–36.

71. May KP, West SG, McDermott MT, et al. The effect of low-dose methotrexate on bone metabolism and histomorphometry in rats. *Arthritis Rheum* 1994;37:201–206.

72. McDonald DJ. Limb salvage surgery for sarcomas of the extremities. *AJR* 1994; 163:509–513.

73. McKillop JH, Etcubanus E, Goris ML. The indications for and limitations of bone scintigraphy in osteogenic sarcoma: a review of 55 patients. *Cancer* 1981;48:1133–1138.

74. Meadows AT, Baum E, Fassati-Bellani F, et al. Second malignant neoplasms in children: an update from the late effects study group. *J Clin Oncol* 1985;3:532–538.

75. Menendez LR, Fideler BM, Mirra J. Thallium-201 scanning for the evaluation of osteosarcoma and soft tissue sarcoma. *J Bone Joint Surg [A]* 1993;75:526–531.

76. Meyers PA, Heller G, Healey J, et al. Chemotherapy for nonmetastatic osteogenic sarcoma. The Memorial Sloan-Kettering experience. *J Clin Oncol* 1992;10:5–15.
77. Miller DR. Acute lymphoblastic leukemia. *Pediatr Clin North Am* 1980;27:269–293.
78. Mirra JM. *Bone Tumors*. Philadelphia: Lea & Febiger; 1989.
79. Nadel HR, Rossleigh MA. Tumor imaging. In: Treves ST, ed. *Pediatric Nuclear Medicine*. 2nd ed. New York: Springer-Verlag; 1995:496–527.
80. Nesbit M, Krivit W, Heyn R, et al. Acute and chronic effects of methotrexate on hepatic, pulmonary, and skeletal systems. *Cancer* 1976;37:1048–1054.
81. Newton WA, Meadows AT, Shimada H, et al. Bone sarcomas as second malignant neoplasms following childhood cancer. *Cancer* 1991;67:193–201.
82. Norton KI, Hermann G, Abdelwahab IF, et al. Epiphyseal involvement in osteosarcoma. *Radiology* 1991;180:813–816.
83. O'Connor MI, Pritichard DJ. Ewing's sarcoma. Prognostic factors, disease control, and the reemerging role of surgical treatment. *Clin Orthop* 1991;262:78–87.
84. O'Flanagan SJ, Stack JP, McGee HM, et al. Imaging of intramedullary tumour spread in osteosarcoma. A comparison of techniques. *J Bone Joint Surg [B]* 1991;73:998–1001.
85. Ohtomo K, Terui S, Yokoyama R, et al. Thallium-201 scintigraphy to assess effect of chemotherapy to osteosarcoma. *J Nucl Med* 1996;37:1444–1448.
86. Oritz SS, Miller JH, Villablanca JG, et al. Bone abnormalities detected with skeletal scintigraphy after bone marrow harvest in patients with childhood neuroblastoma. *Radiology* 1994;192:755–758.
87. Paltiel HJ, Gelfand MJ, Elgazzar AH, et al. Neural crest tumors: [123]I MIBG imaging in children. *Radiology* 1994;190:117–121.
88. Parisi MT, Greene MK, Dykes TM, et al. Efficacy of metaiodobenzylguanidine as a scintigraphic agent for the detection of neuroblastoma. *Invest Radiol* 1992;27:768–773.
89. Parker BR, Castellino RA. *Pediatric Oncologic Radiology*. St. Louis: Mosby; 1977.
90. Parker BR, Margin S, Castellino RA. Skeletal manifestations of leukemia, Hodgkin disease, and non-Hodgkin lymphoma. *Semin Roentgenol* 1980;15:302–315.
91. Piwnica-Worms D, Chiu ML, Budding M, et al. Functional imaging of multidrug-resistant P-glycoprotein with an organotechnetium complex. *Cancer Res* 1993;53:977–984.
92. Podoloff DA. Malignant bone disease. In: Henkin RE, Boles MA, Dillehay GL, et al, eds. *Nuclear Medicine*. 2nd ed. Philadelphia: Mosby Year Book; 1996:1208–1222.
93. Podrasky AE, Stark DD, Hattner RS, et al. Radionuclide bone scanning in neuroblastoma: skeletal metastases and primary tumor localization of 99m Tc-MDP. *AJR* 1983;141:469–472.
94. Quddus FF, Espinola D, Kramer SS, et al. Comparison between x-ray and bone scan detection of bone metastases in patients with rhabdomyosarcoma. *Med Pediatr Oncol* 1983;11:125–129.
95. Ragab AH, Frech RS, Vietti TJ. Osteoporotic fractures secondary to methotrexate therapy of acute leukemia in remission. *Cancer* 1970;25:580–585.
96. Ramanna L, Waxman A, Binney G, et al. Thallium-201 scintigraphy in bone sarcoma: comparison with gallium-67 and technetium-99m MDP in the evaluation of chemotherapeutic response. *J Nucl Med* 1990;31:567–572.
97. Ramanna L, Waxman A, Rosen G. Evaluation of Tl-201 uptake patterns in bone lesions: differentiation of benign from malignant processes [abstract]. *J Nucl Med* 1992;33:869.
98. Raney RB, Hays DM, Tefft M, et al. Rhabdomyosarcoma and the undifferentiated sarcomas. In: Pizzo PA, Poplack DG, eds. *Principles and Practice of Pediatric Oncology*. 2nd ed. Philadelphia: JB Lippincott; 1993:769–794.
99. Rees CR, Siddiqui AR, duCret R. The role of bone scintigraphy in osteogenic sarcoma. *Skeletal Radiol* 1986;15:365–367.
100. Resnick D. Tumors and tumor-like lesions of bone: radiographic principles. In: Resnick D, ed. *Diagnosis of Bone and Joint Disorders*. 3rd ed. Philadelphia: W.B. Saunders; 1995:3613–3627.
101. Resnick D, Kyriakos K, Greenway GD. Tumors and tumor-like lesions of bone: imaging and pathology of specific tumors. In: Resnick D, ed. *Diagnosis of Bone and Joint Disorders*. 3rd ed. Philadelphia: W.B. Saunders; 1995:3662–3697.

102. Rogalsky RJ, Black B, Reed MH. Orthopedic manifestations of leukemia in children. *J Bone Joint Surg [A]* 1986;68:494–501.

103. Rosen G, Loren GJ, Brien EW, et al. Serial thallium-201 scintigraphy in osteosarcoma. Correlation with tumor necrosis after preoperative chemotherapy. *Clin Orthop* 1993;293:302–306.

104. Rosenberg ZS, Lev S. Osteosarcoma: subtle, rare, and misleading plain film features. *AJR* 1995;165:1209–1214.

105. Rufini V, Fisher GL, Shulkin BL, et al. Iodine-123-MIBG imaging of neuroblastoma: utility of SPECT and delayed imaging. *J Nucl Med* 1996;37:1464–1468.

106. Schima W, Amann G, Stiglbauer R, et al. Preoperative staging of osteosarcoma: efficacy of MR imaging in detecting joint involvement. *AJR* 1994;163:1171–1175.

107. Schwartz AM, Leonidas JC. Methotrexate osteopathy. *Skeletal Radiol* 1984;11:13–16.

108. Schweil AM, McKillop JH, Milroy R, et al. Mechanism of ^{201}Tl uptake in tumours. *Eur J Nucl Med* 1989;15:376–379.

109. Shapiro B, Gross MD. Radiochemistry, biochemistry, and kinetics of ^{131}I-metaiodobenzylguanidine (MIBG) and ^{123}I-MIBG. Clinical applications of the use of ^{123}I-MIBG. *Med Pediatr Oncol* 1987;15:170–177.

110. Shimada H, Chatten J, Newton WA, et al. Histopathologic prognostic factors in neuroblastic tumors: definition of subtypes of ganglioneuroblastoma and an age-linked classification of neuroblastomas. *JNCI* 1984;73:405–416.

111. Shulkin BL, Shapiro B, Hutchinson RJ. Iodine-131-metaiodobenzylguanidine and bone scintigraphy for the detection of neuroblastoma. *J Nucl Med* 1992;33:1735–1740.

112. Silberzweig JE, Haller JO, Miller S. Ifosfamide: a new cause of rickets. *AJR* 1992; 158:823–824.

113. Sim FH, Frassica FJ, Unni KK. Osteosarcoma of the diaphysis of long bones: clinicopathologic features and treatment in 51 cases. *Orthopedics* 1995;18:19–23.

114. Simon MA, Kirchner PT. Scintigraphic evaluation of primary bone tumors: comparison of technetium-99m phosphonate and gallium citrate imaging. *J Bone Joint Surg [A]* 1980;62:758–764.

115. Smith FW, Gilday DL, Ash JM, et al. Primary neuroblastoma uptake of ^{99m}Tc methylene diphosphonate. *Radiology* 1980;137:501–504.

116. Sommer HJ, Knop J, Heise U, et al. Histomorphologic changes of osteosarcoma after chemotherapy: correlation with ^{99m}Tc methylene diphosphonate functional imaging. *Cancer* 1987;59:252–258.

117. Stanisavljevic S, Babcock AL. Fractures in children treated with methotrexate for leukemia. *Clin Orthop* 1977;125:139–144.

118. Sty JR, Wells RG, Starshak RJ, Gregg D. The musculoskeletal system. In: Sty J, Wells R, Starshak R, Gregg D, eds. *Diagnostic Imaging of Infants and Children*. Vol. 3. Gaithesburg: Aspen; 1992:233–405.

119. Thrall JH, Geslein GE, Corcoran RJ, et al. Abnormal radionuclide deposition patterns adjacent to focal skeletal lesions. *Radiology* 1975;115:659–663.

119a. Treves ST, Connolly LP, Kirkpatrick JA. Bone. In Treus ST (ed) Pediatric Nuclear Medicine. 2nd ed. New York: Springer-Verlag; 1995:233–301.

120. Triche TJ. Pathology of pediatric malignancies. In: Pizzo PA, Poplack DG, eds. *Principles and Practice of Pediatric Oncology*. 2nd ed. Philadelphia: JB Lippincott; 1993:115–152.

121. Unni KK. *Dahlin's Bone Tumors: General Aspects and Data on 11,087 Cases*. Philadelphia: Lippincott-Raven; 1996.

122. Vanel D, Henry-Amar M, Lumbrosus J, et al. Pulmonary evaluation of patients with osteosarcoma: roles of standard radiography, tomography, CT, scintigraphy and tomoscintigraphy. *AJR* 1984;143:519–523.

123. Warner WW. Kyphosis. In: Morrisy RT, Weinstein SL, eds. *Lovell and Winter's Pediatric Orthopedics*. 4th ed. Philadelphia: Lippincott-Raven; 1996:687–716.

124. Weeks DA, Beckwith JB, Miereau GW, et al. Rhabdoid tumor of the kidney. A report of 111 cases from the National Wilms' Tumor Study Pathology Center. *Am J Surg Pathol* 1989;13:439–458.

125. Wolf EL, Berdon WE, Cassady JR, et al. Slipped femoral capital epiphysis as a sequela to childhood irradiation for malignant tumors. *Radiology* 1977;125:781–784.

126. Woods WG, Lemieux B, Tuchman M. Neuroblastoma represents distinct clinical-biologic entities: a review and perspective from the Quebec neuroblastoma screening project. *Pediatrics* 1992;89:114–118.
127. Young G, L'Hereux P. Extraosseous tumor uptake of ^{99m}Tc phosphate compounds in children with abdominal neuroblastoma. *Pediatr Radiol* 1978;7:159–163.

Index

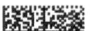